Manual of Drug Safety and Pharmacovigilance

Barton L. Cobert, MD

JONES AND BARTLETT PUBLISHERS

Sudbury, Massachusetts

BOSTON   TORONTO   LONDON   SINGAPORE

World Headquarters
Jones and Bartlett Publishers
40 Tall Pine Drive
Sudbury, MA 01776
978-443-5000
info@jbpub.com
www.jbpub.com

Jones and Bartlett Publishers Canada
6339 Ormindale Way
Mississauga, Ontario L5V 1J2
CANADA

Jones and Bartlett Publishers
International
Barb House, Barb Mews
London W6 7PA
UK

Jones and Bartlett's books and products are available through most bookstores and online booksellers. To contact Jones and Bartlett Publishers directly, call 800-832-0034, fax 978-443-8000, or visit our website, www.jbpub.com.

Substantial discounts on bulk quantities of Jones and Bartlett's publications are available to corporations, professional associations, and other qualified organizations. For details and specific discount information, contact the special sales department at Jones and Bartlett via the above contact information or send an email to specialsales@jbpub.com.

Library of Congress Cataloging-in-Publication Data
Cobert, Barton L.
  Manual of drug safety and pharmacovigilance / Barton L. Cobert.
    p. ; cm.
  ISBN-13: 978-0-7637-3889-1 (pbk.)
  ISBN-10: 0-7637-3889-1 (pbk.)
  1. Drugs--Side effects--Handbooks, manuals, etc. 2. Pharmacoepidemiology--Handbooks, manuals, etc. I. Title.
  [DNLM: 1. Pharmaceutical Preparations--adverse effects. 2. Product Surveillance, Postmarketing. 3. Drug Toxicity. 4. Pharmacoepidemiology. 5. Risk Management. QZ 42 C655m 2007]
  RM302.5.C63 2007
  615'.7042--dc22
                    2006017423

6048

Production Credits
Executive Editor: David Cella
Editorial Assistant: Lisa Gordon
Production Director: Amy Rose
Production Editor: Tracey Chapman
Associate Marketing Manager: Laura Kavigian
Manufacturing and Inventory Coordinator: Amy Bacus
Composition: Paw Print Media
Cover Design: Kristin E. Ohlin
Cover Image: © Mircea Bezergheanu/ShutterStock, Inc.
Printing and Binding: Courier Stoughton
Cover Printing: Courier Stoughton

Printed in the United States of America
10 09 08 07 06   10 9 8 7 6 5 4 3 2 1

Thank You

My sincere thanks to Pierre Biron, MD, retired Professor at the University of Montreal Faculty of Medicine, who reviewed the manuscript, corrected my errors, and improved the text in a multitude of ways. He has been a friend and colleague for many years and represents everything that a great physician and professor should be.

Also my sincere thanks to Paul Fallot, PharmD, friend and colleague of many years who also reviewed the manuscript, gave me a reality check and corrected my errors. Paul combines an encyclopedic knowledge of pharmacovigilance, extraordinary people skills, and wisdom. An unbeatable combination.

Thanks to Chris Davis who published (at another company) the first book Pierre and I wrote and who had faith in this book, too—thank you!

Dedication

To my son Julien, with all my love.

Contents

Introduction

This manual is a practical instruction book on drug safety. It is aimed at newcomers, old-timers, and outsiders to the field who would like a demystification and explanation of what adverse events are and how drug safety departments work. Hopefully, readers, especially those not in the field, will understand that drug safety, as with all other areas of medicine, is as much an art as it is a science.

For newcomers, this is a "Drug Safety 101" course giving a broad overview of how adverse events are handled from start to finish. For old-timers, this book will fill in gaps in knowledge on drug safety. For outsiders not working directly in this field, this book will explain how "side effects" are handled by the industry and by health authorities.

This book is not meant to be an encyclopedia. There are other such books already available. Rather, it is my hope that this will be an approachable book that will give a global overview of the field.

It is expected that after carefully reading and absorbing the contents, the reader will be able to begin work in a drug safety department or, if an outsider, understand what happens in such a department and where listings or adverse events come from.

I have attempted to avoid excess jargon ("This spontaneous SAE is expeditable since it is unlisted.") and make the book approachable by those with limited or no knowledge of medicine or pharmacology.

Housekeeping: In this age of high technology, the references in the text are primarily websites rather than published citations. After much discussion, it was felt that putting URLs directly in the text would be distracting and of little use. Thus they are noted in a table in the back of the book. In addition, accompanying this text is a CD-ROM with the entire contents of the book. This allows for rapid and easy searching for any topics the reader wishes. The URLs are "active" so that with a click or two the reader will be able to jump to that website when using the CD-ROM. The usual disclaimer about links applies: They were all active and correct when this book was prepared but they cannot be guaranteed to be so in the future.

I wish you well in the world of drug safety.

Notice

This book is not meant to be used in the practice of medicine or for the prescription of medicines or drugs. The medications described do not necessarily have specific approval by the FDA or any other health authority for use in the diseases, patients, or dosages discussed. The FDA-approved labeling (the package insert) in the United States and the local labeling for countries outside the United States should be consulted. Because standards for usage change, it is advisable to keep abreast of revised recommendations, particularly those concerning new drugs.

This book is not intended to express opinions about the value of specific products or about their comparative value within a drug class, even when a specific product is used to provide examples of adverse reactions. The content of the book is not meant to be used in choosing one product or another in medical practice. As with all medications, the official approved product labeling should be consulted before prescribing or using.

The opinions in this book do not express those of the Novartis Consumer Health Corporation or of the Novartis Corporation.

The Theory and Definitions of Drug Safety (Pharmacovigilance)

W hat is an adverse event (AE)? A serious AE? An adverse drug reaction (ADR)? A suspected adverse drug reaction (SADR)? A suspected, unexpected, serious adverse reaction? A suspected, expected, serious adverse reaction? What does expected and unexpected mean?

➥ **NOTE:** (Unless otherwise noted the word "drug" or "drug product" should be taken in this book to include "biologics" and "vaccines.")

◼ The Theory

There have been many variants on the terms and definitions used to talk about safety issues over the years. The terminology is somewhat confusing and is explained below in "The Practice" section.

The "official" and accepted definitions in most countries are based on the International Conference on Harmonization (ICH) E2A Guideline and are as follows.

Adverse Event

"Any untoward medical occurrence in a patient or clinical investigation subject administered a pharmaceutical product and which does not necessarily have to have a causal relationship with this treatment" (ICH E2A).

"Any unfavorable and unintended sign (including an abnormal laboratory finding, for example), symptom, or disease temporally associated with the use of any dose of a medicinal product, whether or not considered related to the medicinal product" (ICH E2A).

Adverse Reaction

In the preapproval (i.e., not yet marketed, experimental) phase of a product, the definition is as follows:

"All noxious and unintended responses to a medicinal product related to any dose should be considered adverse drug reactions." This means "that a causal relationship between a medicinal product and an adverse event is at least a reasonable possibility, i.e. the relationship cannot be ruled out" (ICH E2A).

For postapproval (i.e., marketed) products, the definition is as follows:

"A response to a drug which is noxious and unintended and which occurs at doses normally used in man for prophylaxis, diagnosis, or therapy of disease or for modification of physiological function" (ICH E2A).

Serious Adverse Event and Serious Adverse Reaction

"A serious adverse event (experience) or serious adverse reaction is any untoward medical occurrence that at any dose:

- *results in death,*
- *is life-threatening,*

➡ **NOTE:** The term "life-threatening" in the definition of "serious" refers to an event in which the patient was at risk of death at the time of the event; it does not refer to an event that hypothetically might have caused death if it were more severe.)

- *requires inpatient hospitalization or prolongation of existing hospitalization,*
- *results in persistent or significant disability/incapacity, or*
- *is a congenital anomaly/birth defect.*

"Medical and scientific judgment should be exercised in deciding whether expedited reporting is appropriate in other situations, such as important medical events that may not be immediately life-threatening or result in death or hospitalization but may jeopardize the patient or may require intervention to prevent one of the other outcomes listed in the definition above. *These should also usually be considered serious.*

"Examples of such events are intensive treatment in an emergency room or at home for allergic bronchospasm; blood dyscrasias or convulsions that do not result in hospitalization; or development of drug dependency or drug abuse" (ICH E2A).

Suspected Adverse Drug Reaction

A noxious and unintended response to any dose of a drug or biologic product for which there is a reasonable possibility that the product caused the response. In this definition, the phrase "a reasonable possibility" means that the relationship cannot be ruled out (US Food and Drug Administration proposed regulations of March 14, 2003 and ICH E2A).

Serious, Unexpected, Adverse Drug Reaction

An SADR that is serious and unexpected. See the definitions for serious and unexpected.

Serious, Expected, Adverse Drug Reaction

An SADR that is serious and expected. See the definitions for serious and unexpected.

Unexpected

"For a pre-marketed product: Any adverse drug experience, the specificity or severity of which is not consistent with the current investigator's brochure; or, if an investigator brochure is not required or available, the specificity or severity of which is not consistent with the risk information described in the general investigational plan or elsewhere in the current application, as amended. For example, under this definition, cerebral thromboembolism and cerebral vasculitis would be unexpected (by virtue of greater specificity) if the investigator brochure only listed cerebral vascular accidents" (21CFR312.32(a)).

"For marketed products: Any adverse drug experience that is not listed in the current labeling (package insert or summary of product characteristics) for the drug product. This includes events that may be symptomatically and pathophysiologically related to an event listed in the labeling, but differ from the event because of greater severity or specificity. For example, under this definition, hepatic necrosis would be unexpected (by virtue of greater severity) if the labeling only referred to elevated hepatic enzymes or hepatitis" (21 CFR 314.80(a)).

AEs that are "class related" (i.e., allegedly seen with all products in this class of drugs) and are mentioned in the labeling (package insert or summary of product characteristics) or investigator brochure but are not *specifically* described as occurring with this product are considered unexpected.

Expected

As opposed to "unexpected," an event that is noted in the investigator brochure or labeling (package insert or summary of product characteristics).

■ The Practice

In practice, these definitions are rather murky and confusing. There is an attempt now to standardize this nomenclature around ICH/Council for International Organizations of Medical Sciences definitions. This will probably succeed, but all these terms will be used in various places for some time to come.

AEs are unintended "bad things" that occur when taking a drug (or biologic or vaccine, etc.). They may or may not be due to the drug itself (the active moiety), the formulation, excipients in the product (e.g., the inactive ingredients, fillers, etc.), the packaging (e.g., leaching of products from a container into the liquid drug product), a contaminant, manufacturing problems, the underlying disease, or some other unknown cause or causes. Thus an AE does not imply that the drug (i.e., the active component) caused the "bad thing" to occur.

An ADR is an AE in which there is reasonable possibility of a causal relationship between the drug and the AE. Or, as others put it, the relationship cannot be ruled out. The notion of causality is discussed in much greater detail in Chapter 37. Thus an AE possibly/probably due to the drug is an ADR.

The latter term is slowly being replaced by "suspected adverse drug reaction" (SADR), which emphasizes the suspicion that the drug is a/the possible cause of the "bad thing."

Following logically from this, we now have the term suspected, unexpected (unlabeled), serious adverse reaction. The addition of the words "serious" and "unexpected" to the SADR term represent the criteria for submission as expedited reports (see Chapter 39) to government health agencies in many countries of serious reactions from clinical trials.

Suspected, expected, serious adverse reactions usually do not have to be submitted as expedited reports to governmental agencies. They are usually submitted periodically (e.g., yearly) or at the end of the study in the final study report.

Expectedness represents an area that is often highly subjective. An event or reaction is expected if it is found in the product labeling or investigator brochure. Events or reactions that are more specific or more severe, however, are considered to be unexpected. Thus if "pneumonia" is in the brochure or product labeling and the patient has "streptococcal pneumonia," this is considered unexpected because the "streptococcal" designation is more specific. Similarly, "fatal pneumonia" is considered unexpected if only pneumonia is labeled.

sonal allergy drugs should be marketed near the time for the allergy season to hit). The FDA may require that certain phase IV studies be done immediately after marketing as a requirement of NDA approval. This may be to clarify some safety and efficacy issues that remained after phase III but which the FDA believed were not sufficient to prevent or delay marketing of the drug.

Phase IV studies may be marketing or pharmacoeconomic studies to aid in selling the product by studying head-on comparisons with competitor drugs. They may be studies looking at subgroups of the approved group and indication (e.g., a drug approved for diabetes now looking at diabetics who are elderly or are also in heart failure). They may be done in children, not only to evaluate the usefulness and safety but also to obtain, in the United States, additional patent exclusivity.

Phase IV studies may be done for specific safety reasons to investigate an AE or a signal that has unexpectedly occurred after marketing. Such studies may be classical clinical trials or they may be epidemiologic studies done in large databases. The design and size are very variable, ranging from small open-label trials to massive, multicenter, double-blind comparator trials. Sometimes patients are compensated for participation.

So-called market-driven phase IV "seeding studies" are now forbidden in most parts of the world. These were pure marketing projects designed to encourage physicians to prescribe a particular product in place of a competitor's product. A protocol was usually written (to justify calling the endeavor a study) but was often of poor quality. Results were not always collected by the sponsor and, if collected, often not analyzed. Prescribers were sometimes compensated.

Investigator-Initiated Trials or Studies

Investigator-initiated trials (IITs) or studies are usually new ideas thought up mainly by researchers in the academic world or occasionally suggested by the pharmaceutical company. New uses or ways of administering drugs are frequently proposed by academic researchers to pharmaceutical companies. Many companies actually have physicians, PhDs, or pharmacologists on staff (often called "medical liaisons") who travel to academic medical centers and seek out such clever new uses.

This can be instrumental in the scientific development of a drug. The advantages of IITs are that new ideas are found and explored, costs are usually fairly small, and the studies can be done fairly quickly. The disadvantage is that many details that should be determined before doing trials are unanswered (e.g., effective dose, safety in

this population, etc.). An IIT that fails usually ends that idea. Thus, if too low a dose is chosen, one might never know that a higher dose would produce positive results. Funding is usually from the pharmaceutical company in the form of a grant-in-aid, drug supply, protocol, or case report form support. A contract or agreement is usually signed by both parties. The legal sponsor of the study is not the pharmaceutical company but rather the investigator. It is he or she who opens the IND with the FDA (often with the help of the pharmaceutical company). The usual safety provisions are followed: Good Clinical Practices, investigational review boards, and SAE reporting to the FDA by the investigator. Most pharmaceutical companies also require that SAEs be reported to the company (in addition to the health authority) by the investigator so that a full safety database is maintained for all uses of a product by the company. These trials would technically be phase I if a new indication or formulation or delivery is being studied. If not, they would most probably be considered phase IV trials. Not all studies require an IND (if the use of the drug is fully covered within the approved labeling).

In earlier years, there were disputes over ownership of the data and the publication (or rather lack of publication) of negative results. These are resolving, in general, with the "ownership" of the data by both parties and with the right to publish retained by the investigator no matter what the results.

■ The Practice

Study phases are often more hazy than the "official" schema described above. Phase I studies that go beyond the initial dose finding and escalation studies are often done throughout the phases over several years. If a drug does not go beyond phase II because of lack of efficacy (i.e., the company "kills" it), there is little point in doing drug, food, or alcohol interaction studies early in the course of development.

Some companies have been known to try to speed up development (and lower costs) by doing somewhat larger phase II trials that, should they succeed, are submitted to the FDA as combined phase II–III trials for approval. For critical drugs this may be advantageous as long as it does not compromise the safety and efficacy evaluations. In general, the more patients studied, the more comfortable one is with the safety profile of the drug.

Phase I studies are created and supervised in most pharmaceutical companies by a dedicated phase I group (e.g., the pharmacokinetics/pharmacodynamics group) usually run by pharmacologists (PhDs, PharmDs) and physicians. The actual study is often out-sourced to CROs or academic centers (clinical research units) where the actual patient enrollment and dosing occur.

Phases II and III are usually run by "high power" clinical research groups within the company led by physicians (often subspecialists such as cardiologists, oncologists, and pulmonologists). These studies are complex and have large infrastructures supporting them in biostatistics, study site monitoring, in-house data monitors, clinical research associates, regulatory affairs associates, safety monitors, quality control, quality assurance, and so on. Many companies also out-source the trials (or parts of the trials) to CROs. These studies are rigorously done and are likely to be audited by the FDA before approval of the NDA.

Phase IV studies may be done by the phase II/III group or by a separate postmarketing group. If part of the clinical research department, the rigor of the earlier phases usually carries over to the phase IV studies. If done by the marketing department in isolation, the studies may be somewhat more variable in quality and rigor. Some companies now have separate Safety/Epidemiology departments that handle postmarketing clinical and epidemiologic trials (but not the marketing studies).

Some company executives have argued that small phase IV marketing studies or IITs are dangerous because they might discover some safety "problem" and might fail to show efficacy, thus doubly hurting the drug. The safety officers often argue just the reverse; these studies may uncover a previously unknown safety issue that can now be added to the product labeling to better inform prescribers and patients.

Clinical trial registries are now being set up by pharmaceutical companies whereby all research trials are now posted, in fairly great detail, on a website. This practice will spread (as it becomes obligatory), and it is possible that phase IV marketing trials will also be posted. This will most probably raise the standards for all trials and allow for easier data comparisons.

IITs have traditionally posed problems. IITs are usually encouraged by companies by having roving or regional medical professionals visit academic medical centers to seek out new trials. These visiting medical liaisons may or may not be trained in classic clinical research methodology. They may also do "in-service" teaching or training on the company's new product(s) in the medical centers. Thus this role combines a medical and a marketing function. In well-structured pharmaceutical companies, protocols submitted by academics through the roving professionals are reviewed by the clinical research department, the statisticians, and the pharmacovigilance group. A formal contract requiring completion, a final report within a finite period (e.g., 1

year), and SAE reporting is done. Pharmacovigilance departments in companies usually submit the SAEs to their own NDAs or INDs (even if the investigator has said he or she has also done so to the IND). In less well-structured companies, the medical marketing group may be less well connected to the other research groups and details may slip.

New types of outreach programs (sometimes in combination with registries) are also being developed by companies to help patients finish the course of therapy when they are already taking the drug. In particular, for chronic therapy diseases such as cancer, hepatitis, and hypertension, companies have found that it is good medicine and good marketing to encourage patients to stay on their therapy to the end (e.g., until the cancer is in remission or cured, the hepatitis titers drop, etc.). This means continued sales of the drug as well as successful patient treatment. The usual reasons for stopping therapy are AEs, dosing problems, or convenience reasons. Outreach programs with the use of nurses or pharmacists who contact patients every week or month on how to handle AEs and other issues are now common. When done well, the patient's physician is kept informed of issues and progress and works with the patient and the outreach nurse to get the patient over rough patches in the treatment regimen. AE data must be collected by the company, kept in the safety database, and reported to the FDA as required.

■ FAQs

Q: Does the company have to collect *all* AEs from all trials?

A: Basically yes, in one form or another. First, it is good medicine to collect all serious and nonserious AEs so that one fully understands the safety profile of the product. In practice, in clinical trials only SAEs must be collected by the drug safety group and reported either in 7 or 15 days or periodically in yearly reports. Nonserious AEs and some SAEs (e.g., expected SAEs that the sponsor and FDA agree will be reported only at the end of the study) do not get reported until the final study report.

What this means is that in many large pharmaceutical companies there are two databases. There is the drug safety database maintained by the drug safety group for expedited and periodic regulatory reporting and the clinical research database for NDA submissions. The safety database contains all serious clinical trial AEs (as well as all serious and nonserious postmarketing AEs) but not nonserious clinical trial AEs. This database is dynamic and always up to date. The clinical research database contains the case report form information, including all serious and nonserious AEs. Sometimes data are not entered into this database rapidly but rather only when case report forms arrive in the research department, perhaps monthly or even less frequently. This produces two problems. Anyone who needs to do safety analyses must obtain the SAEs from the safety group (their database is up to date) and the nonserious AEs from the clinical research group (which may not be up to date) to have a full data set. In addition, the SAEs in the two safety databases must be reconciled because the same safety data are collected in two different places usually derived from two different forms (the SAE reporting form sent to the drug safety department within 24–48 hours of the SAE and the case report form safety page, which may not be harvested until later or at the end of the study). In any case, signaling investigations should be done using all clinical trial data no matter where they are stored. This may mean the creation of a "data warehouse" to allow access to the data contained in both databases.

A new twist is starting to be seen with the introduction of "electronic data capture," formerly known as "remote data entry," in which either a dedicated computer is installed at each clinical study site for uploading to a company network or each study site logs onto a URL and enters data directly into the company database. This is taking the place of paper case report forms. There are many implications attached to this:

■ Safety data (serious and nonserious AEs) are received in real time.

■ Data entry is now moved from a central location (usually in the company) where it is well controlled in the hands of a few highly trained data entry employees to many remote sites where the data entry person is less well controlled and possibly less well trained.

■ The company drug safety database may not be linked electronically to the electronic data capture database, and new procedures must be developed to get the safety data to the safety group in a timely manner.

■ Source documents (e.g., laboratory tests, x-ray reports) may not be sent to the company now that studies are "paperless." In fact, source documents may now disappear, because the classic case report form no longer exists.

One can envisage the day when the whole of the United States, the European Union, and other medical systems are standardized and on-line. All data, including study data and safety data, are sent electronically to all needed databases at the company, the FDA, the hospital, the insurance company, and so on. Safety data will be accurate and rapidly received everywhere they are needed.

Q: Are phase IV study SAEs reportable to the IND (experimental) or NDA (postmarketing) or both?

A: A tricky question.

■ If a study is done under an IND, then the SAEs that meet reporting criteria are reported to the IND. Many companies believe that the NDA takes precedence over the IND and would report those SAEs to the NDA also.

■ SAEs from studies not done under an IND should be reported to the NDA.

In general, the NDA takes precedence over the IND for reporting purposes. The NDA is continually scrutinized by the FDA in expedited reports, annual reports, and Periodic Safety Update Reports (outside the United States and on a test basis in the United States). The IND dossier, on the other hand, if old and with little activity may be less well scrutinized.

3

Spontaneous Postmarketing Adverse Events

Their pivotal and irreplaceable role in providing signals when a wider population is exposed to a new product. How a clinician detects a signal and unexpected adverse drug reaction.

➡ **NOTE:**(Unless otherwise noted the word "drug" or "drug product" should be taken in this book to include "biologics" and "vaccines.")

■ Background

Before a drug comes to market it is studied in patients in clinical trials that aim to show efficacy of the product for a particular selected disease in a highly selected sample of the population. The clinical trials may be large, covering up to 10,000 patients, or very small, covering dozens to hundreds of patients (e.g., for orphan drugs). The clinical trials also aim to define the safety profile of the drug, at least in this selected population with this selected disease.

These studies, which are (usually) carried out with rigorous and highly regulated methodology, have significant limitations in defining the safety profile. They generally only find frequently occurring adverse events (AEs). For example, if in studying 10,000 patients not a single patient has a particular AE, such as a heart attack, we can be only 95% confident that the chance of having a heart attack based on the data from this trial is less than 1 in 3,333. If we raise the safety threshold to be 99% confident that a heart attack has an incidence of only 1 in 10,000 with this drug, we would need to have no heart attacks in 46,000 patients studied. In other words, studying even 5,000 or 10,000 patients does not give a warm enough or fuzzy enough feeling that the major or rare safety issues have been identified before the drug goes on the market for large-scale use.

This means that the uncommon AEs and even the fairly common AEs (e.g., an incidence of 1 in 500) will not be picked up until the drug is extensively used in the general population after marketing. When, say, a million people start using a new drug in the months after a product launch, a "rare" AE with a 1 in 10,000 incidence rate could be expected in about 100 patients. Should the AE in question be dramatic and rapidly discovered, such as torsades de pointes, aplastic anemia, or rhabdomyolysis (a severe skeletal muscle injury), there will be a torrent of recriminations about why this was not discovered earlier during the clinical testing. The correct response is that the testing of only 5,000 to 10,000 patients could not pick up such a rare event. This response is usually lost in the clamor.

Also of note is the fact that the clinical trials are often done in a narrow group of patients. For example, an antihistamine may be tested in otherwise healthy adults between 18 and 60 years of age with allergies. Even if the drug is only approved for use in this population, physicians have the right (which they freely exercise) to prescribe the drug for anyone. Thus many people with other diseases and at the extremes of the age range (the very old and young) receive the drug and may have AEs that the healthy 18- to 60-year-old study population did not experience in the clinical trials. The elderly, for example, are particularly sensitive to certain AEs (e.g., swallowing disorders) or to certain classes of drugs of psychotropic drugs.

The issue of polypharmacy cannot be adequately treated in the preclinical setting. Although food interaction studies and some drug interaction studies are done before approval, it is not possible to study "real world" patients (often elderly) who take many drugs and have bizarre or irregular eating and drinking habits.

Hence, particular attention must be paid to the time just after a product is first marketed to fully understand the drug's profile. In a sense, the first 500,000 to 1,000,000 patients prescribed the drug after launch are doing the large-scale safety testing.

What this means then is that the entire edifice of the drug safety system as it now stands depends on the good will and energy of nurses, pharmacists, physicians, and consumers to report AEs. Without them, no one would know of the AEs that are appearing as individual cases in isolated areas around the country or the world. These people must take time out of their day to report such events. The report will inevitably lead to a request for supplementary data (laboratory reports, cardiograms, hospital records, etc.) that are time and effort consuming. There is no evident or immediate gain to the reporter. The gain rather is to society at large, which is largely unaware of this noble effort.

■ The Theory

The fundamental underpinning of the system in place to discover AEs with marketed products is the spontaneous reporting system. This system is in place, in one form or another, in over 50 countries around the world, including the United States, Canada, the European Union, Japan, Australia, New Zealand, and South Africa.

The principles are simple. All health care professionals (and consumers in a few countries, including the United States and Canada) are encouraged to spontaneously report AEs with drugs to either the manufacturer or the governmental health care agency or a third party. Standardized forms have been developed (the MedWatch form in the United States) specifically for this purpose and are available on-line, in publications (e.g., the *Physicians' Desk Reference* in the United States), and elsewhere. The form can be folded up and mailed (postage free), faxed, or sent on-line to the health care agencies. Phone reports are also possible to the manufacturer and often to the health agencies.

The forms are one or two pages in length and include the expected information: patient demographics; the AE(s) that occurred; medical history; drugs taken, including the one or more drugs suspected of causing the AE in question; comedications; dose and timing; a narrative summary of the case; and reporter information. In most cases confidentiality is guaranteed by law, regulation, or policy regarding the patient's identity and the reporter's identity. In the United States, information submitted spontaneously is available for a small fee to anyone in the public under the "Freedom of Information Act" (see Chapter 40). The cases are redacted before being released by the US Food and Drug Administration (FDA) to avoid identifying the patient or reporter. In the United States, approximately 20% of the reports go directly to the FDA and the remaining 80% to the manufacturers, who then forward them to the FDA. Most reporters tend to be pharmacists. In 2001 the FDA's Office of Drug Safety noted in its annual report (Web Resource 3-1) that the breakdown of the sources of reports was as follows:

- Pharmacists, 41%
- Physicians, 11%
- Nurses, 11%
- Other health care professionals, 11%
- Unknown, 18%
- Consumers, 8%

The requirements for AE reporting have largely been standardized through the International Conference on Harmonization (ICH). Reporting for health care professionals (and consumers in some places) is usually voluntary and should be more highly encouraged by agencies. There is no time frame for reporting after the occurrence of the AE, but obviously rapid reporting is preferred for public health reasons; in some cases it may save lives. For manufacturers, reporting is obligatory. Any AE that comes into a company, whether through sales representatives, phone calls, or literature reports (which must be actively searched for by the company), must be rapidly reviewed by qualified medical personnel.

For marketed drugs, all serious AEs that are unexpected (i.e., that do not appear in the approved product labeling) must be reported to the agency within 15 calendar days. In the United States, most of the remaining serious and nonserious cases must be reported to the FDA in the New Drug Application periodic reports (quarterly for new drugs and yearly for older drugs). In the European Union and elsewhere (and soon perhaps in the United States), periodic reporting is done as Periodic Safety Update Reports, which are prepared every 6 months, yearly, or every 2.5, 3, or 5 years depending on the age of the drug and the country receiving the report. These reports contain line listings of various cuts of the data as well as medical analyses prepared by medical teams, usually headed by a physician. They look at AEs that are expected and unexpected and indicate which need to be added to the drug labeling as new AEs, warnings, and so forth and which need to continue to be watched with heightened vigilance. These reports are then scrutinized by the regulatory agencies who may agree or disagree with the company analysis and who decide on changes to the drug labeling. There is usually dialogue between the health agency and the company. At the health agency, the data are then entered into a database and reviewed. Analysis of individual AE cases and of aggregates of AE cases is done.

Many countries now send extracts from their spontaneous databases of local AE reports to the Uppsala Monitoring Centre (UMC) in Sweden (Web Resource 3-2). Approximately 72 countries supply AE reports to the Centre, which has over 3,000,000 cases. About half are from the United States. An excellent document from the UMC describing the details of the database is available on its website (Web Resource 3-3). Extracts of the database are available from the UMC for a fee.

■ The Practice

Specifically addressing spontaneous reports, a company must set up a failure-proof system to receive AEs. Time is of the essence, because some of the reports must be sent to the FDA and other health authorities within 15 days. The clock for reporting starts counting down from the moment the first person anywhere in the company hears about the AE.

For phone reports, this means that any phone number in the company is a potential source of AE reports and anyone who answers the phone in the company must be instructed in what to do if an AE report comes into a place where it is not expected. A rapid and painless (to the caller) transfer system must be set up if the information is not immediately written down by the company employee first answering the call. No one wants to be kept on hold or to repeat the same story for the third or fourth time. No AE may be lost, so all efforts must be directed to the proper handling of the call. Because some AEs may need to be reported to the health care agency within 15 days, time is of the essence. The company must be ready to accept calls 24 hours a day, 7 days a week and in multiple languages if that is the normal custom in the country. Some companies that do not maintain 24-hour coverage in the company out-source the AE receiving function after hours to poison control centers or private companies.

Similarly, any e-mail or website in which an outsider can send a message is a source of AEs. Many companies report complaints and AEs arriving on job-posting websites, free sample websites, survey websites, message boards, and so forth.

Sales representatives must also be aware that a physician, pharmacist, or other health care worker they call on may be the source of an AE. Even innocuous off-the-cuff remarks about a possible AE ("Oh, by the way one of my patients took your other drug XXXX and had a heart attack the next day") made to a company representative constitute a report to the company that must be acted on. Even off-hand remarks over the barbecue on a Sunday afternoon in which a neighbor off-handedly relates an AE to a company employee must be reported to the drug safety department!

Many companies have media services that review transcripts of newspapers, television shows, and so forth, looking for anything about their products. Should AEs be noted, they must be sent to the safety department.

Lawsuits often represent the point of entry of AEs. The legal department must be aware that they must also report the AE noted in the suit to the safety department.

Some people still write "snail mail" letters, and the company mail room or mail screeners must be aware that AEs received in the mail are to be sent to the drug safety group immediately (usually by fax and not interoffice mail).

One of the more complex problems companies face is the phone call or letter that notes a product complaint ("the pill was the wrong color") and an AE ("and then I took it and had violent stomach pains") and then wants restitution ("I want my money back now!"). These cases must be handled by three or more departments in the company: the drug safety group to get details and report the AE, the manufacturing or quality group to see why the pill was the wrong color, and the marketing/sales group to refund (or not refund) the money. Companies must set up systems to handle this.

There is now a transition by companies reporting serious AEs to health agencies from paper or fax reporting with MedWatch forms (or CIOMS I forms) to electronic reporting using a standardized electronic format and transmission known generically as "E2B transmissions" after the ICH document of that name. In theory, this transmission is the same to all agencies around the world and simplifies the multiple reporting obligations now in force from country to country. This is also being seen in the trend toward reporting from standardized lists of drug names, medical and surgical history, AE codes, laboratory data, and demographic codes. This allows people to document AE cases in a standardized language and format that is easily translated by the computer into any other language. The only area proving resistant to this computerization is the medical narrative where a case is summarized in prose in a few paragraphs such that the reader can get an understanding of what happened to the patient. Whether a computer-derived narrative will prove to be as useful as a narrative prepared by a health care professional remains to be seen.

Interestingly, English has become the international language of AE reporting. Periodic Safety Update Reports are written in English. Some countries require translation of some or all sections, but this is becoming less prevalent as short time frames and international harmonization are requiring that English be the language of drug safety.

After the report is received in the safety department, it must be logged in and a unique number assigned (either before or after a search for duplicate cases is done). A rapid determination must be made by a medical professional to see whether it is an "expedited" or "alert" report that must be sent to the FDA and other health authorities within 15 calendar days of first arrival in the company. The data must be entered into the database, coded, medically reviewed, quality checked, and dispatched to the FDA and subsidiaries, business partners, and others inside the company such as clinical research physicians who follow the safety profile of the drug in question. Any horrific AEs that might produce immediate regulatory or public health problems must also be identified and acted on urgently.

4

The Theory of Drug Safety (Pharmacovigilance)

Why a company needs a drug safety group and how it is constituted. The mission of a drug safety group within a pharmaceutical company. A brief history of the US Food and Drug Administration's (FDA's) safety duties and functions. The FDA's mission. Pressures on the corporate safety department and the FDA.

> **NOTE:**(Unless otherwise noted the word "drug" or "drug product" should be taken in this book to include "biologics" and "vaccines.")

■ Background

A century or two ago the requirements for the safety and efficacy of drug products were either nonexistent or poorly defined at best. In 1906 the Pure Food and Drugs Act prohibited interstate commerce of mislabeled and adulterated drugs and food within the United States. This covered some safety aspects of drugs but not efficacy. The FDA had, at that time, no jurisdiction or control of efficacy

claims made for drugs. In 1912, the law was changed to cover false and fraudulent claims made for drugs. However, the law did not mandate safety, and in effect unsafe products could be and were marketed. The FDA could not seize unsafe drugs and was limited only to issuing public warnings.

In 1937 a company in the United States marketed elixir of sulfanilamide, which contained diethylene glycol (similar to antifreeze). Over 100 people (including children) died from this product. Because the law did not require safety testing for drugs, the company had done none. As a result of this, the Federal Food, Drug and Cosmetic Act was passed into law in 1938. This law required safety testing to be performed and submitted to the FDA in a New Drug Application (NDA). Additional laws were passed in the 1940s requiring testing for purity, strength, and quality of many drugs.

The next major event was the thalidomide disaster of the early 1960s, when the NDA for thalidomide was valiantly opposed by Dr. Frances Kelsey at the FDA because of insufficient safety information despite strong pressure to approve it. Though never marketed in the United States, thalidomide was extensively used in the investigational setting, and by 1962 the terrible teratogenic (birth defect) aspect of the drug became known as babies were born with severely deformed arms and legs. In 1962 the Kefauver-Harris amendment became law and introduced the modern era of drug regulation. Drug manufacturers now had to demonstrate to the FDA both safety and efficacy before marketing a new drug. In 1971, the National Drug Experience Reporting System was begun, as was the publication of "The FDA Drug Bulletin" to alert physicians and pharmacists to drug issues. In 1985 the regulations on adverse event (AE) reporting for marketed drugs were strengthened, and new requirements for Investigational New Drug Applications (INDs) were introduced. Over the years, the FDA has had multiple reorganizations and alterations in its structure and function as the overseer of drug safety and efficacy in the United States. The result is the complex system of AE collection, analysis, and reporting that we know today. See a brief history of the Center for Drug Evaluation and Research (CDER) on the FDA's website (Web Resource 4-1).

■ The Theory

The regulations, laws, guidances, rules, and other relevant documents covering drug safety are detailed, arcane, and scattered throughout multiple places in the Code of Federal Regulations for the United States and the various European Commission venues for European Union (EU) documents. Each individual country in the EU and most others in the world have their own set of local laws, regulations, and guidances (often available only in the local language). Most are updated fairly frequently.

Suffice it to say, most countries' regulations are fairly similar in requiring all or almost all serious AEs and some nonserious AEs to be reported quickly if there appears to be a potential impact on public health and at periodic intervals for more routine AEs. Although the rules are similar throughout the world, they are sufficiently different in detail ("the devil is in the details") to be infuriating and well nigh impossible to track, categorize, and keep up to date. The major documents for the United States and EU are listed below. Those with an asterisk are the ones that should be read and digested by anyone doing drug safety for a living. The contents of these documents are topics of this book.

The US regulations do not explicitly state that a department or group must exist to deal with drug safety. Rather there are sponsor obligations that are spelled out. To do this adequately, an organized system or department is necessary.

The EU regulations are more specific and do require that a formal pharmacovigilance system be put in place (from Volume 9—Pharmacovigilance. Rules Governing Medicinal Products in the European Union, published by the European Commission, Directorate Enterprise, Regulatory Framework and Market Authorisations [Version June 2004], page 13):

> "The marketing authorisation holder must ensure that it has an appropriate system of pharmacovigilance in place in order to assure responsibility and liability for its products on the market and to ensure that appropriate action can be taken, when necessary.
>
> The marketing authorisation holder should have permanently and continuously at its disposal, in the European Economic Area (EEA), a qualified person responsible for pharmacovigilance. This person should have experience in all aspects of pharmacovigilance and if not medically qualified should report to, or have access to a medically qualified person."

The US Regulations and Guidances

Drug safety in the United States is covered under several sections of the Code of Federal Regulations.

*The US Code of Federal Regulations, Title 2, Chapter 312 covers INDs. 21CFR312.32 covers IND safety reports, including expedited 7- and 15-day reports. Section 21CFR33 covers the IND annual reports. The NDA regulations are found in section 21CFR314.80. A searchable version of 21CFR is available on the FDA's website (Web Resource 4-2).

Updates to regulations are published in the Federal Register and viewable on its website (Web Resource 4-3). The Food, Drug and Cosmetic act is available at Web Resource 4-4.

A summary page of the regulations developed and enforced by CDER is found on CDER's website (Web Resource 4-5). All CDER guidances are also found on its website (Web Resource 4-6).

The Center for Biologics Evaluation and Research has some safety information available on its website (Web Resource 4-7). They refer the reader to the MedWatch website (Web Resource 4-8).

*MedWatch has an automatic e-mail notification system that sends out free safety updates periodically. Information is available on its website (Web Resource 4-9).

*In 1992 the FDA issued a "Guideline for Postmarketing Reporting of Adverse Drug Experiences." This is somewhat out of date but is worth reading for some details on the FDA's philosophy on sending in MedWatch forms (then known as 1639 forms). It can be found at the MedWatch website (Web Resource 4-10).

*In August 1997 the FDA issued a short Guidance for Industry entitled "Postmarketing Adverse Experience Reporting for Human Drug and Licensed Biological Products: Clarification of What to Report." This document covers the four data elements needed for an AE report, solicited information, and nonserious labeled cases. See the CDER website (Web Resource 4-11).

*In March 2001 the FDA published a Guidance for Industry entitled "Postmarketing Safety Reporting for Human Drug and Biological Products Including Vaccines." This document has not been formally issued as a final regulation, however. It is worth reading to better understand the FDA's more or less current thinking on safety reporting. See the CDER website (Web Resource 4-12).

*CDER has a 1999 guide for FDA field inspectors on what to look for when doing inspections on safety matters. It is worth reading and can be found on the CDER's website (Web Resource 4-13).

*In March 2003, the FDA published proposed new regulations markedly altering the reporting requirements in 21 CFR parts 310, 312, 314, 320, 600, 601, and 606. These proposals have been nicknamed "The Tome." They have not been issued yet and remain as proposed rule changes. For the complete text, see the FDA's website (Web Resource 4-14).

For Risk Management documents, see Chapters 14–17.

For International Conference on Harmonization documents, see Chapter 26.

For Council for International Organizations of Medical Sciences documents, see Chapter 25.

The EU Directives, Regulations, and Guidances

A summary of safety documents for the EU can be found at the Eudravigilance website (Web Resource 4-15).

The major document covering safety in the European Union is a 385-page document entitled as follows:

*"Volume 9—Pharmacovigilance. Rules Governing Medicinal Products in the European Union, published by the European Commission, Directorate Enterprise, Regulatory Framework and Market Authorisations (Version June 2004)." See the Eudravigilance website (Web Resource 4-16).

➡ **NOTE:** Note that in December 2006 a revision of Volume 9, now called Volume 9a, was released with comments requested through March 2006.)

Detailed guidances on AE collection in clinical trials from April 2004:

Detailed guidance on the collection, verification, and presentation of adverse reaction reports arising from clinical trials on medicinal products for human use. See the Eudravigilance website (Web Resource 4-17).

Detailed guidance on the European database of serious, unexpected, suspected adverse reactions (Eudravigilance, Clinical Trial Module). See the Eudravigilance website (Web Resource 4-18).

Other documents of interest for EU safety reporting:

One of the earliest of the documents on drug safety in the European Union. It preceded the creation of the European Medicines Evaluation Agency (EMEA) in 1995. See the Eudravigilance website (Web Resource 4-19).

The 1995 regulation on reporting of suspected unexpected adverse reactions from the European Union and outside the European Union. See the Eudravigilance website (Web Resource 4-20).

This 2004 regulation setting out the procedures for safety within the European Community. See the Eudravigilance website (Web Resource 4-21).

A directive covering clinical trial Good Clinical Practices in the European Union. The so-called Clinical Trial Directive. See the Eudravigilance website (Web Resource 4-22).

■ The Practice

Pharmaceutical companies in the United States are obliged to capture AEs, analyze them, and report them to the FDA and to other health authorities (HAs) or to companies abroad for submission to their HAs if there are formal corporate arrangements for sales and trials outside the United States. Thus, a company needs to create a safety team or department equipped to handle spontaneous and clinical trial AEs (as required) or to outsource this function. If the company is based purely in one country, the department may be relatively small and uncomplicated and report only to the HA in their territory. If, however, AEs can come from subsidiaries or affiliates in other countries or from business partners with which the company has contractual relationships, the complexity of the needs and requirements grows enormously.

Different languages, time zones, government requirements, reporting due dates, reporting documents and formats, electronic transmission, and so forth must be taken into account. Standard operating procedures, MedDRA (*Medical Dictionary for Regulatory Activities*), and training systems must be in place. An electronic safety database must be built (an enormous task) or purchased (still a complex and costly endeavor).

Health care personnel, including physicians, nurses, and pharmacists, and a support staff must be hired. The business relationships with other concerned departments within the company, such as regulatory affairs, sales and marketing, legal, clinical research, and others, must be established. In other words, creating a safety department is a complex and expensive endeavor that must be done absolutely correctly.

After an AE report is received in the safety department, it must be entered into the database, which is used for storage, retrieval, analysis, and reporting of the data. Although such databases may start out in small companies as spreadsheets with the data typed onto MedWatch forms, most companies respond to this need by purchasing an expensive (up to hundreds of thousands of dollars depending on the number of users) dedicated safety database and creating complex departments with tight standard operating procedures to ensure that the company remains in full compliance with all laws, regulations, and guidelines and will withstand inspections and audits from the FDA, EMEA, and other HAs; business partners; outside auditing companies; and others.

There is usually a vice president for drug safety (an experienced physician) to oversee the entire group. Within the drug safety group there are usually separate groups to handle:

■ Case triage and processing by (nonprofessional) data entry personnel;
■ Case evaluation by medical professionals;
■ Coding of AEs in MedDRA (sometimes this group is separate from drug safety);
■ Coding of drugs in *WHO-Drug* or another drug dictionary;
■ Quality review;
■ Medical review by physicians;
■ Submission to HAs, subsidiaries, business partners, and so on.

To support the drug safety group there is often a dedicated informatics (computer) group, a signaling/pharmacovigilance group, a training group, a standard operating procedure group, an epidemiology group, and more. These groups may be within or separate from the drug safety department. Sometimes a medical report writing group also falls under drug safety to prepare Periodic Safety Update Reports, NDA periodic reports, IND annual reports, and so on.

Similar groups often exist within HAs. Some authorities (FDA) receive reports directly from health care professionals, and consumers and groups that are similar to those noted above in companies must be created within the agency to receive, enter, and evaluate data and make medical judgments on the cases. The volumes in companies may run to the tens or even hundreds of thousands of cases per year. The FDA received over 422,000 postmarketing reports in 2004. See its website (Web Resource 4-23).

This is a large task and is performed in many countries throughout the world. Because most serious cases tend to be reported to most health agencies, there is enormous duplication of effort in creating multiple databases in agencies and companies throughout the world. In practice, only HAs in large countries with advanced pharmacovigilance practices are able to maintain relatively complete databases and do meaningful signal analyses.

The efforts of the Uppsala Monitoring Centre (UMC) in Sweden and the European Eudravigilance database are attempting to centralize data collection to create large repositories of safety information. In time it is likely that three major databases with large but not total overlap will exist for postmarketing AEs: the FDA in the United States, the Eudravigilance database in the EMEA (London), and the Vigibase at the UMC in Sweden.

Clinical trial AEs tend to be more scattered and far less transparent than AEs for marketed products because most of the information on drugs not yet on the market is proprietary and guarded as secret information both by companies and HAs. There is now a move in the United States by pharmaceutical companies and the FDA to have safety and efficacy data from clinical trials placed in "registry" websites. These websites, as of this writing, tend to contain serious AEs from the trials but little summary or aggregate information as contained in investigator brochures. How this will evolve and the level of transparency attained remains to be seen.

The mission of the drug safety group must be clearly defined and made known to all employees of the company, in particular to senior management and marketing and sales.

The mission of the drug safety group, whether in a company or a health agency, is first and foremost to protect the public health by maintaining accurate, up-to-date, and complete safety information. Medical analyses must be done with patient safety in mind, not only "product protection." Secondary goals within a company's safety department relate to such corporate functions as the preparation of regulatory reports (NDA periodic reports, Periodic Safety Update Reports, IND annual reports, etc.) for submission to HAs and consultation within the company on safety issues.

There is often enormous pressure on the safety group to minimize or wait on safety issues until they are proven beyond the shadow of a doubt. The attitude that the "drug is innocent until proven guilty" and that safety warnings should not be issued to the FDA or the public until this point is reached is not appropriate in the world of safety. Rather, each safety issue must be evaluated and acted on because of its own merit and criticality in a timely fashion. Some problems must be addressed on Friday at 5 p.m.

In the corporate world this attitude runs contrary to the prevailing fiduciary obligation of a corporation ("to increase stockholder value by making more profit"). The personnel in the drug safety department need a fair amount of masochism and a thick skin to work in this very nonglorious field, unlike the world of clinical research or sales where there are congratulations (and monetary bonuses) for completing a study, getting an NDA approved, or selling more drug. Rather, drug safety personnel need strong backbones to be able to say to management that a product has a safety problem that must be acted on immediately. Good and wise corporate management understands this and welcomes "straight talk" from the safety unit. Bad management buries or delays. This is becoming more and more dangerous as the penalties (commercial, regulatory, and legal) are becoming more and more severe. Corporate executives are now realizing that a safety problem hidden in the short run may, in the long run, appear on the front page of the *NY Times*, on CNN, or the 6 o'-clock news. They may need to explain their actions to congressional panels and to the multiple lawsuits—class action, civil, and criminal—that now pop up in the United States on any safety-related issue.

Similarly, the role of drug safety in the FDA is difficult. The primary mission is similar to the corporate safety role: protect the public health. However, the profit-making motive is not present. Instead, there are always intense budget pressures to save money as well as the need to answer to multiple demanding constituencies: the Secretary of Health and Human Services, the US Congress, the public, the press and media, the health professions, and the companies (and lobbies) the HA regulates. Employees at the FDA often make less money and have fewer of the corporate "perks" than their counterparts in the industry. This is one reason why some of them leave the FDA after several years of service and join a big pharmaceutical company, whereas the reverse path is rarely seen.

FAQs

Q: Why would anyone want to work in drug safety?

A: Good question. Once the decision is made by a health care professional to move out of the clinical world and into industrial medicine, it is noted that certain personality types tend to go to drug safety. Unlike the "glamour" of clinical research where new and exciting drugs are tested, drug safety tends to have a different atmosphere, dealing with the problems of the new and exciting (and old and dull) drugs.

There is much more detective work and medical analysis in working hard to obtain all the clinical facts available, perform a defensible medical analysis, and come to a medically sound conclusion often based on incomplete data. The work can be quite academic when one is working up a complex signal. And as always in medicine, one never has enough information. There is always one more test or examination one could do to get closer to the truth. Yet given the data available, one must come to the medically proper conclusion and convey this in a cogent way to both medical and nonmedical people. The work is challenging and very fulfilling when done well.

There is also much drama and excitement. Much can be routine, but the next fax or e-mail may bring a disaster with widespread consequences if the signal bears out. The adrenaline level rises and the "crisis" team mobilizes. Those who do perform drug safety as a career are often passionate about it. Few decide at the outset of a pharmaceutical career that they want to "do side effects." Rather, they want to discover new drugs or do clinical research or study the pharmacology of drugs. Many come into drug safety after trying other areas in the industry and discover they love it.

Q: Is there not an inherent conflict of interest in asking a company to police itself?

A: In a sense yes, especially when money is involved. Most regulated professions have some level of self-policing, including aviation, the food industry, medicine, and law. Still, there must be some level of outside oversight to try to ensure that the self-policing is done correctly. Finding the right balance is always the trick. In practice, there is far too much to do and oversee in the pharmaceutical industry to have total outside oversight from the FDA. Rather, practicalities force the system to police itself with regulations, periodic reports, monitoring, reviews, audits, and other mechanisms looking over the industry's shoulder to "keep them honest."

Adverse Events with New Chemical Entities, Generics, Excipients, and Placebos

Are some adverse events (AEs) created more equal than others? Are some AEs more important than others? Why AEs with generics and older drugs are important. What to do with other manufacturers' AEs. Why AEs with new chemical entities are critically important. Why AEs due to excipients are so hard to pick up. Why AEs with over-the-counter drugs are also important. Why AEs before taking the drug can matter.

> ➡ **NOTE:** (Unless otherwise noted the word "drug" or "drug product" should be taken in this book to include "biologics" and "vaccines.")

■ Background

The reporting requirements for AEs and drugs are generally thought of as being critical for the safety evalua-

tion of new chemical entities (NCEs) newly approved for marketing. NCEs by definition have not been on the market before. Their safety profile is known only from limited laboratory, animal, and human testing under an Investigational New Drug Application (IND) or equivalent. Clearly, AE reporting is critical in this period, and companies and agencies pay particular attention to the spontaneous AE reports received shortly after launch (known as the Weber Effect: a large number of AEs/adverse drug reactions reported just after launch that decrease after some months to a lower more steady state number of reports [see Chapter 7]). Rare AEs that were not seen in the trials are often picked up in the weeks to months after launch in major markets with good AE reporting structures, such as the United States or Europe. Regulations on AE reporting are written with this in mind.

Given the large number of AEs that drugs can produce and given the limited number of resources that the US Food and Drug Administration (FDA), companies, and health care professionals can devote to reporting and processing AEs, there is an ongoing debate about what AEs are most cost-effective and medically important to collect to protect the public health.

◼ The Theory

The FDA MedWatch program collects safety information about "prescription and over-the-counter drugs, biologics, medical and radiation-emitting devices, and special nutritional products (e.g., medical foods, dietary supplements and infant formulas)." See the FDA's website (Web Resource 5-1).

Generics

The current regulations from the FDA do not address generics in and of themselves. Any drug under a New Drug Application (NDA) or an Abbreviated NDA must meet the AE reporting requirements in 21CFR314.80. This includes generics and NCEs.

Excipients

An excipient is a theoretically inactive ingredient added to a drug to provide bulk or to give it form or consistency. In regard to excipients, there are many types, including binders, fillers, diluents, lubricants, sweeteners, preservatives, flavors, printing inks, colors, and others. The most common ones used in the United States include magnesium stearate, lactose, microcrystalline cellulose, silicon dioxide, titanium dioxide, stearic acid, sodium starch glycolate, gelatin, talc, sucrose, povidone, pregelatinized starch, hydroxyl propyl methylcellulose, shellac, calcium phosphate (dibasic), and others. Standards are set by committees of the US Pharmacopeial Convention and published in the US Pharmacopeia and the National Formulary.

Excipients became a major issue in the United States when a sulfonamide elixir was diluted in diethylene glycol (automobile antifreeze) and killed about 100 Americans, including children. It led in 1938 to the Food, Drug and Cosmetic Act.

An excipient for drugs is approved for use in the United States by one of three mechanisms:

1. It meets the requirements of being "Generally Recognized as Safe" under 21CFR182, 184, 186.

2. The FDA approves a petition as a food additive under 21CFR171.

3. It is referenced in an approved NDA for a particular function for that drug.

Excipients for over-the-counter products must comply with section 21CFR330.1(e) as "safe in the amounts administered and do not interfere with the effectiveness of the preparation...."

Please refer to the excellent website run by the International Pharmaceutical Excipients Council (Web Resource 5-2) for further information.

The FDA definition of an adverse drug experience refers to "any AE associated with the use of a drug" (21CFR314.80(a)) without indicating whether the event is associated with the active ingredient (moiety) or an excipient. Should the submitter have some reason to suspect an excipient to be the cause of the AE, this should be noted in the report and the appropriate investigations and follow-up done. In the European Union, Volume 9 only refers to excipients in regard to altering Periodic Safety Update Report cycles. There is no direct comment on AEs possibly related to fillers or excipients. Excipients in one country may be considered active ingredients in other countries and vice versa.

Placebo

In the United States, placebo AEs from trials do not generally have to be reported as expedited reports. However, many blinded trials do have AEs (including serious AEs) that are reported as blinded events during the trial either as expedited reports or in periodic or annual reports. At the end of the study, the unblinding reveals some of them to be associated with placebo and not active drug. In addition, in preparing final study reports, integrated safety sections for NDAs, dossiers for marketing approval in the European Union and elsewhere, and comparisons of AEs on active drug and placebo must be reported if there is a placebo arm of the trial. Thus, all placebo AEs should be recorded and tracked in the safety database.

In the European Union, some countries require reporting of all AEs related to the "biomedical research," not just to the taking of the active study drug. In this case placebo cases need to be reported as expedited reports and in periodic summary reports. The EU Clinical Trial Directive (2001/20/EC of April 4, 2001) defines an "investigational medicinal product" as "a pharmaceutical form of an active substance or placebo being tested or used in a clinical trial..." and requires certain serious AEs to be reported as expedited reports. Thus many have read this as a requirement for placebo reporting.

Other Manufacturers' AEs

The US regulations are not clear on this point. There is a section 21CFR314.80(1)(iii) on how to handle 15-day expedited serious AEs that are received by a company whose name appears on the product as a packer, distributor, or manufacturer but who is not the applicant (holder of the NDA). This section allows the nonapplicant to submit the serious AE to the FDA or to transmit it within 5 calendar days to the applicant who will then submit it to the FDA. Some have extrapolated from this section to mean that AE reports that are received but are clearly those of another company's product should be sent to the other company.

■ The Practice

In practice, companies collect all AEs that come to them whether the drug in question is their drug, a generic, or a placebo or if excipients are suspected. The data are usually handled in the usual way and entered into the database. During the workup the issues of generic, placebo, and so forth are sorted out.

Placebo

The practice for placebo is variable depending on whether or not a company breaks the blind when reporting 7- and 15-day expedited reports to health authorities. If a company breaks the blind routinely for all serious, unexpected, possibly related AEs from a trial and the product in question is placebo, this case is usually not reported to the FDA but kept in the company's database for listing in the final study report. If, however, the company does not unblind and thus reports blinded cases to the FDA and other health authorities as 15-day reports, when the blind is broken at the end of the study the company must submit a follow-up noting whether the patient received drug or placebo. Health authorities in the European Union do not want blinded expedited reports.

Excipients

It is very difficult to pick up AEs due to excipients. The reasons are many. Most drug safety personnel do not pay much attention to excipients and may not even know what excipients are in which drug. Excipients often vary from formulation to formulation of the same drug and may vary in quantity from dose strength to dose strength (e.g., higher doses of the same active ingredient may be larger tablets or capsules and have more fillers and excipients) and may vary from country to country.

Manufacturers often change excipients and production methods (with the appropriate Good Manufacturing Practice change control and notification to the regulatory

agencies) without telling the drug safety department. There may thus be hundreds to hundreds of thousands of individual products with varying excipients manufactured by a large company. These are usually not easily computerized, updated, and searchable. A problem with one excipient in one or only a handful of lots or formulations may go undetected unless there is an obvious and unusual AE and a high level of suspicion on the part of the reviewer.

Manufacturers also often change vendors for excipients, and this too may produce issues if product quality or characteristics change. For companies with many products and formulations manufactured in many countries, tracking formulations is impossible for the drug safety group.

The author recalls a product that contained lactose as a filler and that had much more lactose in the US version than in the Canadian version. When it was discovered that the incidence of diarrhea in the United States was higher than in Canada, the signal investigation revealed the lactose dose difference to be the cause. A very high level of suspicion must be maintained to keep open the possibility of an excipient causing an AE. It is particularly difficult if the AE is common, like diarrhea, or may be caused by the active ingredient itself.

Generics

In general, if an AE is reported and the product is identified by the reporter of the AE as a generic and the manufacturer is known, this AE is reported to that manufacturer (see above) rather than to the FDA directly. It would be the responsibility of the manufacturer of the product in question (the generic) to report it to the FDA. If the AE is not known to be from the sponsor's drug or from a generic, then the sponsor receiving the report must treat it as if it were that company's product and handle it in the usual manner for submission to the FDA. It can be noted in the report that the manufacturer is unknown.

It is obviously important that the correct manufacturer of a drug be identified. Problems might occur with one company's drug and not another's. Causes could relate not just to the active compound itself but also to manufacturing issues (product quality complaints), different excipients, impurities, supplier issues, and so on. Thus when a company receives a spontaneous AE for a product it must make a concerted effort to determine who the manufacturer is if other versions are marketed to ensure that the report is attributed to the correct drug.

■ FAQs

Q: So for products with generic formulations and/or several branded formulations of the same chemical entity, the FDA and other health authorities receive multiple reports from multiple manufacturers at varying time points, some of which may be duplicates reported to different NDAs and/or INDs. This doesn't seem, shall we say, optimal. Is there not a better way to do this?

A: Another fine question. Clearly, there is multiple reporting of cases to different countries, reporting of AEs for a particular chemical entities to separate and unrelated INDs and NDAs at the FDA, and then retransmission, often with recoding of AEs, to other databases (e.g., World Health Organization's Uppsala Monitoring Centre in Sweden). It is nearly impossible to sort out duplicates, excipient effects, and other subtle causes of AEs. We are not aware of any central or complete database that lists a product's excipients of all or multiple manufacturers. Each company keeps its own AE database usually not linked to a formulations database.

The solutions are straightforward but not easily done. A single, enormous, worldwide database or well-linked multiple databases, updated frequently in which all drugs (generic, branded, branded generics, etc.), formulations, excipients, registration numbers, dose, and so on are maintained would be the optimal solution. The likelihood of this happening in the near to mid future is nil due to multiple reasons, including cost, lack of ownership, lack of a complete dataset, and lack of a perception that this is really needed. In reality, with thousands of pharmaceutical manufacturers worldwide, it is unlikely we will ever attain a complete database. More likely is that the major players (United States, European Union, China, Japan, India, and a handful of others) representing the large majority of manufacturers and users of drugs will set up some degree of database linking. This will go a long way to resolving many of these issues.

Q: If resources are limited and demand infinite, should we even bother looking at all generics and excipients? Shouldn't we concentrate on the newest or most used or most dangerous products and concede such things as excipients problems in little used products?

A: Yes, you are probably right. It is impossible to track everything. Rather, a triage strategy needs to be developed should there ever be a rational use of pharmacovigilance resources and not duplicative work from agency to agency and company to company. One might wish to look at a particular excipient in only, say, five products in five countries periodically to see whether there are any safety issues. One must also decide whether to be proactive and do such investigations periodically and in anticipation of potential safety issues or whether to be reactive and start an investigation only after a problem or signal arises.

Q: What about generics? Shouldn't they be all grouped under one NDA or something like that for AE and signaling purposes?

A: Yes, that is probably a good idea but very difficult to do under the current laws and regulations around the world. Rather, the same result could be attained (and is, in fact, done) at the database level where data are combined or analyzed over multiple products with the same chemical entity.

Acute and Chronic (Late Occurring) Adverse Events, Adverse Events That Disappear (Bendectin™), and Diethylstilbestrol

➤ **NOTE:**(Unless otherwise noted the word "drug" or "drug product" should be taken in this book to include "biologics" and "vaccines.")

■ Background

Adverse events (AEs) seen shortly after starting or stopping drugs are common and relatively easy to recognize (though if it were that easy, there would be little need for this book). There is usually a high index of suspicion, a close temporal relationship, and often biologic and pharmacologic plausibility.

This is not the case for AEs that occur weeks, months, or even years after stopping the drug ("long latency period"). There may be no medical record available, the memory of use of the product by the patient may be hazy, the index of suspicion is low or nonexistent, and there may be no logical, biologic, or pharmacologic reason for this AE to be associated with the drug. Examples are common in long latency diseases. Examples include cigarette smoking and cancer of the lung many years later, asbestos inhalation producing pleural mesotheliomas decades after

exposure ended, or the classic example of vaginal cancer in the offspring of women taking diethylstilbestrol (DES).

It is now more and more recognized that drug therapy as well as other therapies (radiation therapy) can produce late AEs. Usually, it takes a very insightful clinician or a good epidemiologic study to show that a particular drug caused (or is associated with) a particular AE years later. Such a proposal is often met with disbelief and even ridicule. However, public health demands that all contingencies be kept in mind and examined when appropriate.

Finally, to keep us humble, an example of what looked like a clear and related AE and that turned out not to be such is presented (Bendectin™).

■ The Theory

From empirical observations, the latency period from starting or stopping of a drug to the onset of the AE is very variable. AEs can be seen immediately after starting to take a drug, shortly thereafter, or even after weeks or months of taking the drug with no problems. AEs can also be seen long after stopping the drug. Examples noted below are examples of AEs seen long after starting or stopping a drug.

■ The Practice

Adriamycin

Examples of drugs producing late AEs include Adriamycin, which may produce cardiac problems years after therapy has ended.

> "Myocardial toxicity manifested in its most severe form by potentially fatal congestive heart failure may occur either during therapy or months to years after termination of therapy. The probability of developing impaired myocardial function based on a combined index of signs, symptoms and decline in left ventricular ejection fraction (LVEF) is estimated to be 1 to 2% at a total cumulative dose of 300 mg/m^2 of doxorubicin, 3 to 5% at a dose of 400 mg/m^2, 5 to 8% at 450 mg/m^2 and 6 to 20% at 500 mg/m^2.* The risk of developing congestive heart failure (CHF) increases rapidly with increasing total cumulative doses of doxorubicin in excess of 450 mg/m^2. This toxicity may occur at lower cumulative doses in patients with prior mediastinal irradiation or on concurrent cyclophosphamide therapy or with pre-existing heart disease" (Package Insert for Adriamycin, Pharmacia, 2005).

Gene Therapy

An area of increasing concern is the possibility of late-occurring AEs seen after gene therapy. The US Food and Drug Administration (FDA) has cited this as an issue in gene therapy:

> "Many of the potential adverse effects of concern in gene therapy patients are the same as those of concern for other therapies; however, gene therapy raises some concerns that are relatively unique. Perhaps the greatest area of concern is that of late-occurring toxicities. By permanently altering the genetic makeup of the recipient cells, some forms of gene therapy may cause toxicities that do not manifest themselves until years later. Additionally, some gene therapies use viral vectors with the potential to form latent infections that may emerge clinically years later" (Center for Biologics Evaluation and Research Publication: Gene Therapy Patient Tracking System, Final Document, June 27, 2002). See the FDA's website (Web Resource 6-1).

Antiretroviral Drugs

It is now well recognized that many human immunodeficiency virus drugs can produce late toxicity. The FDA has issued a guidance noting that long-term follow-up should be done in clinical trials:

> "Because multiple adverse events have been observed with chronic administration of antiretroviral therapy, mechanisms should be used for systematically evaluating adverse events over prolonged periods following traditional approval. Controlled comparisons and prospectively evaluated cohorts may be helpful in characterizing and defining drug associations for late-occurring adverse events. Therefore, after traditional approval, the Division strongly encourages sponsors to continue to collect safety data in key randomized studies or other treatment cohorts for prolonged periods (3–5 years)" (Guidance for Industry, Antiretroviral Drugs Using Plasma HIV RNA Measurements—Clinical Considerations for Accelerated and Traditional Approval, Center for Drug Evaluation and Research, October 2002). See the FDA's website (Web Resource 6-2).

Diethylstilbestrol (DES)

Perhaps the most interesting and striking example of delayed-onset AEs is that of vaginal cancer in the offspring of women who took DES. This is examined in detail.

DES is an estrogen first synthesized in 1938. In 1941 DES was approved for human use by the FDA. In 1947 the agency approved the use during pregnancy for the treatment/prevention of spontaneous abortion (miscarriage) based largely on the work of Harvard researchers, George and Olive Smith, work that eventually proved to be wrong; the drug did not prevent miscarriages.

The suspicion of a problem arose in 1970, when clinicians observed a rare vaginal cancer occurring in women aged 14 to 22 years. This cancer, clear cell adenocarcinoma (CCA), was classically seen only in women in their seventies. No explanation seemed apparent until the mother of one of the young cancer patients mentioned that she had taken DES to prevent a miscarriage. Questioning of the other mothers revealed that they too had taken DES, and Dr. Arthur Herbst confirmed the association between DES and CCA in a case control study in 1971.

Delayed Onset of Malignancy (Long Latency)

The delay in the appearance of the adverse drug reaction after the last dose (the latency period) is among the longest ever seen. The delay in detection has several explanations:

- The AE did not occur in the women who took DES but in their female offspring exposed during the critical window of vaginogenesis.
- The AE was not visible in the female offspring at birth.
- The AE was not evident until after puberty during a gynecologic examination.
- Obstetric problems (see below) appeared only when a pregnancy occurred

The spontaneous reporting consisted of a publication of the first series of cases and by a case-control study.

The reported risk of developing CCA in DES-exposed women is approximately 1 in 1,000 from birth to 34 years of age. The risk increases rapidly from the onset of puberty until the late teens and early twenties. Subsequently, the risk drops dramatically, although a few cases have been reported in women in their forties. Other less serious but more frequent obstetric and gynecologic problems in the DES-exposed progeny have also been commented on in the medical literature:

- Vaginal adenosis, cervical ectropion (normal, albeit misplaced, columnar epithelium);
- Structural anomalies such as cervical hoods, hypoplastic, and T-shaped uterus;
- Functional problems such as decreased fertility, ectopic pregnancy, spontaneous abortions (relative risk, 92:1), and preterm births (relative risk, 5:1);
- Possible abnormalities in children of daughters whose mothers received DES (i.e., third generation);
- Benign malformations, such as small testicles and epididymal cysts in males exposed in utero.

Actions Taken

In 1971, the FDA banned the use of DES in pregnant women (FDA Drug Bulletin, 1971). In the same year, a Registry was established with Dr. Arthur Herbst as the Chairperson, and in 1978 the DESAD Project was developed to study DES-exposed women with adenosis. In 1973 the US National Institutes of Health notified medical schools and gynecologic oncologists about increased cancer risk. In 1977 France withdrew the obstetric indication. A movement known as DES Action was created in the United States in 1977, in Canada in 1982, in France in 1987, and in the United Kingdom in 1989. See its website (Web Resource 6-3).

In 1999, the US Congress directed the National Cancer Institute to fund a 3-year DES National Educational Campaign housed at the Centers for Disease Control and Prevention (Herbst, *N Engl J Med* 1971;284:878–881; Wilcox, *N Engl J Med* 1995;332:1411; Giusti, *Ann Intern Med* 1995;122:778; *DES Action VOICE*, Summer 2000 [section adapted from Cobert and Biron, *Pharmacovigilance from A to Z*]).

Bendectin™: A False Alert

Bendectin™ is a fixed combination of three active ingredients used for the treatment of nausea and vomiting of pregnancy:

1. Doxylamine, an H_1 antihistamine that acts as an antinausea and antivomiting agent;
2. Pyridoxine, vitamin B_6;
3. Dicycloverine, removed from the product shortly before market withdrawal of Bendectin™.

This product was incorrectly suspected of causing congenital abnormalities. Several case-control studies were performed, and their results formed the basis for the exoneration of this product. It had been on the market for about 27 years and was taken by some 33 million pregnant women in the United States, representing 20–40% of all pregnant women. It was voluntarily withdrawn from the US market and never returned even after its exoneration. It was sold under the name of Debendox™ in other countries (Fleming *BMJ* 1981;283:99; CSM/MCA, *Current Problems in Pharmacovigilance* 1981;6; *Lancet* 1984;2:205; *BMJ* 1985;271:918).

Return to the Market in Canada

A laboratory was authorized to sell a product containing doxylamine and pyridoxine under the name of Diclectin™. To reduce the remaining suspicions held by obstetricians, it was specified in the product labeling that the therapeutic category for which this combination was approved was "Anti-nausea agent for the nausea and vomiting of pregnancy." A group of Canadian experts published a statement on August 11, 1989 affirming that this fixed association was safe. The British authorities had also expressed the same opinion. The Canadian government has thus maintained a marketing authorization for this product for a Canadian manufacturer (CSM/MCA, *Current Problems Pharmacovigilance* 1981;6; *Lancet* 1984;2:205; Medico-Legal Committee Opinion, *J Soc Obstet Gynaecol Can* 1995;17:162; Koren, *Can J Clin Pharmacol* 1995;2:38).

There is an enormous literature on Bendectin™, and it is maintained by some that this is the most-studied drug in pregnancy ever. There are several books and hundreds of references available. The Reprotox® database has several references and brief summary of the data on Bendectin™. See its website (Web Resource 6-4).

The Future

An academic Canadian group has studied late-occurring AEs and other ill effects that occur long after stopping treatment with biotherapeutics. They have proposed the creation of a registry to track such events throughout Canada: Post-Market Surveillance of Biotherapeutics for Late Health Effects—A Systematic Review and Recommendations on Active Surveillance in Canada. See its website (Web Resource 6-5).

■ FAQ

Q: This seems to put the practitioner in an impossible position. How can one even begin to make a rational attempt to determine whether a particular sign or symptom or AE is due to a drug (or drugs) taken weeks, months, or even years ago? The patient may not even remember or know precisely what he or she was taking. And how can we even approach the issue of AEs due to the drugs a parent took a generation ago?

A: A valid point. The finding of very-long-term or skipped-generation AEs remains primarily in the domain of epidemiology and observational studies. There is a tendency to run the safety arm of clinical trials for longer periods of time after the acute study is over. However, even that will not pick up the rare AE due to the small number of patients involved and the difficulties of long-term observational studies of safety where all patients will have AEs (and will die) if you follow the patients long enough. That is, there are confounding and coincidental events that make interpretation of the long-term results very difficult. It may well be that a more formal health authority–driven review of large databases in an ongoing manner will be the wave of the future, as suggested by the Canadian proposal.

Spontaneous reporting by astute clinicians remains the next best approach based on the examples seen to date. From the practitioner's point of view, a high level of suspicion must be maintained. The patient should be quizzed on both recent and remote drug history, including over-the-counter medications. Beyond that, we must await better techniques and methodology for tracking drugs taken and AEs that occur.

The Mathematics of Adverse Events

➥ **NOTE:** (Unless otherwise noted the word "drug" or "drug product" should be taken in this book to include "biologics" and "vaccines.")

◼ Background

This chapter is by no means intended to be a reference on statistics, epidemiology, or the technical mathematical aspects of data analysis. Rather, it is meant to give a very elementary and selective overview of some of the "numbers" used in pharmacovigilance and show why, in our view, they have not been very useful in clinical medicine and pharmacovigilance.

When a new adverse event (AE) begins to be reported in association with a new product, the two fundamental questions raised in the eyes of the regulator and the manufacturer are about rates (Will it?) and causality (Can it?).

Suppose that spontaneous reports of a liver injury under drug X start coming in at the safety center. First, what is the estimated causality link between the liver problem and that suspect drug? Were the patients exposed to only the suspect drug or were they simultaneously taking other products? Was the time to onset short

enough to be very suggestive or was it so long that suspicion is rather low? Was the patient in perfect health or was he or she at high risk of developing viral hepatitis? According to these and other diagnostic criteria, the clinician will roughly assess causality: definite, probable, possible, or unlikely. When enough details are available in a case report and when the report is complete enough, these judgments are feasible and they matter. We then say these reports are valid, of high quality.

The next question is the rate of occurrence of this reported AE; in other words, what is the probability of the next patient exposed to product X developing severe liver disease? One in 10, 1 in 100, 1 in 1,000? It is obviously important to know.

Over the years, many attempts have been made to apply statistics and epidemiologic methods to case series of AEs, primarily with spontaneously reported AEs. The results have been disheartening.

It is necessary to differentiate between AEs received in clinical or epidemiologic trials and those received spontaneously or in a solicited manner. Broadly speaking, the use of statistics is well described and defined for data generated in formal clinical trials. The patient populations to some degree are under the control of the investigator or researcher. The methodology for efficacy and safety analysis is well described and largely agreed on. Placebo and comparator controlled trials give clear pictures of occurrence rates of AEs, and significance values and confidence intervals can be determined and used to draw conclusions. The data are usually very solid, because data integrity is good to excellent. In addition, the data collected are usually complete. As patients are seen by the investigator at periodic intervals and as the investigator and his or her staff questions the patient on AEs, it is believed that few AEs are missed, especially serious or dramatic AEs. Incidence rates calculated from these data are held to be believable and useful.

Spontaneous reports are a different situation entirely. The data are unsolicited and may come from consumers and/or health care professionals. In the current system, some 80% of AEs in the United States initially arrive at pharmaceutical companies' safety departments and 20% at the US Food and Drug Administration (FDA). Follow-up is variable, and source documents (e.g., laboratory reports, office and hospital records, autopsy reports, etc.) are not always obtained due to privacy issues, busy physicians, or pharmacists unable to supply records from multiple sources, patients not wanting to disclose information, and so on. Hence, the data integrity is variable and inconsistent.

Spontaneously reported data respond to two broad phenomena: the Weber Effect and secular effects, described below.

Weber Effect

The Weber Effect, also called the product life cycle effect, describes the phenomenon of increased voluntary reporting after the initial launch of a new drug. "Voluntary reporting of adverse events for a new drug within an established drug class does not proceed at a uniform rate and may be much higher in the first year or two of the drug's introduction" (Weber, *Advances in Inflammation Research*, Raven Press, New York, 1984, pages 1–7). This means that for the period of time after launch (from 6 months to as long as 2 years), there will be a large number of spontaneously reported AEs/adverse drug reactions (ADRs) that taper down to steady-state levels after this effect is over. It is to be distinguished from secular effects.

Secular Effects

Drug safety officers live in dread of reports of celebrities or politicians using a particular product, especially if an AE is reported. This phenomenon is also called "temporal bias" and reflects an increase in AE reporting for a drug or class of drugs after increased media attention, use of a

medication by a celebrity, a warning from a health agency, and so on. "Overall adverse drug reaction reporting rates can be increased several times by external factors such as a change in a reporting system or an increased level of publicity attending a given drug or adverse reaction" (Sachs and Bortnichak, *Am J Med* 1986;81[suppl 5B]:49).

Perhaps the most difficult problem with spontaneous and stimulated reporting is the incompleteness of the data. Ideally, one would like to calculate incidence rates for a particular AE with a particular drug where

$$\frac{\text{Numerator}}{\text{Denominator}} = \frac{\text{AEs that occurred}}{\text{Patients exposed}}$$

However, the number of reports of an AE is always less than the true number of occurrences, because not all AEs are reported. It is estimated that in the United Kingdom only 10% of serious ADRs and 2–4% of nonserious ADRs that occur are reported (Rawlins, *J R Coll Phys Lond* 1995;29:41–49). In the United States the FDA estimates that only 1% of serious suspected ADRs are reported (Scott, Rosenbaum, Waters, et al., *R I Med J* 1987;70:311–316). These figures are cited by the FDA in a continuing medical education article from the FDA entitled, "The Clinical Impact of Adverse Event Reporting" (October 1996) available on its website (Web Resource 7-1). The number of uncaptured AEs is therefore quite variable. This renders the numerator in the proportion quite suspect.

In addition, the denominator, patient exposure, is unknown. Although one can obtain prescription data and one can know how many tablets or capsules or tubes were sold, it is hard to know how many people actually took the product in the manner and for the length of time prescribed. Should one count the patient who took one tablet once in the same way as someone who took three tablets a day for a month?

This could be patients exposed, patient-months of exposure (number of patients times number of months each patient took the drug), tablets sold, kilograms sold, kilograms manufactured, prescriptions written or filled, and so on.

Nonetheless, by obtaining these data, crude estimates of reporting rates can be made. However, the numbers are often not terribly meaningful. The author recalls one very widely used product for which 12 cardiac arrhythmia reports were received for what was calculated to be 9 billion (9,000,000,000) patient years of exposure. This works out to 12/9,000,000,000 or a reporting rate of 0.0000000013 cardiac arrhythmia events/patient-years of exposure, which is not a very meaningful number, particularly to a clinician who needs to make a decision on whether a particular patient should be given this drug.

The manufacturing data (kilograms made) are available from the company producing the product, and the prescription information and the patient exposure data are obtained from various private companies that track such things (e.g., a company named IMS Health Incorporated; see its website [Web Resource 7-2]).

These data can be broken down by gender, age, and other demographic characteristics. Trends over time in usage can be observed.

In summary, as Dr. David Goldsmith has said, "the numerator is bad; the denominator is worse and the ratio is meaningless." Hence, one cannot calculate the incidence rates for a particular AE based on spontaneous data. Period.

■ The Theory

The reader is referred to the many excellent textbooks at all levels available on epidemiology and statistics in medicine and pharmacology, including the following:

Brian Strom: *Pharmacoepidemiology*. 1994. John Wiley Inc.

Ron Mann and Elizabeth Andrews: *Pharmacovigilance*. 2002. John Wiley Inc.

Abraham Hartzema, Miquel Porta, Hugh Tilson: *Pharmacoepidemiology*. 1998. Harvey Whitney Books.

Joseph Ingelfinger, Frederick Mosteller, Lawrence Thibodeau, James Ware: *Biostatistics in Clinical Medicine*. 1987. McGraw-Hill.

David Streiner, Geoffrey Norman: *PDQ Epidemiology*. 1996. BC Decker.

David Streiner, Geoffrey Norman: *PDQ Statistics*. 2003. BC Decker.

Douglas Altman: *Practical Statistics for Medical Research*. 1990. Chapman & Hall/CRC.

Beth Dawson, Robert G. Trapp: *Basic & Clinical Biostatistics (LANGE Basic Science)*. 2004. McGraw-Hill.

Another interesting book is not about medicine or statistics or pharmacology but is about the concept and history of financial risk. It gives a broad and well-written overview on the role of risk in society:

Peter Bernstein: *Against the Gods—The Remarkable Story of Risk*. 1996. Wiley.

Many concepts have been examined over the years. One area where mathematical and statistical methods have been somewhat useful is in signal screening. In these meth-

ods, large amounts of data are examined statistically to see if any signals "pop out." They are evaluated and if of interest (however that is determined) they are further evaluated clinically. There are many methods, and they are excellently summarized by Clark, Klincewicz, and Stang in *Pharmacovigilance* by Andrews and Mann (pp. 247–271).

Bayesian analysis, also called probabilistic causality, is a technique used to analyze causality in which conditional probabilities are used and which are modified as new information is obtained to obtain a final causality. The method was tried in the 1980s and 1990s with moderate success. In practice, this method has not been found to be useful in the analysis of case series due to the inability to obtain AE rates in exposed (the true ADR rate + the background AE rate) and unexposed populations (the natural background AE rate).

See the following references:

Clark JA, Klincewica SL, LaFrance NL. A Bayesian method for the evaluation of case series of adverse drug reactions (Abstr). *Pharmacoepidemiology and Drug Safety* 2000;9(suppl):S33.

Clark JA, Klincewica SL, Stang PE. Spontaneous adverse event signaling methods: classification and use with health care treatment products. *Epidemiol Rev* 2001;23:191–210.

Cobert B, Biron P. *Pharmacovigilance from A to Z*. Blackwell Scientific 2000, pp. 23–24.

Mann R, Andrews E. *Pharmacovigilance*. John Wiley Inc. 2000, pp. 240–243.

■ The Practice

In practice there are few statistics applied to case series of spontaneous AEs. The most commonly used "numbers" include a ratio of AEs reported in the numerator to a denominator reflecting some sort of exposure.

The International Conference on Harmonization document E2C (Periodic Safety Update Report preparation, see Chapter 26) notes that "The most appropriate method [for patient exposure] should be used and an explanation for its choice provided. This includes patients exposed, patient-days, number of prescriptions, tonnage sold etc." The E2C addendum notes "It is acknowledged that this data is often difficult to obtain and not always reliable. If the exposure data does not cover the full period of the PSUR, extrapolations may be made. A consistent method of exposure calculations should be used over time for a product."

Various methods are being developed and used for looking at spontaneous reports. The methods go under the general heading of "data mining." They tend to be used for signal generation and not really for analysis of case series where a signal has already been found. These methods are as follows:

1. Proportionality methods (or disproportionality methods): These methods do not use exposure data but rather rely on the proportion of a particular AE or series of AEs for a specific drug compared with the same AE or series of AEs for other drugs either in the same database or in a larger database. Using the example above of cardiac arrhythmia events, one would compare the number of such AEs for drug X with the number of such events for the rest of the database (excluding drug X) to see whether there is a larger proportion of such events seen with drug X. At best this is usually suggestive of a signal, but it is hard to draw any real causality or frequency information from this number. There are many issues to consider:

   - Are the other drugs in the database cardiac drugs?

   - Are there a disproportionate number of cardiac patients in the drug X group versus the rest of the database?

   - Are the rest of the demographics for the remaining database patients the same as the drug X patients?

   - Is the coding "tight and crisp" for all the AEs?

   - The methodology is less useful if the number of (expected) AEs in question is very small.

2. Bayesian methodology to determine causality: Bayesian causality is the analysis of the causality of an ADR using conditional probabilities that are, in turn, modified with each new piece of information obtained, successively altering the preceding causalities to come up with a final causality. It is also called "probabilistic causality." This approach, which is based on probabilities, has also been applied to the differential diagnosis of medical conditions. Thomas Bayes (1702–1761), a Protestant minister and amateur mathematician, developed a theorem on conditional probabilities that supplied the theoretical basis for this approach. However, it took an additional two centuries for this concept to actually be applied to medical diagnosis in general and ADRs in particular (Bayes, *Phil Trans R Soc Lond (Biol)* 1763;53:370–375, reprinted in *Biometrika* 1958;45:296–315).

   It represents a partial model for diagnostic reasoning. Its rigorous use is possible, however, only in the context of a research project. It is not practical to use in pharmacovigilance or in clinical medicine because its use in individual cases can take many weeks of research to develop the incidences in exposed and unexposed populations. It is more useful to consider this approach as a conceptual method of clinical reasoning (Davidoff, *Med Care* 1989;29:45).

   Each judgment takes the form of a ratio whose numerator represents the drug etiology hypothesis and whose denominator represents the alternative nondrug etiology. The clinician must therefore start by choosing the most suspect drug among those possibly taken by the patient and the most likely alternative explanation in terms of the patient's medical condition. Then the relevant information is broken down into two main categories of criteria:

   - Prior, predictive
     - General prior odds (drug's background knowledge)
     - Case-specific prior odds, modified by history (risk factors)
   - Likelihood ratios of AE characteristics
     - Temporal (timing, rechallenge, etc.)
     - Nontemporal (site of application etc.)

   The Bayesian equation is composed of a series of relationships expressed as fractions that are multiplied together to obtain a final fraction that quantifies causality on a scale of 0 to 1.

   This methodology is now being developed for use in computerized programs and is in use by the Uppsala Monitoring Centre and others. The FDA is also actively looking at these techniques. See the following references:

   Empirical Bayesian data mining for discovering patterns in postmarketing drug safety: Conference on Knowledge Discovery in Data. Proceedings of the Ninth ACM SIGKDD International Conference on Knowledge Discovery and Data Mining. Washington, DC, Fram D, Almenoff J, DuMouche W. ACM Press, New York, 2003.

   Bate A, Lindquist M, Edwards IR, Orre R. A data mining approach for signal detection and analysis. *Drug Safety* 2002;25:393–397. This article reviews the Uppsala Monitoring Centre's approach.

   Hauben M. Early postmarketing drug safety surveillance: data mining points to consider. Published online in *The Annals of Pharmacotherapy*, 10 August 2004, www.theannals.com (Web Resource 7-3).

8

Organizations: The US Food and Drug Administration and MedWatch

➥ **NOTE:** (Unless otherwise noted the word "drug" or "drug product" should be taken in this book to include "biologics" and "vaccines.")

■ Background

In the last 20 or so years the number of organizations that are devoted to drug safety has increased markedly, in particular outside the United States. This chapter deals with the US Food and Drug Administration (FDA) and focuses on the major players involved in handling drug safety.

■ The Theory

The "granddaddy" of drug safety regulatory agencies dates back to 18th century Japan when the 8th Shogun, Yoshimune Tokugawa (1716–1745), upon recovering from an illness, awarded 124 medicinal traders in Osaka special privileges to examine medicines throughout the country. However, the safety of the medicines was difficult to guarantee despite these efforts. A shrine in Osaka, called Shinno-san, was created and dedicated to Shinno, the

guardian of the pharmaceutical industry and the divine founder of medicine from China. This information was found at the Osaka tourism website (Web Resource 8-1).

The FDA handles safety in several different areas. The two largest areas touching drug safety are the Center for Drug Evaluation and Research (CDER) and MedWatch.

CDER

This is the prime center in the FDA for handling drugs. In a nutshell, CDER handles new drugs from the Investigational New Drug Application (IND) stage (when a product first moves into human study) to the evaluation of the New Drug Application (NDA) for approval or rejection of the request to market the product in the United States. CDER then continues in its evaluation of the postmarketing safety of the product. Although simple in theory, the actual practice is complex and has evolved over time. It continues to change and should be viewed as a work in progress.

The organization chart is posted on-line and is quite useful giving names, addresses, and contact information (Web Resource 8-2). There are over 20 "offices" in CDER covering many areas, including biotechnology, new drug evaluation, counterterrorism, pediatric drug development (the latter two in the same office in 2005), generic drugs, compliance, and, of course, drug safety. There are also advisory committees that consist of outside experts who meet periodically to review data and advise the FDA on various issues, including drug approvals and policy issues. See CDER's website (Web Resource 8-3). There is a fairly new advisory committee on Drug Safety and Risk Management that looks at safety issues.

The FDA reorganized in May 2006. The Office of the CDER Center Director has under it the Office of Surveillance and Epidemiology and the Office of Safety Policy and Communication Staff. The Office of Surveillance and Epidemiology has under it three divisions: 1) Drug Risk Evaluation, 2) Surveillance, Research and Communication Support, and 3) Medication Errors and Technical Support. The Office of Safety Policy and Communication Staff has the MedWatch group and the Drug Safety Oversight Board. These are the primary groups that deal with drug safety. They handle postmarketing drug safety and work with the reviewing divisions on specific products. There has been criticism to the effect that these groups are not sufficiently independent of the reviewing groups to make safety decisions.

In May 2005, the FDA announced the creation of a new Drug Safety Oversight Board "to develop and disseminate important emerging drug safety information concerning marketed drug products to healthcare professionals and patients." See CDER's website (Web Resource 8-4). The goal is to make the FDA's review and decision-making policies more independent (of the scientists in the reviewing decisions who approve new drugs) and more transparent. The board includes members from the CDER, the Center for Biologics Evaluation and Research (CBER), the Center for Devices and Radiological Health, and other departments such as the Department of Defense, the Veterans Administration, and the National Institutes of Health. They call on outside experts and patient and consumer groups as needed. There is no industry involvement.

To improve communications the FDA is also creating a new "Drug Watch" website in which information on emerging drug safety issues is posted. Of most interest are postings that include information on signals that are being investigated by the FDA that in the past were not made known to the public. Examples of proposed postings from the FDA's guidance are as follows:

> "FDA is investigating postmarketing reports of renal failure in elderly patients treated with Drug A, but a causal relationship has not been established. We are continuing to analyze these reports to determine whether the occurrence of these adverse events affects the risk/benefit assessment of Drug A therapy."

> "Drug B has been associated with serious skin reactions in patients allergic to eggs. Prescribers should consider this information when treating patients with these allergies."

> "The sponsor for Drug C has determined that Drug C can cause liver damage in patients with impaired liver function. The sponsor has advised prescribers to check a patient's liver enzymes before the drug is prescribed and at regular intervals thereafter."

The manufacturer of a product will be told about the posting shortly before it occurs, but this appears to be for informational purposes only and not for discussion. Manufacturers are notified in the guidance that using this site for claims in advertising and promotion is not permitted.

The FDA has a very extensive website that is very useful, although the information tends to be scattered and difficult to find. There is a search engine. The main CDER website (Web Resource 8-5) lists late news and provides a jumping off point to other CDER information, including regulatory documents in force (Web Resource 8-6), postmarketing drug safety commitments (Web Resource 8-7), and the Freedom of Information reading room (Web Resource 8-8) where information on disqualified investigators, warning letters, advisory committees, and other useful nuggets are found. There is a miscellaneous section (Web Resource 8-9) on drug safety that has a few useful articles. There is an on-line directory (Web Resource 8-10) of all FDA employees. CDER provides an e-mail update service (Web Resource 8-11) that is well worth subscribing to. There is a site (Web Resource 8-12) that gives information, including safety information, on specific drugs by trade and generic names.

Risk Management

There is extensive information on risk management initiatives. This is covered in Chapters 15–17.

MedWatch

The MedWatch program is the FDA's national pharmacovigilance program. Formally called the "Safety Information and Adverse Event Reporting Program," it provides clinical information about safety issues involving prescription and over-the-counter drugs, biologics, medical and radiation-emitting devices, and special nutritional products (e.g., medical foods, dietary supplements, and infant formulas). See the MedWatch site (Web Resource 8-13).

Medical product safety alerts, recalls, withdrawals, and important labeling changes are disseminated to the medical community and the public on its website and via an e-mail notification system, the MedWatch E-List. See the website (Web Resource 8-14).

The MedWatch website (Web Resource 8-15) has an enormous amount of safety information, including safety alerts and labeling changes dating back to 1996, recalls, medication errors, drug shortages, vaccine safety information, blood products, biologics, devices, dietary supplements, infant formulas, medical foods, and cosmetics. There is also information on the four FDA safety databases:

- Adverse Event Reporting System (AERS) (Web Resource 8-16) AERS collects information about adverse events (AEs), medication errors, and product problems on marketed drug and therapeutic biologic products. Its database of spontaneous reports is one of the largest of its kind. Quarterly (noncumulative) data files since January 2004 are available for downloading as zipped SGML files. Data include information on patient demographics, the drug(s) reported, the adverse reaction(s), patient outcome, and the source of the reports. The actual files can be downloaded directly.

- Vaccine Adverse Event Reporting System (VAERS) (Web Resource 8-17) VAERS is a cooperative database from the Centers for Disease Control and Prevention and the FDA. VAERS collects information about AEs that occur after the use of licensed vaccines.

- The Special Nutritionals Adverse Event Monitoring System (Web Resource 8-18) AE (illness or injury) reports associated with use of dietary supplements, infant formulas, and medical foods (1993–1998 data).

- Manufacturer and User Facility Device Experience Database (Web Resource 8-19) This database contains device information on voluntary reports since June 1993, user facility reports since 1991, distributor reports since 1993, and manufacturer reports since August 1996.

The MedWatch site also has extensive information on the voluntary submission of reports of AEs (reactions) from the general public (Web Resource 8-20) and health care practitioners (Web Resource 8-21). The submission can be done directly on-line by filling in an electronic form (Web Resource 8-22). It is then submitted to the FDA, and an e-mail is returned acknowledging receipt. A submission can also be done by downloading a "3500" form, which is then filled in manually and faxed or mailed to the FDA.

Additional information on vaccine, device, and veterinary reporting is given (Web Resource 8-23).

There is also a link (Web Resource 8-24) to a section covering the privacy issues of Health Insurance Portability and Accountability Act (HIPAA) and voluntary reporting. It notes that the HIPAA law recognizes that safety reporting is vital to the country and that it permits "covered entities" that usually require consent or authorization to disclose private information to do so for AE reporting.

Finally, there is an excellent page (Web Resource 8-25) that covers mandatory reporting by drug and biologic manufacturers, distributors, and packers. There are hyperlinks to the applicable federal regulations:

- Drugs
  - 21CFR310.305: (Web Resource 8-26) Records and reports concerning adverse drug experiences on marketed prescription drugs for human use without approved NDAs.
  - 21CFR312.32: (Web Resource 8-27) IND safety reports.
  - 21CFR314.80: (Web Resource 8-28) Postmarketing reporting of adverse drug experiences.

- Biologics
  - 21 CFR 312.32: (Web Resource 8-29) IND safety reports.
  - 21 CFR 600.80: (Web Resource 8-30) Postmarketing reporting of adverse experiences.

In addition, the guidances in force for industry, FDA field staff, the E2B pilot for AE submission, International Conference on Harmonization documents, and Federal Register publications on postmarketing reporting are referenced in pdf and/or text format.

CBER

The CBER website contains less information regarding product safety than the CDER site because the regulatory responsibility for approval and postmarketing evaluation of many CBER products was transferred to CDER in 2003. The products remaining in CBER include cellular products (e.g., pancreatic islet cells for transplantation, whole cells, cell fragments, or other components intended for use as preventative or therapeutic vaccines); allergenic extracts used for the diagnosis and treatment of allergic diseases and allergen patch tests; antitoxins; antivenins; venoms; blood; blood components; plasma-derived products (e.g., albumin, immunoglobulins, clotting factors, fibrin sealants, proteinase inhibitors), including recombinant and transgenic versions of plasma derivatives (e.g., clotting factors); blood substitutes; plasma volume expanders; human or animal polyclonal antibody preparations, including radiolabeled or conjugated forms; certain fibrinolytics such as plasma-derived plasmin; and red cell reagents. More extensive information on this subject can be found at the CBER website (Web Resource 8-31).

Prescription Drug User Fee Act (PDUFA)

In 1992 the Prescription Drug User Fee Act was passed and then renewed in 1997 and 2002. This Act allowed the FDA to collect a fee from the manufacturer whenever the manufacturer submitted an NDA. In addition, companies pay annual fees for each manufacturing establishment and for each prescription drug product marketed. Previously, taxpayers alone paid for product reviews through budgets provided by Congress. In the new program, industry provides the funding in exchange for FDA agreement to meet drug-review performance goals, which emphasize timeliness. Questions have been raised about the appropriateness of what is, in effect, industry funding of the NDA approval process. See the website for further details (Web Resource 8-32).

What Is Expected from Drug Companies by the FDA

The federal regulations noted above describe what the FDA expects to receive from pharmaceutical companies in regard to the reporting of drug safety information. In all cases companies are expected to do follow-up with due diligence to get complete information on (serious) cases:

- Clinical trials—AEs reported to the IND
  - In 7 calendar days: deaths/life-threatening serious, unexpected, associated with the drug
  - In 15 calendar days: serious, unexpected, associated with the drug
  - In annual periodic reports: summary of all studies, tabular summary of the most serious and most frequent serious AEs, deaths, discontinuations due to AEs, and the 15-day reports submitted since the last report

- Marketed drugs—AEs reported to the NDA
  - In 15 calendar days: serious, unexpected. Note that all spontaneous reports are considered to be "associated with the drug." The reasoning is that if the reporter did not believe there was at least some level of association (causality) with the drug he or she would not have reported it.

- In 15 calendar days: reports from the medical literature that are serious and unexpected.
- In the quarterly or annual periodic reports: A narrative summary and analysis of the 15-day alert reports submitted since the last report plus all other reports that are not serious and not unexpected. Foreign nonserious AEs do not have to be reported. In general, clinical trial AEs do not have to be reported to the NDA.
- Solicited reports: AEs that are received from disease management programs, patient support programs, and such should be reported as 15-day reports to the NDA if they are serious, unexpected, and associated with the drug. It is the latter causality assessment that differentiates solicited reports from spontaneous reports (FDA Guidance for Industry, August 1997, on the MedWatch website [Web Resource 8-33]).

What Is Expected from Consumers and Health Care Professionals by the FDA

Reporting is purely voluntary but strongly encouraged. Reports may be made to the FDA directly via MedWatch (mail, on-line, fax, etc.) or to the pharmaceutical company manufacturing, selling, or packing the product. Most reports sent directly to the FDA come from pharmacists and only a few come from physicians (FDA's Office of Drug Safety noted in its 2001 annual report). See the FDA website (Web Resource 8-34).

Product Safety News

The FDA's home page (Web Resource 8-35) has an "FDA News" section in which new and breaking information (not just on safety) is headlined with hyperlinks to the specific information. In addition, in this section there are links to product alerts, withdrawals, and recalls (drugs and food). There is also a "hot topics" page (Web Resource 8-36) that has information on specific products (drugs, biologics, foods, vaccines, devices, dietary supplements, and more). The MedWatch home page also has late breaking news on specific issues (Web Resource 8-37).

■ The Practice

The FDA's influence on life in the United States is extensive. The FDA ("The Agency") oversees and regulates drugs, biologics, vaccines, dietary supplements, radiation-emitting devices, food, and cosmetics. They cover both human and veterinary products. Attempts to extend FDA regulation to include tobacco products and "health foods" have failed but remain on the agenda of many people in and out of the government. FDA's influence outside the United States is obviously less strong than within the United States but nonetheless is felt through direct and indirect actions in international entities (e.g., International Conference on Harmonization, Council for International Organizations of Medical Sciences), interactions with other health agencies (Europe, Canada, etc.), and as a thought and action leader (e.g., a drug withdrawal in the United States must be addressed, in practice, rather quickly elsewhere).

For those in industries regulated by the Agency, the FDA has an impact on actions every moment of the day in just about all areas of business:

- Approval of INDs and NDAs, 510Ks, and so on;
- Regulations covering all aspects of manufacturing (Good Manufacturing Practices), clinical research (Good Clinical Practices, animal research (Good Laboratory Practices), quality systems, and so on;
- Inspections (often unannounced) of factories, clinical trial sites, safety divisions, clinical trial divisions, and so on;
- Drug safety;
- Product labeling and packaging;
- Product advertising and sales promotion;
- Advice to the public.

The FDA has multiple "clients" to which it must answer: the Secretary of Health and Human Services (in the President's cabinet), the Congress (which provides funding and oversight), the American public in general, activist groups (consumer groups, lobbies, etc.), the media (press, TV, internet, etc.), and the pharmaceutical industry and, indirectly, foreign health agencies.

Pharmaceutical companies also have multiple clients but different ones: The stockholders (owners) of the company, the American public, activist groups, the media, the FDA, and if multinational companies, other health agencies, insurance companies, and foreign media.

The FDA's fundamental viewpoint and raison d'être differ from those of pharmaceutical corporations. The FDA's prime concern is the protection of the American public (and animals). They are, in theory, not concerned with the viability or profitability of corporations or market share, whereas companies, again in theory, have a primary fiduciary goal of increasing shareholder value. Obviously, a company would not want to increase its stock price at the expense of the public health. But, in practice, decisions on what is good or bad for public health are al-most never black or white. Rather, they are the subject of debate on the risks and benefits that fall somewhere in the gray area between the extremes.

Other factors come into play. In general, salaries and bonuses, particularly for professionals, are better in the private sector companies than in the FDA or academia. On the other hand, benefits, pensions, and retirement packages are often better in government service. Also broadly speaking, private sector companies tend to have more resources (people, computers, parking space, etc.) than government agencies.

As with other federal agencies, there is often a steady flow of personnel leaving the agency to go to the private sector and, with the FDA, occasionally vice versa. This is generally viewed as a good phenomenon because it allows government workers to understand the functions and pressures in private industry and for private industry personnel to understand how government agencies function. Many people enter the industry or the FDA from academia but primarily just after finishing training (in medicine, pharmacy, nursing, pharmacology, toxicology, statistics, etc.).

There is a continuing debate, which varies in intensity and persistence over time, on whether the FDA works too slowly ("drug approval lag") or too quickly ("releasing dangerous drugs onto the market without adequate evaluation") and on whether there are too many regulations ("pharmaceuticals is one of the most regulated or overregulated industries in the United States").

Most pharmaceutical companies live with a low level dread of the FDA coming into their safety departments (or other departments) to do an unannounced audit. The audit may be a routine one done periodically (often every 1 to 2 years) or "for cause" (where the FDA has a suspicion that all is not right). The audit may last from a few days to months if major issues are found. The FDA may audit sites outside the United States if appropriate. Conversely, the European Medicines Evaluation Agency and other agencies abroad may audit in the United States (see Chapter 45).

There has been much controversy after the withdrawal of Vioxx from the US market for apparent safety reasons. Some (both from within the FDA and from the outside) have accused the FDA of not sufficiently protecting the American public from "dangerous drugs." There have been accusations of too rapid approval of drugs or insufficient analysis of data submitted to the FDA or companies not submitting complete or sufficient data to the FDA and other charges. Similar controversies have been seen with other regulatory agencies. The FDA has commissioned the Institute of Medicine to convene a committee of experts to do an independent assessment of the current system of postmarketing drug safety and to make recommendations to improve risk assessment and the safe use of drugs (see its website [Web Resource 8-38]).

■ FAQ

Q: Is there too close a relationship between the FDA and the pharmaceutical industry? Are they in bed together?

A: The answer depends on whom you ask.

The FDA (would most probably) say that they are not compromised by maintaining correct and formal communications with the industry. The industry supplies FDA with 80% of the postmarketing safety data and almost all of the premarketing safety data. There must be communication between the industry and the Agency to clarify ambiguous points, get further information on critical cases, and so forth. The FDA also encourages meetings with the industry in the course of the development of drugs (in the IND phases) and in postmarketing situations where safety issues arise. It is a professional-to-professional exchange of information to ensure the safety of the American public.

The industry would say that its influence on the FDA is slight. The companies go out of their way to be sure the FDA gets what it needs (and wants) and that the companies usually submit more (e.g., so-called desk copies of data) than is actually required by regulations to be sure that the FDA gets what it wants. The industry often (privately) believes that the FDA is rather tough and tends to not give the industry a fair shake or a level playing field.

The consumer groups and activists believe that the FDA is indeed in bed with the industry and point to the various "fiascos" in safety that have occurred, such as Vioxx (Web Resource 8-39), Fen-Phen (Web Resource 8-40), suicide in pediatric patients on antidepressants (Web Resource 8-41), among others (see Chapters 47–50). The FDA and the industry would (probably) counter by saying, quite the contrary, that these episodes have shown that the drug safety system in place is indeed functioning and functioning well and that the challenge is to identify these problems earlier.

This is a fascinating and controversial area that is a work in progress. Much will evolve over the next several years in drug safety.

Organizations: European Medicines Agency

➡ **NOTE:**(Unless otherwise noted the word "drug" or "drug product" should be taken in this book to include "biologics" and "vaccines.")

■ Background

In 1995 the European Medicines Evaluation Agency (EMEA) was created and based in the Canary Wharf section of London, England. Now, over a decade later, the face of drug regulation in Europe has totally changed. In 2004 a new directive changed the name of the EMEA to the European Medicines Agency (EMA, also called, like the US Food and Drug Administration [FDA] and Central Intelligence Agency, "The Agency"). See its website (Web Resource 9-1).

Like the FDA, its main responsibility is the protection and promotion of public and animal health through the evaluation and supervision of medicines throughout the European Union comprising 25 countries (Member States) and their 42 national authorities. There is also representation from three additional European countries that are not members of the European Union: Norway, Lichtenstein, and Switzerland.

The EMA is headed by an executive director who has five divisions reporting to him or her, including two that touch on drug safety: The sections on "Pre-Authorization Evaluation of Medicines for Human Use" and the "Post-Authorization Evaluation of Medicines for Human Use" have a subsection on the "Safety and Efficacy of Medicines."

There is a senior-level committee handling human medicines called Committee for Medicinal Products for Human Use. This committee has created a pharmacovigilance committee called the Pharmacovigilance Working Party that has experts from each member state. They meet for 2 to 3 days each month to discuss major safety issues such as standard operating procedures, guidance documents, "points to consider" documents, new procedures, class or product specific safety issues, International Conference on Harmonization (ICH) documents, and interactions with other bodies (e.g., the Uppsala Monitoring Centre and non–European Union organizations). In addition, urgent or emergency safety matters may also be brought to the Working Party. Their yearly work schedule is usually published in advance.

In 2001, a European Union–wide central database, called the Eudravigilance System, was created (Web Resource 9-2). This database is meant to capture data on suspected, unexpected, serious adverse reactions

(SUSARs). Mandatory electronic reporting (i.e., no further paper reporting) of SUSARs became effective November 2005. The latest version of the *Medical Dictionary for Regulatory Activities* must be used as well as the *Eudravigilance Medicinal Product Dictionary*. All these are works in progress, and the pharmacovigilance scene in the European Union is changing almost day to day. It is expected that over the next several years the major operational efforts of obtaining safety data (SUSARs, Periodic Safety Update Reports, and other post- and premarketing safety reports) will continue and finally stabilize. In addition, the European Union has created the European Clinical Trials Database, which is also becoming operational. The reader is referred to the EMA website (Web Resource 9-3) for further information as well as to the Eudravigilance database (Web Resource 9-4).

In addition, each European country has its own national health authority (HA) (or authorities) that handle drug safety. The European Union is still in the midst of defining itself in political terms. The interplay between the central authority (primarily in Brussels but with various agencies scattered throughout the European Union such as the EMA in London and The European Central Bank in Frankfurt, Germany) and the individual countries has not been fully worked out. For drug safety, some functions are primarily centralized in London and some remain in each member state. There are currently (2006) 25 member states in the European Union with the possibility of others joining over the next decade. This division and in some cases duplication of labor along with the multitude of languages involved in the European Union produces a challenge for safety reporting both for the pharmaceutical industry and for the member states themselves. The comparison with other countries, particularly the United States, where the drug safety function is clearly centralized, is striking. The closest analogy would be if each of the 50 states in the United States had its own mini-FDA and used languages other than English.

■ The Theory

In terms of pharmacovigilance the EMA has largely harmonized along the lines of ICH. In addition, the member states of the European Union, which formally had radically different requirements for the handling and submission of adverse events (AEs), have also largely harmonized.

The basic reporting rules date back to one of the original documents—E2A (see [Web Resource 9-5]). The requirements are as follows:

Preapproval (before the marketing authorization is granted)

- Any fatal or life-threatening unexpected adverse drug reaction (an AE believed to be reasonably associated with the use of the drug, i.e., causality is possibly due to the drug): report within 7 calendar days to the HA.

- Any serious and unexpected adverse drug reaction that was not fatal or life-threatening: report within 15 calendar days to the health authority.

- Information that could materially influence the benefit–risk assessment of a medicinal product or that would be sufficient to consider changes in a medicinal product administration or in the overall conduct of a clinical investigation.

Postapproval (after the marketing authorization is granted)

- Any serious and unexpected AE (whether it is believed to be associated with the drug or not): 15 calendar days.

The complications in the European Union occur because each member state has one or more HAs in addition to the EMEA. The complexities of the system are beyond the scope of this work but can roughly be summarized as below. The requirements vary depending on how the drug was approved:

- Local authorization (or local or national approval) means that an individual country approved that drug for that country only. There can be local approvals in multiple countries. This is the case for older drugs.

- Mutual recognition authorization means approval primarily by one member state ("the reference member state") with approval in some or all of the other member states.

- Central authorization refers to approval for all countries in the European Union.

With the arrival of the Eudravigilance system (see below) the following requirements are becoming outmoded:

Reporting for locally authorized drugs

- All spontaneously reported serious AEs (expected and unexpected) that occur in a member state must be reported (transmitted) to the HA of that country. Spontaneously reported cases are always considered to be associated with the drug ("possibly related"). Some countries may have additional local requirements.

- All spontaneous serious and unexpected AEs that occur outside the European Economic Area (EEA = 25 European Union member states plus Liechtenstein, Iceland, and Norway) must also to be reported to the local HA.

Reporting for mutually recognized products
- Same as above for locally authorized products *plus*:
- All spontaneously serious AEs (expected and unexpected) that occur inside the other EEA countries to the HA of the reference member state.

Reporting for centrally authorized products
- All spontaneous serious AEs (expected and unexpected) that occur in that member state to the HA of that country.
- All spontaneous, serious, unexpected AEs that occur outside the EEA to all the EEA member states and the EMA.

Eudravigilance

On November 20, 2005, in accordance with EC Regulation 726/2004, adverse drug reactions have to be transmitted electronically in the European Union. Because of this, the reporting rules for spontaneous cases are changing. All non-European cases are sent to the EMA only and no longer to each individual member state. Submissions to local HAs can be made by using the EMA hub. Investigational drug cases (whether in the premarketing phase or whether for new indications of drugs already approved) are also submitted electronically.

The EMA serves as a "clearing house" to ensure that all appropriate cases are transmitted to the appropriate member states. The EMA has created the Eudravigilance system (Web Resource 9-6) that supplants the local databases and allows for a single European database accessible to the member states' HAs and possibly to the public and the industry (at least to some degree). The mode of transmission of cases is electronic transmission via the E2B mechanism (see Chapter 26) rather than paper mailings or fax.

Risk Management

The EMA, like the FDA and the Japanese HA, is moving heavily into risk management, covering the entire lifespan of a drug to minimize safety problems. This is an evolving field. The EMA issued guidances on risk management. See the following:

- The report of the ad-hoc working group on risk management strategy (Web Resource 9-7)
- The action plan on risk management (Web Resource 9-8)
- The document on establishing a risk management strategy (Web Resource 9-9)
- Chapters 14–18 on risk management

Qualified Person

Volume 9, "Rules Governing Medicinal Products in the European Union," states that the Marketing Authorization holder should have permanently and continuously at its disposal residing in the European Union a qualified person (QP) responsible for pharmacovigilance at the European level.

This person should have experience in all aspects of pharmacovigilance and if not an MD, should report to or have access to an MD. This person is responsible for the establishment and maintenance of the data collection and reporting system. This system (database) must be accessible from at least one point in the European Union. The QP is also responsible for the preparation of adverse drug reaction reports (e.g., 15-day expedited reports), Periodic Safety Update Reports, and postauthorization clinical study reports. Finally, the QP is responsible for ongoing pharmacovigilance evaluation and risk management for that company's products.

The QP has personal liability. That is, any fines or penalties for failure to comply with duties cannot be paid by the company but must be paid by the individual.

Individual member states of the European Union may have additional requirements for QPs at the national level. In Germany this person is called the "Stufenplanbeauftragter."

This position then puts an individual in the position where he or she is responsible for the proper functioning of all drug safety activities. This can be a potentially difficult position if the QP works for a non-European-based company in which the QP does not have real control and input into pharmacovigilance, signaling, label changes, drug withdrawal, and so forth. This may put the QP in the awkward position of having responsibility but no authority if his or her needs are not heard and handled in the safety department thousands of miles away at headquarters.

In December 2005 a revised version of Volume 9 was released, entitled Volume 9a. Comments were requested from the public. This revision markedly increases the responsibilities of the QP, holding him or her further responsible for almost all aspects of pharmacovigilance.

This has elicited significant comments from the industry regarding the practicality of the position as it is now constituted. How this will be handled in the final document remains to be seen.

■ The Practice

The operational issues involved in drug safety in the European Union are far more complex than those in the United States, as noted above. The type of approval (local, mutual recognition, or central) determines to a large degree what is submitted and where. The closest analogy in the United States would be if there were a requirement to submit AEs to the FDA and some of the AEs to agencies in each of the 50 states, sometimes to several of the states and sometimes to all of the states and sometimes not in English. In addition, a QP would need to live in each state to which cases were submitted. Fortunately, this seems to be changing toward a more consistent and simpler system.

Remaining in compliance with all of the ever-changing reporting requirements, new drug approvals, safety issues, and such in the 25 European Union member states plus the EMA plus the affiliated countries presents enormous practical and logistical problems. The European Union, like the United States and Japan, is now and will continue to undergo changes in many aspects of AE reporting (electronic reporting, new risk management initiatives, a new drug dictionary, etc.). The EMA and the member states are also becoming much more active in auditing companies' drug safety practices both on a routine basis and on a "for cause" basis both within the European Union and outside the European Union if that is where the primary safety department is located (see Chapter 45).

In practice, what this means now is that any company that does studies or which sells (or distributes) products within the European Union must either have subsidiary or affiliated offices within the European Union (and sometimes even within each country in which they sell or study). Failing this, the company needs to engage, with a written contract, a company (i.e., a contract research organization) to handle these functions for it. There must be a QP physically living in the European Union, and he or she must have direct and immediate access to the database to deal with the EMA's and individual member states' issues and requests for information. Language issues also oblige a company to be sure it has personnel who can deal with local HAs and others in the language of the country.

The cost of doing business within the European Union has increased significantly. Conversely, European companies wishing to do business in the United States and in Canada must also open offices in these countries.

The listing of the websites for the HAs for the member states of the European Union can be found at the EMA's website (Web Resource 9-10). The websites are usually available in English as well as the national language and are of variable completeness and usefulness. Many appear to be works in progress, particularly for the newest members of the European Union.

To keep up to date with happenings in the European Union, it is worthwhile taking courses given periodically by the Drug Information Association in Europe as well as various private organizations that give courses several times a year. Some of these organizations include the following:

- Drug Information Association in Europe (Web Resource 9-11)
- IBC Inc. (Web Resource 9-12)
- IIR Inc. (Web Resource 9-13)
- Marcus Evans Inc. (Web Resource 9-14)
- PERI (Web Resource 9-15)

■ FAQ

Q: Is it likely that the European Union, the United States, and the rest of the world will "settle down" and stabilize its rules and regulations anytime soon?

A: Probably not. There are several factors at work. First, the entire world of drug safety and risk management is in a state of flux. New technology and regulations are being put in place as a result of many influences, including

- Consumer awareness
- Political pressures and globalization
- Economic pressures and outsourcing
- Changes in the structure of HAs (e.g., the European Union is likely to expand beyond its current 25 members)
- The evolution of the theory of drug safety, including data mining
- The response to some major drug safety issues in the United States and European Union (e.g. Vioxx®)
- Guidelines from international organizations (Council for International Organizations of Medical Sciences, ICH)

Where Data Reside

➡️ **NOTE:**(Unless otherwise noted the word "drug" or "drug product" should be taken in this book to include "biologics" and "vaccines.")

■ Background

There is an enormous amount of data collected in the course of doing pharmacovigilance work. Much of it is real, reliable, and verified, but much is not. The problem is obtaining access to the data, verifying that it is real and correct, ensuring that no duplicates occur, getting it into a database accurately, and making valid clinical judgments at the individual patient level and at the aggregate (public health) level. As with everything else in drug safety, this is a moving target.

■ The Theory

Adverse event (AE) data are collected all over the world by many people and groups. There is little standardization in the way they are collected, how they are measured and graded, how they are stored, and how they are used. Some of the data are collected as a matter of public health,

and some are collected by pharmaceutical companies or other companies who process the data and sell them to others. In theory, with the International Conference on Harmonization, Council for International Organizations of Medical Sciences (CIOMS), *Medical Dictionary for Regulatory Activities* (MedDRA), and other standards, we should be moving toward better and better use of these data.

■ The Practice

AE data reside in several places. The two main resources are:

US Food and Drug Administration

The US Food and Drug Administration (FDA) has a very large amount of data stored in four publicly accessible databases of primarily postmarketing safety data as well as other proprietary databases containing clinical trial information. The FDA drug database, the Adverse Event Reporting System (AERS), is discussed here.

AERS collects information about AEs, medication errors, and product problems on marketed drug and therapeutic biologic products. Quarterly (noncumulative) data files since January 2004 are available under the US Freedom of Information Act for downloading as zipped SGML files. Data include information on patient demographics, the drug(s) reported, the adverse reaction(s), patient outcome, and the source of the reports. The actual files can be downloaded directly. The data can be difficult to manipulate, and various companies offer services that include periodic updates, data searches, or repackaging of the data in a more user-friendly form.

This database is rather large, with over 3 million cases as of late 2002, and is growing by hundreds of thousands of cases per year. It contains primarily post-marketing data from prescription drugs and over-the-counter drugs with a New Drug Application sold in the United States, but it also contains some foreign reports of AEs for these drugs. The majority of the data (~80%) is supplied from pharmaceutical companies making obligatory reports using MedWatch 3500A forms or direct electronic transmission via E2B. The remainder represents direct reports to the FDA from health care professionals and consumers. It is coded in MedDRA. It is of very variable quality ranging from full due diligence inquiries and follow-ups with complementary data (laboratory reports, electrocardiograms, etc.) to lay consumer reports not validated by a medical professional. There are few clinical trial data in this database. The clinical trial data are proprietary and are generally not available, although some advocacy groups would like to see a change in this. Some can be found in Summary Basis of Approval documents that the FDA sometimes releases after a drug is approved, and some may soon be found on the new Drug Watch website.

AERS data (excluding attachments) can be obtained as noncumulative quarterly reports dating back to 2004. There is a variable lag of weeks to months between AEs being reported to the FDA and their making it into the quarterly report. The quarterly data, after being uploaded into a database (or spreadsheet), can be manipulated and provide line listings. Should further information be desired, the full MedWatch form (anonymized to protect the reporter and patient) can be obtained using the unique identification number assigned to each case by the FDA. Data can be obtained directly from the FDA under the Freedom of Information Act (see the FDA's website [Web Resource 10-1]) or from private companies. Using the latter ensures the anonymity of the requester.

Although getting and using the data can be difficult, it can be very rewarding because large amounts of detailed data are available, particularly for newer products. The full MedWatch forms are available, and the narratives can be read to obtain clinical summaries of the cases.

The Uppsala Monitoring Centre

Vigibase (Web Resource 10-2). The Uppsala Monitoring Centre (UMC, on behalf of the World Health Organization) has over 3 million AE case reports from 75 countries. The data are supplied by national health authorities. Most of the data are from the United States and are supplied by the FDA. The UMC does not review or assess the individual cases put into the database, but it does pharmacovigilance analyses and signaling. Not all of the supplying countries allow their data to be released. The database does not contain all the data found in the MedWatch or CIOMS I form. In particular, there are no narratives.

Customized searches are available directly on-line from the UMC (for a small fee) or indirectly from third-party vendors (e.g., Galt Associates' Halo™ product [Web Resource 10-3] and Lincoln Technologies QScan™ [Web Resource 10-4]).

Signals and Signaling in the Context of Risk Management

➡ **NOTE:**(Unless otherwise noted the word "drug" or "drug product" should be taken in this book to include "biologics" and "vaccines.")

■ Background

Enormous efforts are made, in terms of people, time, cost, and technology, to collect adverse event (AE) data in companies, governments, and elsewhere. The collection of vast amounts of data is meaningless in and of itself. It is only when these data are organized and analyzed for new safety issues (which are then acted on in the context of risk management) that the true value of this effort becomes apparent. The hunt for meaning is known as "signaling."

■ The Theory

The Signal

The Uppsala Monitoring Centre defines a signal as follows:

"Reported information on a possible causal relationship between an adverse event and a drug, the relationship being unknown or incompletely documented previously. Usually more than a single report is required to generate a signal, depending upon the seriousness of the event and the quality of the information."

They comment further:

"This describes the first alert of a problem with a drug. By its nature a signal cannot be regarded as definitive but indicates the need for further enquiry or action. On the other hand it is prudent to avoid a multiplicity of signals based on single case reports since follow up of all such would be impractical and time consuming. The definition allows for some flexibility in approach to a signal based on the characteristics of individual problems. Some would like a 'signal' to include new information on positive drug effects, but this is outside the scope of a drug safety Programme" (see Delamothe, *Br Med J* 1992;304:465 and [Web Resource 11-1]).

Not everyone agrees that all signals based on single cases should not be pursued. Sometimes rare events are picked up after a single case.

Signals may be "qualitative" (based on spontaneously reported data) or "quantitative" (based on data mining, epidemiologic data, or trial data). The signal may be a new issue never before seen with this product, or it may be the worsening or changing of a known AE or problem (e.g., a previously unaffected patient group is experiencing this problem or it is now fatal in those it attacks, whereas before it was not or the incidence has increased, etc.). As noted above, qualitative signals may be based on one single striking case or on a collection of cases.

The term "signal" is primarily used to refer to marketed products, although the term is occasionally used for new issues in clinical trials too. Some people use the term "potential signal" to indicate an issue with minimal data (e.g., only one case report), whereas others use the term "weak signal."

Just identifying signals, however, is not enough. The signal must be further investigated by doing what is variously called a "signal workup," a "signal inquiry," or a "pharmacovigilance investigation." The ultimate goal and true raison d'être of signal discovery and investigation is to determine whether the newly identified problem is indeed due to the drug and of sufficient severity and frequency in relation to the benefit to require the alerting of physicians, nurses, pharmacists, and patients via a change in the product labeling, television, internet, and other announcements or, in more severe cases, recall of the product or stopping of a clinical trial.

Signal Generation

Signals are looked for in multiple ways. The oldest method is essentially passive and relies on the collection in pharmaceutical companies or government health authorities or in third-party organizations (academic centers, medical registries) of spontaneous AE reports. They are then reviewed individually and in aggregate looking for "striking" or "unusual" or "unexpected" AEs. Medically qualified people (physicians, nurses, pharmacists) examine large quantities of data, attempting to find the proverbial needle in the haystack and discuss the "potential signals" found during group meetings. This technique is elegantly known as "global introspection." This technique is quite time-consuming and laborious, but in the hands of astute and clever clinicians does indeed pick up major problems and remains the cornerstone of signal generation and identification around the world. It obviously relies on the good will and astuteness of the reporting physicians, nurses, pharmacists, and patients to send AE reports into the companies or health authorities (without

remuneration) and on the goodwill and competence of the data analysts.

It is most sensitive when

- The signal is very unusual and rarely seen in general (e.g., aplastic anemia).
- The signal is rarely seen with that drug class (pulmonary fibrosis with beta-blockers, e.g., practolol).
- The signal is rarely seen in that cohort of patients (cataracts in young nondiabetic patients).
- The signal is fatal, particularly in patient groups who classically do not have high mortality rates (e.g., deaths in 20 year olds).
- The signal is expected to be seen because it has been reported in other drugs in the same class (e.g., rhabdomyolysis with a new statin).
- The signal is expected because it is due to an exaggeration of the drug's pharmacologic effect (e.g., fainting in patients taking an antihypertensive).
- The AE in question is seen almost exclusively with drugs (e.g., fixed drug reaction).
- The causality is crystal clear (e.g., the tablet is large and sticky and gets stuck in the oral pharynx, producing obstruction; or when immediate swelling and itching is seen at the site of a drug being injected).
- No other drugs are being taken by the patient(s) in question.
- The drug is being taken for a short time and there are no or few confounders.
- The patients are otherwise healthy and have no other medical problems beyond the one being treated with the drug in question.
- There is a positive rechallenge (reaction reappears upon drug reintroduction after a positive dechallenge).

It is least sensitive when

- The signal has a high background incidence in the general population (e.g., headaches, fatigue).
- The signal has a high background incidence in the population being treated (e.g., myocardial infarctions in elderly hypertensives).
- The signal represents a worsening of the problem being treated (e.g., fialuridine, producing worsening and fatal hepatitis in patients being treated for hepatitis; see Chapter 47).
- The patients are taking multiple drugs (polypharmacy, intensive care unit).

- The patients have major underlying medical problems producing disease, signs, and symptoms (e.g., oncology patients).

- The drug is taken chronically, and many intercurrent illnesses and problems occur over time (confounders).

- There is a negative dechallenge (reaction continues even after stopping drug), or the drug in question is not stopped in the patient and the AE disappears by itself anyway.

Increased Frequency

This is a technique that has been on again, off again. It has been in favor and out of favor. It basically relies on a statistical calculation of reporting frequency in the current period versus a previous period (e.g., 2005 vs. 2004) and seeing if there is an increase in reporting of a particular AE. The technique is easy to do and can be computerized and run for all reported AEs for a drug. It has, in practice, turned out to be not very useful. Although signals are, by definition, generated by this process (some AEs go up [i.e., a signal], whereas some go down and some remain the same), they have, in general, turned out to be false alarms, meaningless, or were easily picked up by other means. It is recommended that frequency analyses be done in Periodic Safety Update Reports by the International Conference on Harmonization (see Chapter 26). The US Food and Drug Administration (FDA) also required frequency analysis until 1997 in its New Drug Application periodic reports but ended that because it was found to be of little practical use. The FDA has, however, proposed reinstating its use in the proposed regulations published in 2003 ("The Tome").

Data Mining

This term is used, sometimes somewhat pejoratively, to describe various automated or semiautomated techniques to generate signals from existing databases. One example of this is called fractional or proportional reporting rates:

- For each AE, the calculation of the proportion of that AE as a function of all AEs reported for a drug is calculated and compared with the proportion of that AE for all other drugs in the database.

- For example, liver failure for drug X was reported 95 times out of the 1,418 total AEs for drug X.
  - The proportion is $95/1,418 = 0.067$ and can be called the "score" or "statistic."

- For the entire AE database of all drugs (except drug X) the score of liver failure was, for example, found to be 0.054.

- Thus for drug X, compared with the rest of the database, there is a higher proportion of liver failure reports ($0.067/0.054 = 1.24$). If the proportion was the same, the number would be 1.00. If there were proportionally fewer liver cases with drug X, the score would be <1.00.

- The level at which one considers a signal to be generated could be chosen as anything >1.00, although this will probably produce many false positives. In practice, one might take a score above, say, 1.2 or 1.4. Alternatively, one might look at the top 10 or 20 scores.

For further details, see Evans SJW, Waller PC, Davis S. Use of proportional reporting ratios for signal generation from spontaneous adverse drug reaction reports. *Pharmacoepidemiology and Drug Safety* 2001;10:483–486.

There are other data mining techniques described and under development in an attempt to determine as early as possible, using the least amount of data, which signals need to be aggressively followed up and which signals are background noise. Examples that the FDA refers to in its Guidance (see below) include the multi-item gamma Poisson shrinker algorithm and the neural network approach. Whether these or other methods will ultimately prove useful remains to be seen.

Signal Workup

Once a signal has been identified, it should be prioritized among all the signals for workup. A signal is usually one or more individual case reports ("case series"). Some signals, usually those that are new, fatal, or medically severe or those that may represent tampering, should be considered for immediate high-priority workup. Others that are mild and have little effect on the public health can be worked up after the high priority signals are done. The efficacy of the suspect drug and the severity of the disease treated should always be taken into account; for example, a new mild and self-limited skin eruption associated with a new chemotherapeutic agent that saves lives in a usually recalcitrant form of cancer does not warrant an intensive safety investigation. A formal written process for signal handling should be put in place. This process involves data collection, evaluation by medically trained experts, further follow-up if needed, recommendations for action, and a senior responsible person or group to take action:

- Intensive follow-up of the individual cases is needed to obtain the maximum amount of clinical information.
- The cases should be arranged into an aggregate document such as line listings to allow comparison of the cases at a glance along with the MedWatch (or CIOMS I) forms as an appendix to the document.
- Causality (association) should be assigned with the drug in question. There are many scales available, and no single scale has emerged as a standard. The scale should be simple and clearly defined using words (e.g., related, probably related, possibly related, unrelated, not enough information, with each of these terms defined) or numeric (e.g., 1–5, with 1 being unrelated and 5 being definitely related). The assignment should be done by medical professionals (usually physicians skilled in signal analysis) along with risk management and epidemiology colleagues either as individuals or in committee or both. The cases should then be grouped or separated ("lumpers and splitters") in a medically logical manner and then examined by causality to see how many of the cases in the series are believed to be related, possibly related, or weakly related. The reviewers should come to a conclusion or conclusions for recommendation to the decision maker or safety committee (see below). The conclusions may be along the lines of

  - Not a signal—no further investigation needed.
  - Weak signal—continue watching; no further action at this time.
  - Signal warranting further investigation and follow-up of the current cases (e.g., for outcomes); to be reexamined in 60 days.
  - Signal warranting intensive follow-up and further investigation in the form of a clinical trial, an epidemiologic trial, outside consultation, and so on.
  - A signal warranting immediate action to protect public health. These actions may be temporary (if the signal is ultimately determined to be unfounded) or permanent.

- A senior safety/risk management committee should be in place. There should be a formal written procedure to review and adjudicate signals on a regular basis. There should be a decision maker either in the form of a person or a committee. For emergency signals, the committee should be able to meet within 24 hours (or even sooner). In a pharmaceutical company this could be a senior safety committee composed of the chief medical officer, chief safety officer (if not the same person), and heads or senior people from drug safety/pharmacovigilance, regulatory affairs, labeling, clinical research, the legal department, preclinical (animal) toxicology/pharmacology, risk management, epidemiology, and other corporate subject matter experts as needed (e.g., formulations). If the product is marketed outside the home country, the needs of these countries should also be represented on the committee. The marketing and sales and similar departments should *not* be represented on this committee. In occasional instances, outside expert consultants, as neutral as possible given that they are paid consultants to the company, may be invited to join if appropriate.

In a health authority, the committee structure should be constituted in a similar manner with senior medical, toxicology, pharmacology, labeling, risk management, epidemiology, and legal subject matter experts as well as any other members needed depending on the structure of the health authority.

- The safety committee needs to come to conclusions in regard to issues presented to it. It should never routinely request more data at successive meetings for a particular problem to delay a decision. Relevant data should be requested and rapidly obtained and decisions made. These decisions should be documented in minutes. The outcomes should consider the public health and risk management and what, if anything, needs to be done:

  - Label change for marketed drugs (e.g., new AE, warning, precaution, etc.), dear doctor/health care professional letter, drug withdrawal and, if so, to what level (consumer, pharmacist, wholesaler), and communication plan to the public and health care professionals.
  - Further study and consultation regarding this signal.
  - If in clinical trials, stop or change studies to enhance patient protection, changes in the investigator brochure, and informed consent.
  - Notification of the FDA and other health agencies by phone, fax, or letter.
  - Other follow-up actions and further review by the committee at a later date.

When the committee is in a health agency, depending on legal responsibilities and regulations, the committee needs to decide on label changes, withdrawal, and study cessation in the same manner as noted above for companies.

The FDA Guidance on Good Pharmacovigilance Practices of 3/05

In March 2005 the FDA (Center for Drug Evaluation and Research and Center for Biologics Evaluation and Research) released a Guidance for Industry entitled "Good Pharmacovigilance Practices and Pharmacoepidemiologic Assessment." This is an excellent document and summarizes the current FDA thinking on the topic. It also, to a large degree, reflects current practices in the industry. It references three guidances initially issued in May 2004 and revised and reissued in May 2005 (see Chapters 15–17):

1. Premarketing Risk Assessment
2. Development and Use of Risk Minimization Plans (RiskMAP Guidance)
3. Good Pharmacovigilance Practices and Pharmaco-epidemiologic Assessment

Key parts of this document in regard to signaling are as follows:

Identifying and describing safety signals: From case report to case series.

- Case reports. The FDA recommends that sponsors make a reasonable attempt to get complete information for case assessment during initial and follow-up contacts. Companies should use trained health care practitioners. If the report is from a consumer, it should be followed up with contact with the health care practitioner. The most aggressive efforts should be directed at serious AEs, particularly those not previously known to occur with the drug.

- Case series. After an initial postmarketing spontaneous case report is found, additional cases should be sought in the sponsor's database, the FDA Adverse Event Reporting System database, published literature, and other databases. Cases should be evaluated and followed up for additional information where needed and where possible. Of importance are data that would support or reject a causal association with the drug. Although the FDA notes that there is no internationally agreed on causality classifica-

tions, they do note that *probable*, *possible*, and *unlikely* have been used. Cases with confounders should be analyzed too and not routinely excluded.

- After such a review, the cases that support the signal's further investigation should be summarized in a table or other manner to describe the important clinical characteristics.

- The FDA refers to the use of data mining techniques but notes that their use "is not a required part of a signal identification or evaluation."

- The FDA then gives guidance as to which signals should be further evaluated: new unlabeled serious AEs; an apparent increase in the severity of a labeled event; occurrence of serious AEs that are extremely rare in the general population; new drug–drug, drug–food, or drug–dietary supplement interactions; identification of a previously unrecognized at-risk populations; confusion about a product name, label, package, or use; concerns about product usage (e.g., use at higher than labeled doses); concerns that the current risk management plan is not adequate; or "other."

- Calculation of reporting rates. In a somewhat controversial section, the FDA recommends that the sponsor calculate the crude AE reporting rates using the number of reported cases of that signal AE in the United States as the numerator and the estimate of US patient exposure (as patients or patient-time) as the denominator. Where feasible, the reporting rates over time or versus similar products or drug classes or versus estimates of the background rate for this even in the general population may be useful. The FDA does warn, however, that these figures are generally used for exploratory purposes or for hypothesis generation. They note that reporting rates are not incidence rates.

In practice, use of these figures is fraught with danger. The numerator is bad because there is always under-reporting of an unknown degree; the denominator is worse because it is hard to know how many patients truly took the drug (as opposed to filling the prescription) and for how long. Thus the ratio is often meaningless. A high reporting rate may suggest that the signal is real, but a low reporting rate does not exonerate the drug.

Investigating a Signal

- Pharmacoepidemiologic studies are cited by the FDA. There are various types of nonrandomized trials that can be done, including cohort (prospective or retrospective), case-control, nested case-control, and others. They can be done at any time (before or after marketing), although they are often done after a signal has been suggested by postmarketing adverse events. The FDA suggests that bias be minimized and that confounding be accounted for. They also suggest that "it is always prudent to conduct more than one study, in more than one environment and even use different designs."

- Registries. The FDA defines a registry as "an organized system for the collection, storage, retrieval, analysis and dissemination of information on individual persons exposed to a specific medical intervention who have either a particular disease, a condition (e.g., a risk factor) that predisposes [them] to the occurrence of a health-related event, prior exposure to substances (or circumstances) known or suspected to cause adverse health effects." A control or comparison group should be included where possible.

- Surveys. Without clearly defining a survey, the FDA recommends that they be done when information gathering is needed. For pharmacoepidemiologic studies, registries, and surveys, the FDA encourages consultation with the agency before beginning.

Interpreting a Signal

The FDA recommends that the sponsor conduct a case level/case series review and also use data mining and calculation of reporting rates where feasible. Then the sponsor should consider a further study to establish whether a safety risk exists.

When the sponsor believes a safety risk is possible, a synthesis of all information should be prepared and submitted to the FDA, including the following:

- Cases (spontaneous and literature) with exposure information;

- The background rate for the event in general and the specific patient population(s);

- Relative risks, odds ratios, or other pharmacoepidemiology study results;

- Biologic effects from animal work and pharmacokinetic and dynamic studies;

- Safety data from controlled clinical trials;

- General marketing experience with similar products.

The sponsor should provide an assessment of the risk-to-benefit balance for the population as a whole and for at-risk groups (if any). The FDA notes that this is an iterative process, and not all actions described in the guidance are done at all times. Proposals on further steps should also be provided along with risk minimization actions. The FDA then makes its own judgment based on the data.

The FDA recommends that sponsors develop and continually reevaluate their risk management plan. In some cases, postmarketing reporting of spontaneous AEs will suffice. In other situations much more may be needed. The FDA notes it may bring potential safety risks to its Drug Safety and Risk Management Advisory Committee or the specific advisory committee dealing with the product in question.

■ The Practice

The actions described above represent a careful, step-by-step, well-planned proposal for investigating a signal that allows a thoughtful and logical response to a signal. In many and probably most situations, especially those for nonserious signals or drugs not in the public eye, this process unfurls as described above. However, for the situations that make the public eye (e.g., Vioxx®, Phen-fen) the pressures are enormous to act before all the evidence is in.

Signal review does not occur in a vacuum. There are multiple influences that play a role:

- Changes in personnel in the company and the FDA may cause loss of continuity in a signal investigation.

- Publicity from consumer groups, the media, and other companies, some of which may be premature or unnecessarily scary and inflammatory.

- Lawsuits.

- Actions by other health agencies outside the United States.

- The time needed to prepare and carry out whatever actions are proposed, such as registries, studies, data mining, and surveys.

- Further spontaneous reports or lack thereof during the investigation ("Oh no, we just got another case!").

- Pressures from various areas to continue marketing or to stop marketing.

- Extreme positions based on little data.

- Sponsor marketing and financial pressures (lost market and money).
- Pressures on the FDA (Congress, companies, consumer groups, media).
- Pressure to do interim analyses or to stop ongoing trials (often for different indications) of the drug in question, which jeopardizes the integrity of the study.
- Privacy and data protection issues

In addition, the points of view ("agendas") of the protagonists in the drama are clearly different in many regards, although everyone really does want to protect the public health and not hurt people. Here are the points of view using some of the language each group might use to make its case:

- The **company** wishes to protect its (enormous) investment in a product that took years to develop and to market and that is paying the salary of hundreds or thousands of employees. A "handful" of not clearly proven cases with causality in doubt should not be made public and should not be allowed to "destroy" the drug before the full scientific and medical investigations are completed. The drug is clearly helping the "vast majority" of the patients using it, and the possible occurrence of AEs (even serious ones) should not deprive the rest of the public of the product. Because the drug has a finite life (i.e., patent expiration), the company believes it must protect it as much as possible. The investigation of the signal should be done in private without release of the "debate" to the public. Even if the drug is totally exonerated after the signal investigation, there is usually lost market share and harm to the drug. Within the company, no one wants to be the one to "kill the drug," because this can be a career-ending and a stock price–destroying event. Lawsuits will doubtless follow (often no matter what the result of the signal investigation), and the personal and financial liability can be enormous. When lawsuits occur, employees move into defensive mode, spending more and more time with attorneys. In summary, the company will, of course, do the right thing, but only when the data are in and the science is clear. It will not act prematurely.
- The **FDA** wishes to protect the public health as its primary goal. It wants to do this as early as possible

to minimize the risk to the public. Better to err on the side of patient protection than to allow a toxic product to stay on the market (or remain inadequately labeled) for too long. The agency cannot appear to be too cavalier with the data or to "be in the pocket of the drug companies." It is also far easier to take the position against the "big bad drug companies." In some senses, the drug should be considered guilty until proven innocent. Primum non nocere ("Above all do no harm") is an aphorism originally attributed to the ancient Greek physician Galen but which more likely arose in the 17th century. If something bad happens, the Congress, the Secretary of the Department of Health and Human Services, the media, and the consumer groups will attack the companies and the FDA unmercifully.

With the new Drug Watch regulations, more data (much unconfirmed and incomplete) will be released earlier. This will both help the agency protect itself and get the information before the public, but it will also change the shape of the investigation and diminish the use of the drug, perhaps prematurely.

- **Consumers** want totally safe and totally effective drugs with no risk. When bad things occur (because the companies may have withheld data or did not do their job or the FDA may have acted too quickly and did not do its job), someone is at fault and someone must pay and be punished. All data should be available, and the entire process should be transparent. In general, better to err on the side of stopping the use of the drug than continuing its sale and use. And drugs are indeed guilty until proven innocent.
- The **media** is delighted when the spectacle plays out, especially with data dribbling out over time and errors with alleged misdeeds by the company or the FDA surfacing. The more sensational, the more errors or inappropriate or illegal actions, the more individuals hurt, the more the story captivates the public moving into websites and blogs and selling papers and TV time.
- For other competitor pharmaceutical companies there are mixed feelings. Clearly what is happening to another company could happen to them at any time too with one of their products. On the other hand, the competitors are not unhappy if more patients now switch to their drugs rather than using the one undergoing a signal investigation. And finally there is an element of Schadenfreude (from the German meaning pleasure taken from someone else's misfortune) that is common in human nature.

All of this suggests that rather than thinking of the signal investigation process as a careful, rational, well-planned program done in a timely and deliberate manner, one should rather think of the process, for dramatic or serious issues, as the "fog of war" with multiple pressures (some known and some unknown to each player) acting to force rapid and urgent "action" to protect the public.

The consequences of whatever action is taken may have far-reaching and irreversible effects. Drugs that are withdrawn rarely return to the market even if the signal has subsequently been disproven (see Chapter 6). Label changes adding a new safety warning, AE, or other are rarely taken out of the label even if disproven. The change in medical practice to the use of different drugs (which may be more or less expensive, available, effective, safe, etc.) is similarly hard to reverse.

■ FAQ

Q: Again, why would anyone want to work in drug safety for a living?

A: For many reasons. Signal detection and analysis is usually a fascinating exercise requiring medical, investigative, tactical, logical, and political skills. One really is acting to help the public health. Most signals, perhaps the vast majority, are rather unextraordinary and nonserious and can be worked up in a thoughtful and timely manner. In these instances it is very satisfying. Similarly, even in the dramatic instances, the right thing usually does end up being done, and that also is quite satisfying. The probability of one of the horror scenarios is less likely, but that is the risk one takes in this business. As with signaling (and most of life), it all boils down to a benefit-to-risk analysis.

12

Data Privacy and Sharing

Who should know what and when? United States versus European Union. Who owns the data? What can it be used for?

➡ **NOTE:**(Unless otherwise noted the word "drug" or "drug product" should be taken in this book to include "biologics" and "vaccines.")

■ Background

Approximately 20 or 30 years ago with the advent of personal computers, the question of personal privacy and the limiting of access to data first appeared as a controversy in medicine. With the Internet and identity theft, the issue of who has access to what data is now in the forefront of people's minds.

For many years medical data were believed to be the property of the treating physician or hospital, and they were kept confidential by those parties. There was no right to privacy as defined by federal law. The law that was in place was state law, which varied from state to state and offered inconsistent levels of protection.

That viewpoint has largely changed, and a person's health data are now believed to be owned by that person. There are now clear limitations on what third parties (physicians, hospitals, companies, and the government) can and cannot do with the data.

For the purposes of drug safety and pharmacovigilance, there are two major governmental acts that are worth studying in detail: the US Health Insurance Portability and Accountability Act (HIPAA) and the European Union (EU) Data Privacy Directive. Both are reviewed here and the implications and affects on drug safety discussed.

■ The Theory

HIPAA

In 1996, HIPAA became law and gave Congress until August 21, 1999 to pass comprehensive health privacy legislation. Congress failed to do this, and thus another provision in HIPAA allowed the Department of Health and Human Services (HHS) to create privacy protections by regulation. After much discussion, the final rule went into effect at the end of 2000.

The regulation covers health plans, health care clearinghouses, and those health care providers ("covered entities") who conduct certain financial and administrative transactions electronically. All medical records and other individually identifiable health information held or disclosed by a covered entity in any form, whether communicated electronically, on paper or orally, are covered. Further information on HIPAA can be found on the HHS website (Web Resource 12-1), some of which is summarized here:

- **Patient education on privacy protections.** Providers and health plans are required to give patients a clear written explanation of how they can use, keep, and disclose their health information.

- **Ensuring patient access to their medical records.** Patients must be able to see and get copies of their records and request changes and corrections. In addition, a history of most disclosures must be made accessible to patients.

- **Getting patient consent to release information.** Patient authorization to disclose information must be obtained before sharing their information for treatment, payment, and health care operations purposes. In addition, specific patient consent must be obtained for other uses, such as releasing information to financial institutions determining mortgages, selling mailing lists to interested parties such as life insurers, or disclosing information for marketing purposes by third parties (e.g., drug companies).

- **Consent must not be coerced.**

- **Providing recourse if privacy protections are violated.**

- **Providing the minimum amount of information necessary.** Disclosures of information must be limited to the minimum necessary for the purpose of the disclosure.

Covered entities are held to the following stipulations:

- **Adopt written privacy procedures.** These must include who has access to protected information, how it will be used within the entity, and when the information would or would not be disclosed to others. They must also take steps to ensure that their business associates protect the privacy of health information.

- **Train employees and designate a privacy officer.** Covered entities must provide sufficient training so that their employees understand the new privacy protections procedures, and designate an individual to be responsible for ensuring the procedures are followed.

- **Establish grievance processes.** Covered entities must provide a means for patients to make in-quiries or complaints regarding the privacy of their records.

- **Psychotherapy.** Psychotherapy notes (used only by a psychotherapist) are held to a higher standard of protection because they are not part of the medical record and are never intended to be shared with anyone else.

- **Penalties.** Failure to comply may lead to civil or criminal penalties, including fines and imprisonment.

Information may be released in the following circumstances:

- Oversight of the health care system, including quality assurance activities;
- Public health;
- Research approved by a privacy board or institutional review board;
- Judicial and administrative proceedings;
- Certain law enforcement activities;
- Emergency circumstances;
- Identification of the body of a deceased person or the cause of death;
- Activities related to national defense and security.

This regulation clearly has implications for pharmacovigilance. Much discussion occurred, and the Food and Drug Administration (FDA) issued a clarification of the issue.

The FDA fully recognized that pharmaceutical companies are required by law and regulation to maintain databases of adverse events occurring in individuals who have taken their products reported by health professionals. The data identify the person making the report and may or may not identify the individual. The data come both from clinical trials of new products and from the postmarketing data of drugs already on the market.

Although there is no specific patient identification (e.g., name and address), there is sufficient patient data such that it would be possible in many cases, with only minimal effort, to identify the patient based on the known data (e.g., hospital, dates of hospitalization, age or birth date, patient initials, sex, diagnosis, treatment, and hospital course). These data are often required to be submitted to health authorities and are necessary for the clinical and epidemiologic evaluation of the adverse event and safety profile of the drug. It is vitally important to know that certain events occur in special populations (e.g., only in children, females, or the elderly, etc.). There is a broad consensus in the industry and in the health authorities that these data are vital for the maintenance and protection of public health. Removal of these demographic data would make the data much less useful for safety and epidemiologic analyses. Identification of safety problems occurring with both new and old drugs would suffer if the flow of these data were hindered.

The FDA addressed this in the March 2005 Guidance for Industry: Good Pharmacovigilance Practices and Pharmacoepidemiologic Assessment. See the FDA website for the Guidance (Web Resource 12-2). The FDA notes: "It is of critical importance to protect patients and their privacy during the generation of safety data and the development of risk minimization action plans. During all risk assessment and risk minimization activities, sponsors must comply with applicable regulatory requirements involving human subjects research and patient privacy."

The FDA further notes: "The Privacy Rule specifically permits covered entities to report adverse events and other information related to the quality, effectiveness, and safety of FDA-regulated products both to manufacturers and directly to FDA (45CFR164.512(b)(1)(i) and (iii), and 45CFR164.512(a)(1))."

Thus there is a broad understanding that safety data may be reported to manufacturers (sponsors) and to the FDA.

The EU Privacy Directive

In October 1995 the European Commission proposed "Directive 95/46/EC on the protection of individuals with regard to the processing of personal data and on the free movement of such data." All member states in the EU had 3 years to implement local laws and regulations covering the contents of this directive. With some delays, essentially all member states did so. Laws and regulations vary from country to country, and some are stronger (more protective of privacy) than the directive itself. It has had an impact on drug safety, although less than originally feared. A full analysis and history of this effort is well beyond the scope of this book. A brief summary is put forth here, and reference to the directive and various websites is provided. The directive itself can be found at (Web Resource 12-3).

A good summary of the EU Privacy Directive 95/46 can be found at "Directive 95/46/EC on the protection of personal data." Wikipedia 2005 at Answers.com (Web Resource 12-4), GuruNet Corp. Accessed 10 February 2006.

The directive covers all personal data, whether electronic or on paper, and is not limited to health information but broadly covers all other areas of personal data involving trade union, cultural, financial, credit card, criminal, and so forth. The directive refers to the "processing" of personal data. Processing refers to "any operation...which is performed ...such as collection,

recording, organization, storage, adaptation or alteration, retrieval, consultation, use, disclosure by transmission, dissemination...."

Data may not be processed except in the following circumstances:

- The person in question has given consent.
- The processing is necessary for the performance of a contract.
- The processing is necessary to meet a legal obligation.
- The processing is needed to protect the vital interests of the person in question.
- The processing is needed to carry out a task that is in the public interest or is done in exercise of official authority.

The person in question has the right to be informed when his or her data are processed. The person has the right to see all the data processed about him or her as well as the right to changes and corrections for data that are not correct or are incomplete. The data must be accurate and relevant to the purpose they are collected for and should not contain more information than is necessary and should not be kept longer than necessary.

Data may not be transferred to a third country where there is an inadequate level of data protection. The United States is not considered to have, in all instances, adequate levels of protection for EU data. There are various methods of transfer of data to the United States that are available to stay within the EU requirements. See the EU's data protection page (Web Resource 12-5).

The entire situation in the United States and the EU is still in a state of flux. Changes continue to occur. Different companies, industries, and countries are approaching data protection and privacy differently. Research (both clinical and epidemiologic) has been affected and "work-arounds" developed. Most large companies in the United States now have "privacy officers" as counterparts to some degree of the EU-mandated "data controllers." Companies and agencies transmitting data should check with their appropriate personnel to ensure that all privacy and data protection requirements are met. And they should probably recheck periodically because this is a moving target.

■ The Practice

In practice, the data protection and privacy acts in the United States, EU, and member states have fortunately not had a major effect on pharmacovigilance and signaling. The practical steps that have occurred are as follows:

- MedWatch, CIOMS I, and other forms and data transmission to the United States are "anonymized" or "de-identified" in regard to the patient and the reporter. That is, any information that might allow the reader to identify the patient is removed. This includes patient initials, date of birth (age is okay, however), locale of birth (country is okay, city and zip code are not), specifics such as the name of the hospital and date of admission, personal numbers such as telephone or health insurance numbers, and so forth. The reporter is similarly not named but rather his or her occupation is noted (e.g., consumer, physician, pharmacist, health care professional, attorney).

- Attachments such as medical records, laboratory reports, procedure or surgical reports, and autopsy or death certificates must have all identifying information removed or obliterated. This can be tedious and time consuming but nevertheless must be done. For example, if a multipage narrative report refers to the patient by name in several places and in the headers and footers, all such identifiers must be removed or obliterated.

- Case report forms sent to the drug safety department must also be carefully anonymized at least in regard to the patient information. The reporter information (such as the investigator) may be sent in some cases, because this is part of the clinical trial and agreed to by the investigator.

- It is important to note that non-anonymized data may move within an EU country or between EU countries because these countries have (in theory at least) adequate data protection. It is the movement outside the EU that has caused this concern.

- Some EU countries have even more strict data protection rules and laws than the EU directive, and this makes follow-up and data collection more difficult.

- The issue of US data leaving the United States and going to the EU or elsewhere has not been a significant issue. In general, the precautions taken for data entering the United States have been adopted by many in the United States for data leaving the United States.

- The privacy and confidentiality of MedWatch reporting is protected under US law. The FDA has addressed this on the back of the MedWatch form:

"The patient's identity is held in strict confidence by FDA and protected to the fullest extent of the law. FDA will not disclose the reporter's identity in response to a request form the public, pursuant to the Freedom of Information Act. The reporter's identity, including the identity of a self-reporter, may be shared with the manufacturer unless requested otherwise."

The FDA has also reinforced this in other statements on its website (Web Resource 12-6):

"Confidentiality: The FDA acknowledges that health professionals have concerns regarding their confidentiality as reporters, and that of the patients whose cases they report. In order to encourage reporting of adverse events, FDA regulations offer substantial protection against disclosure of the identities of both reporters and patients. This was further strengthened on July 3, 1995, when a regulation went into effect extending this protection against disclosure by preempting state discovery laws regarding voluntary reports held by pharmaceutical, biological and medical device manufacturers."

13

The Roles of Academia, Companies, Government Health Authorities, Non-Governmental Organizations (NGOs), Consumer Groups, and Gadflies in the World of Pharmacovigilance

➡ **NOTE:** (Unless otherwise noted the word "drug" or "drug product" should be taken in this book to include "biologics" and "vaccines.")

■ Background

The players in the world of pharmacovigilance are many. The interactions are complex. Alliances are formed and severed as issues or interests change. The groups are active in various causes in the medical and pharmaceutical world, touching not just on safety but on health care costs, drug prices, and health care availability.

■ The Theory

Patients who take medicines and suffer from adverse events (AEs) are the first and primary group involved in drug safety. Health care professionals make up the next category and include those who prescribe, sell, or dispense the medications and who must also help deal with the AEs. Other participants in the medical world include pharmaceutical companies, pharmacies, pharmacy/formulation committees (in hospitals, insurance companies, and other institu-

tions), and drug benefit managers and others who decide which medications are made available or reimbursed or not.

In government there is, of course, the US Food and Drug Administration (FDA) and equivalent agencies abroad (whose actions outside the United States may still play a big role within the United States), the Department of Health and Human Services (and the equivalent Ministries of Health outside the United States), the US Congress and other federal departments and agencies that work in or provide health care and medications (e.g., Veterans Affairs, the Armed Forces, the Centers for Disease Control and Prevention, Medicare), and state and local health departments including boards of health, Medicaid in the states, and others. In Canada things are somewhat simpler: The federal government approves new drugs, applies some form of price control, and the provinces decide which ones are reimbursed.

Nongovernmental organizations (NGOs) play major roles in health care in the United States and abroad, including the World Health Organization on drug policies and its offshoot, the Uppsala Monitoring Centre in Sweden, on drug safety; various foundations that fund health care initiatives (e.g., the Gates Foundation); and others.

The media of all sorts, including television, radio, newspapers, blogs, and websites, play active roles from all perspectives of the political and medical scene. Lobbies or professional organizations, NGOs from many domains (e.g., Pharmaceutical Research Manufacturers of America [PhRMA], International Society of Pharmacoepidemiology, the Centers for Education & Research on Therapeutics, the American Association of Retired Persons), over-the-counter (OTC) drug manufacturers, generic manufacturers, hospital groups, physician groups, nursing groups, pharmacy groups, consumer groups, disease groups, and advocacy groups such as Public Citizen (WorstPills.org) also play roles in drug safety.

These groups often petition or file position papers to influence legislation and perceptions at the local, state, and national levels as well as in litigation and in the media. The groups work from all parts of the spectrum, including some who strive to increase profits, speed up or slow down drug approval, and increase or decrease governmental oversight and regulation.

Litigators, insurance companies, and companies that provide health care for their employees also play a role in the system. A brief summary of some of the interactions of these players in regard to safety follows in the next section.

■ The Practice

Patients suffer the consequences of adverse drug reactions directly and personally, sometimes suffering dearly or even dying. Many patients are becoming more and more sophisticated and research the drugs they take or will take on the Internet or in printed media. Yet patient perceptions are quite variable. Sometimes there might be a perception that every AE that occurs is due to the drug, and at other times there is not a real awareness or level of suspicion by the patient that a particular sign or symptom could be due to one or more drugs being taken.

It is often presumed (sometimes incorrectly) that a drug cannot produce an adverse reaction if it has been taken safely for months or even years. Drug–drug, drug–food, and drug–alcohol interactions, manufacturing issues, and so on are almost never thought of by patients as explanations of problems. Patients often do not think of OTC products, "health foods," "nutraceuticals," or "herbals" (which may contain drugs or interact with drugs) as culprits in adverse reactions. Physicians too often forget to ask about them when doing the medical history. Many patients who are receiving multiple drugs, particularly the elderly, who are often "polypharmacy" patients, cannot recall the drugs or the doses they take. In some societies or cultures there has been a perception that AEs are the fault of the patient and represent a weakness or a shameful act on the patient's part and that they need to "tough it out." This attitude is changing as the dissemination of information occurs but is still seen in some older patients.

Health care practitioners prescribe, dispense, and administer drugs. When AEs or reactions occur, it may not be the same prescriber, dispenser, or administrator who has to deal with the medical consequences of the drug. Emergency rooms may not be able to get immediate access to the patient's medical records or drug history, for example. Some patients do not want to tell their physicians or health care providers about AEs, feeling embarrassed or ashamed and preferring to "tough it out."

Pharmaceutical companies play a major role in the world of safety. In the United States, most AEs on marketed drugs are reported to the manufacturers. The companies, through PhRMA (see below) and International Conference on Harmonization, have worked with the FDA, the European Union, and Japanese regulators to harmonize the safety reporting procedures, requirements, formats, documents, and expectations. This effort has been very successful because the requirements for reporting certain serious AEs from clinical trials and postmarketing situations are clear, consistent, and quite rigorous (7 or 15 calendar days). The major efforts underway, with varying degrees of harmonization and cooperation between the industry and government, are now in the areas of electronic transmission and standards (e.g., formats for transmission of health care documents, laboratory tests, cardiograms, etc.). These efforts in regard to "mechanics and operations" may well go beyond the pharmaceutical industry as the FDA and the Department of Health and Human Services standardize the transmission of health care data among other entities (hospitals, doctors, pharmacies, laboratories, insurance companies, etc.) and produce significant additional benefits for the public. Most dealings between scientific personnel in the industry and the FDA, European Medicines Agency, and other agencies are cordial and correct with the goal of protecting the public health and helping each do his or her job more efficiently and more rapidly given limited resources.

The reverse of this coin, however, is represented by controversies about specific medical products and safety issues. Some people (consumer groups in particular) believe there is too much cordiality and warmth between the regulators and the regulated, allowing the companies to "get away" with many things to increase profit at the expense of public health. They point out that people move from the government to industry (as in other regulated industries) and vice versa, like revolving doors. They claim that this may compromise the safety of the public because regulators will be hesitant to cross or oppose a company they may shortly wish to work for. There are clearly professional and medical differences between and within the companies and the industry. Many of these "battles" occur behind closed doors or via written or telephonic communications. Most of these communications are privileged and not available to the public.

Pharmaceutical companies play a major role by promoting their products to health care professionals and the public (direct to consumer advertising). Sometimes the promotion is not balanced in the eyes of the FDA, and warning letters are sent to companies by the FDA's Division of Drug Marketing, Advertising, and Communications. See the Warning Letter section of the FDA's website at Web Resource 13-1.

Physicians and other health care workers are also "detailed" by pharmaceutical representatives on products for their patients. The detail should contain balanced information and include the AE profile. The approved prescribing information should also be supplied.

One very public venue where differences are aired, often with full media coverage, is represented by public meetings of the FDA advisory committees. See the FDA's website at Web Resource 13-2. These are standing committees called by the FDA to discuss and recommend courses of action in controversial or unclear areas. Members include the FDA and academia (but not industry). They receive, well in advance, data from the FDA and the industry and then meet in public to discuss the issues involved. The companies are usually well represented and often make presentations themselves. The discussions are usually very scientific and technical but can become adversarial and even quite heated. Some sessions may be held behind closed doors and are not open to the public. Transcripts of the public sessions are usually available shortly afterward—often on the FDA website. This is a good example of transparency in the world of pharmaceuticals.

Broadly speaking, the professionals working in the drug safety area of government and industry tend to be more aligned and better able and motivated to share ideas than are professionals in other areas (research, marketing, legal, etc.) of the industry, being less constrained by legal restrictions and by competitive issues. The sharing of ideas about "what works" is very common and is seen with operational issues (drug coding, conventions for the *Medical Dictionary for Regulatory Activities* coding of AEs) and, now, risk management.

It is in everyone's interest for AEs to be sent to the FDA and other health authorities in a timely, complete, and correct manner. Companies do, in fact, want their competitors to have well-run and efficient safety departments so that the competition's AEs are sent to the FDA in a timely and complete manner too!

PhRMA is the industry organization for pharmaceutical companies. See its website (Web Resource 13-3). Not all companies are members, especially the smaller companies and those that do not do research. There are approximately 33 US companies and 7 international affiliates as members. PhRMA, which is based in Washington, DC, has multiple functions, including lobbying for the industry's position on public issues and legislation, outreach to the public, assistance with patient assistance programs, and representing US industry in the ICH. Their goal is to "encourage discovery of important new medicines for patients by pharmaceutical/biotechnology research companies."

There are multiple other organizations representing OTC manufacturers, generic manufacturers, and device manufacturers that interact with other organizations and lobbies representing physicians (American Medical Association), hospitals (American Hospital Association), nurses, insurance companies, and so forth. The permutations and combinations of interactions are many and complex as the groups sometimes work with each other and sometimes against each other. As attributed to Benjamin Disraeli, "There are no permanent allies, no permanent friends, only permanent interests."

The government entities involved directly or indirectly in drug safety are complex. At the federal level, the executive cabinet (ministry) level Department of Health and Human Services controls the FDA and other health-related agencies and entities. The US Congress controls the budget for the FDA and also has legislative oversight of FDA and other health matters. Other federal level groups with major interests in health care and pharmaceuticals include the Veterans Administration (Web Resource 13-4), which maintains hospitals, clinics, and pharmacies; the US Armed Forces, which also maintain hospitals clinics and pharmacies; the National Institutes of Health (see its website [Web Resource 13-5]), and the Centers for Disease Control and Prevention (see its website [Web Resource 13-6]).

At the state and local level, there are state and local health departments, Medicaid offices (the program that supplies health care to the indigent and certain others), state budget, and formulation offices. One of the recent controversies has been the push by state and local governments to aid consumers in importing prescription drugs from outside the United States.

Academia in the United States and Canada plays a surprisingly small role in drug safety. There are at most a handful of departments of pharmacology, medicine, or epidemiology in North America that play major roles in the drug safety world. Although academics sit on FDA advisory committees, many more make speeches (for a fee paid for by the pharmaceutical companies' "speakers bureaus") around the country regarding drug therapy. In addition, many academics perform clinical trials paid for by the pharmaceutical companies, thus removing them as neutral observers or consultants on safety. Pharmacovigilance is rarely taught to medical or nursing students. On the positive side, pharmacy schools seem to be incorporating drug safety concepts into their curriculum. This is in marked contrast to Europe, where academic institutions play a major role in drug safety, often working with the government and health authority. The best example of this is in France where there are over 30 drug safety centers located at regional university hospitals and medical schools around the country that play an active role in signaling, signal workups, and pharmacovigilance. They work in cooperation with the central health authority, the Agence Française de Sécurité Sanitaire des Produits de Santé. See its website (Web Resource 13-7) and the website of one of the French regional pharmacovigilance centers (Web Resource 13-8) (both in French). A brief summary in English prepared by Prof. Nicholas Moore of the Bordeaux Regional Center is available (Web Resource 13-9).

Consumer groups, insurance companies, employers paying health insurance, health maintenance organizations, retired persons groups, and others also play roles, sometimes direct and sometimes indirect in drug safety. Broadly speaking, many or all of these groups favor, to some degree or another, lower cost (or even "free") drugs, limited formularies ("no need for me-too drugs"), generics, OTC status for many more drugs, and a lessening of the influence of pharmaceutical companies. Many of these groups have very strong lobbies in Washington, DC and at the state levels.

Views on drug safety by all of the players may sometimes be simplistic and polarized, especially if they are conveyed in short sound bites. One may hear that the FDA should approve safe drugs only after careful and thorough study. Side effects, if any, should be mild, reversible, and of limited duration. Some supposedly neutral observers refuse to admit a drug to a formulary for cost reasons rather than for medical reasons and justify this with either lack of efficacy or increased safety concerns. Others believe that there should be no more than two or three products in any particular class of drugs because the me-too drugs add no value to the public health. Others disagree. Consumers often believe that if any re-

ally bad side effects do occur, someone should be made to pay. At the extreme end, some of these groups assume malevolence and ill will on the part of the drug companies whose goal is only to make money and helping the ill is a "side effect" of making profit. As the rhetoric heats up, the science and clarity disappear.

The rhetoric has tended to cloud some of the very real areas of controversy and concern:

- How much secrecy should be permitted in the competitive area of drug development and drug safety? How much transparency should there be?
- What is the role of the industry in patient and health care professional education?
- Is direct to the consumer advertising a good or bad thing for drug safety?
- Is a single-payer system for drugs a good or bad thing for drug safety?
- Is the current drug safety system in the United States adequate? Should the universities be more heavily involved? Should there be a single national formulary?
- Should me-too drugs be limited?
- Should drug safety be separated from the FDA, which would only handle drug approvals?
- Should some level of drug imports by consumers from abroad be tolerated or even encouraged?

Litigation plays a major role in safety decisions made regarding drugs. Any significant episode of AEs produce a flurry of lawsuits, often numbering in the thousands. They may take years to resolve, and costs run into the billions of dollars. The issues usually revolve around who knew what about the drug's toxicity, when it was known, whether it was adequately publicized, and whether remedial actions were taken in a timely fashion.

And finally, there are the unfortunate patients and sometimes unfortunate individual doctors, pharmacists, and nurses who deal on one-to-one levels and who must wade through the controversy, politics, and unclear and equivocal safety information ("the following AEs have been reported with this drug but causality cannot be determined") to come to good decisions for individual patients.

The bottom line is this: Drug safety is a high stakes, multiparty, politicized, highly controversial affair with multiple players involved with multiple agendas. Data are often soft, incomplete, and skewed in one direction or another. One should look at multiple sources for information and keep an open mind on the ultimate outcome of safety issues with drugs. Usually, the "truth will out," although it may take a long time.

■ FAQ

Q: So then how should the individual in the doctor's office, hospital, drug company, FDA, or elsewhere act? What can the individual do to help sort this out?

A: In general, act as a good scientist, an honest person, and do not prejudge until there is a good amount of evidence examined from multiple sides. Trust but verify.

Company safety personnel should always act with the public health foremost in their mind and the company profits secondary. This may be difficult because there are always pressures to "protect the drug" or "hold off on this signal until the data are stronger." Safety workups and signaling should always be done with due diligence and an open mind. Sometimes those terrible-looking serious AEs really do melt away after all the data are in. When the results are bad for the drug, these data must be conveyed to management and the FDA and other health authorities in a timely and correct manner.

Practitioners, pharmacists, nurses, and patients should maintain a healthy skepticism regarding data whether they are from the company, academia, the FDA, or the media—especially during the acute controversy when the "fog of war" is at its height. They should seek out data from all sides and from neutral authorities (if such exist). Health care practitioners must always act in the best interest of the patient.

Patients should find honest caring health personnel and trust them to act in their best interest. Nonetheless, verification (looking at the *Physicians' Desk Reference*, looking on the Internet, being treated at major or academic medical centers, etc.) is also well worth doing.

Risk: What Is It?
Risk Management
and Assessment

Benefit/risk analyses. Limitations in measurement and assessment. Limitations on what is knowable.

➡ **NOTE:** (Unless otherwise noted the word "drug" or "drug product" should be taken in this book to include "biologics" and "vaccines.")

■ Background

Risk is a very broad concept and applies to everything in life. We take risks when we drive a car, go to work, eat a meal, and take a drug. Risk analysis of drugs is now very much in vogue to aid the patient and health care professional as well as the US Food and Drug Administration (FDA) and drug companies in decision making. This chapter looks at risk first in a global manner and then as applied to drug therapy.

■ The Theory

Risk can be defined in many ways:

■ Exposure to a possibility of loss or damage;
■ The quantitative or qualitative possibility of loss

that considers both the probability that something will cause harm and the consequences of that something;

■ The probability of an adverse event resulting from the use of a drug in the dose and manner prescribed or labeled or from its use at a different dose or manner or in a patient or population for which the drug is not approved;

■ The exposure to loss of money as a result of changes in business conditions, the economy, the stock and bond markets, interest rates, foreign currency exchange rates, inflation, natural disasters, and war.

■ The Practice

Over the last 5 to 10 years many in the pharmaceutical world (as elsewhere) have been thinking about risk assessment and management. The FDA first published a document on its thinking in May 1999 entitled "Managing the Risks from Medical Product Use & Creating a Risk Management Framework." It addressed pre- and postmarketing risk management and the FDA's role. It is available at the FDA's website (Web Resource 14-1). Further publications have extended and elaborated the FDA's position.

First some clarifications. FDA "approval" means that a product is safe and effective for the approved indications under the labeled conditions of use. "Safe" means that the beneficial actions outweigh any harmful or undesirable side effects that might occur. Safe does not mean the absence of risk. These points are often forgotten when the phrase "this drug is safe and effective" is used. The implication is that it is always effective no matter when or how used and is without risk. This is not the case.

The FDA has published three guidances for industry on risk management (see Chapters 15–17):

1. Premarketing Risk Assessment (Web Resource 14-2)
2. Development and Use of Risk Minimization Action Plans (RiskMAPs) (Web Resource 14-3)
3. Good Pharmacovigilance Practices and Pharmacoepidemiologic Assessment (Web Resource 14-4)

The first guidance on premarketing risk assessment focuses on measures companies might consider throughout all stages of clinical development of products. For example, a section on special safety considerations describes ways that risk assessment can be tailored for those products intended for use chronically or in children.

General recommended risk assessment strategies include the use of long-term controlled safety studies, enrollment of diversified patient populations, and phase III trials with multiple-dose levels. Some key components of the guidance include

- Providing specific recommendations to industry for improving the assessment and reporting of safety during drug development trials;
- Improving the assessment of important safety issues during registration trials and providing best practices for analyzing and reporting data that are developed as a result of a careful preapproval safety evaluation;
- Building on (but not superceding) a number of existing FDA and International Conference on Harmonization guidances related to preapproval safety assessments.

The second guidance on RiskMAPs describes how industry can address specific risk-related goals and objectives. This guidance also suggests various tools to minimize the risks of drug and biologic products. Key components of the guidance include

- Establishing consistent use and definition of terms and a conceptual framework for setting up specialized systems and processes to ensure product benefits exceed risks;
- Broader input from patients, health care professionals, and the public when making recommendations about whether to initiate, revise, or end risk minimization interventions;
- Evaluating RiskMAPs to ensure that risk minimization efforts are successful.

The third guidance on the postmarketing period identifies recommended reporting and analytical practices to monitor the safety concerns and risk of medical products in general use. Some key components of this guidance include

- Describing the role of pharmacovigilance in risk management. Pharmacovigilance refers to all observational postapproval scientific and data gathering activities relating to the detection, assessment, and understanding of adverse events with the goals of identifying and preventing these events to the extent possible.
- Describing elements of good pharmacovigilance practice from identifying and describing safety signals, through investigation of signals beyond case review, and interpreting signals in terms of risk.
- Describing development of pharmacovigilance plans to expedite the acquisition of new safety information for products with unusual safety signals.

These guidances are critically important in how the FDA and many other health authorities as well as companies actually handle risk. Each guidance is summarized and commented on in a separate chapter.

The US Food and Drug Administration's Premarketing Risk Assessment Guidance of March 2005

➡ **NOTE:** (Unless otherwise noted, the word "drug" or "drug product" should be taken in this book to include "biologics" and "vaccines.")

■ Background

In March 2005 the US Food and Drug Administration (FDA) issued three guidances, which were years in the making, summarizing the agency's views on risk management. These documents are of critical importance in conveying how the FDA (and other health agencies) views risk. Each guidance is examined in detail in this chapter and in Chapters 16 and 17. Note: Exceptionally in this chapter, comments are included below *in italics* by the author.

■ The Theory and the Practice

Premarketing Risk Assessment

The document can be found at the FDA's website (Web Resource 15-1). The sections of this very important doc-

ument are reviewed in the sections below. See the document itself for further detail. The FDA begins by noting that routine risk assessment is already being done. It notes that this guidance is not aimed at use on all products but rather only on those that "pose a clinically important and unusual type or level of risk."

The adequacy of assessment of risk depends on quantity (number of patients studied) and quality ("the appropriateness of the assessments performed, the appropriateness and breadth of the patient populations studied, and how results are analyzed").

"Providing detailed guidance on what constitutes an adequate safety database for all products is impossible." Each product is weighed on its own merits.

The FDA's comments here are consistent with current practice in the industry. Some drug products require extensive additions to the usual safety and risk procedures and others do not. Routine or "me-too" drugs may require less, whereas new chemical entities or drugs that are teratogenic or highly toxic in animals and/or humans in early studies may require more.

Size of the Safety Database

The number of patients studied depends on the novelty of the drug, the availability and safety of alternate therapies, the intended population, the condition being treated, and the duration of use. Safety databases for life-threatening diseases, especially where there are no satisfactory alternate treatments, are smaller than the databases for products to treat less serious diseases where there are alternate treatments available. The FDA recommends end of phase I meetings between the sponsor and the agency to agree on the extent of the phase II trials.

The FDA does not give safety database size advice for products for short term (<6 months use) but does make suggestions for products aimed at treatment over 6 months. For these, the FDA and the International Conference on Harmonization (ICH) recommend 1,500 subjects in total with 300 to 600 exposed for 6 months and 100 exposed for 1 year using doses in the therapeutic range. Higher numbers of patients may need to be studied if

- Specific safety issues arise from animal studies
- Similar drugs or the class of drugs suggests a specific problem
- Pharmacokinetic or pharmacodynamic properties of the drug are associated with certain adverse events (AEs)
- It is important to quantitate the occurrence of low-frequency AEs
- The benefit from the product is small and one wants to be very sure there are no rare AEs that will not be picked up unless large numbers of patients are studied
- The benefit is experienced by only a fraction of the treated patients (i.e., the benefit is "rare" and thus the same reason as above to look for rare AEs)
- The benefit is unclear (e.g., surrogate endpoints used)
- Statistical power requires larger number of patients to show that an already high background rate of safety issues will not be unduly raised even more due to the drug
- The proposed treatment is for healthy populations (e.g., preventive vaccines)
- A safe and effective alternate treatment is available

The FDA again emphasizes both the utility of a meeting with the agency to work out issues such as these early in the development and also the need to take as much care with the safety section of a New Drug Application (NDA) as with the efficacy section. The *Medical Dictionary for Regulatory Activities* (MedDRA) should be used to ensure that information is not obscured or distorted. All patients who left the study (deaths and dropouts for any reason) must be followed up and evaluated for safety issues.

In practice this has been done for quite some time. The ICH/FDA figures above are somewhat arbitrary and may need to be higher depending on the drug and population being studied. Often, statistical needs for power or significance drive sample size and may produce higher numbers of patients studied in short-term trials. What is noteworthy above is the requirement for longer term exposure (6 months and 1 year) for drugs that are being used for 6 months. Even these suggestions may be conservative, and some drugs have had much longer follow-ups (e.g., Adriamycin, diethylstilbestrol) where chronic toxicity is expected or suspected to occur.

Long-Term Controlled Safety Trials

The FDA notes that in many clinical programs, uncontrolled, single-arm, long-term safety studies are done. Although useful, the use of a control or placebo (if possible) is preferable, especially where the AEs in question are relatively common in the treated population (e.g., sudden death in patients with ischemic heart disease) or where the AE might mimic the disease being treated, such as asthma exacerbations due to inhalation treatments given for asthma (see fialuridine and hepatitis, Chapter 47). Long-term safety studies are also very useful if the toxicity worsens with cumulative exposure.

Uncontrolled studies are useful in picking up certain AEs that (essentially) never occur spontaneously. The FDA gives examples of aplastic anemia and severe hepatocellular injury (though not stated, one presumes they mean noninfectious hepatitis).

This section highlights a fundamental difference between FDA and European Union (EU) views on comparators. The FDA has long believed that placebo-controlled trials are the gold standard for characterizing a drug's safety and efficacy. Sponsors often avoid doing head-to-head trials with competitors for fear of getting unexpected bad results against a competitor or even the sponsor's own comparator (e.g., an older drug the sponsor wishes to discontinue). Sometimes, of course, placebo trials cannot be done for medical or ethical reasons, especially now due to changes in the Declaration of Helsinki.

The EU and most medical practitioners generally prefer to see trials against the current standard of therapy, arguing that practitioners do not treat with placebo in the real world but rather with something already out on the market. It is further argued that showing a new treatment to be superior (or inferior) to an old one is a significant public service. Companies obviously fear losing such head-to-head comparison trials.

Sometimes placebo trials are necessary. Examples in the past include duodenal ulcer trials in which H2 blockers showed 40-80% healing rates when compared with each other. Only when a placebo arm was added was it shown that the placebo healing rates were also in the 40% range, demonstrating that some of the active treatments were not very active at all. On the other hand, many now argue that the utility and ethics should put an end to most placebo trials (Moerman and Jonas, Ann Intern Med 2002;136:471-476). The article can be found at Web Resource 15-2.

Diversity

The premarketing safety database (mainly in phase III studies) should represent, as much as possible, the expected target population. The FDA argues that, where possible, inclusion criteria should be fairly broad to include elderly (and in particular "the very old") patients with concomitant diseases and patients taking concomitant medications.

Another fundamental area of potential conflict is between sponsors (companies) and the FDA. Sponsors generally like "very clean" studies in homogeneous patients so that efficacy (and safety) can be evaluated without extraneous "noise" (confounders) and that sample size can be kept "reasonable." The FDA, knowing that the drug will be used in the general population, only some of which resembles the test population, would like to see a much broader selection of patients tested before marketing.

Exploring Dose Effects

Normally, if one is skilled and lucky, the phase II trials establish the clinical dose that is then studied in large numbers of patients in phase III studies. The FDA argues for the study, in phase III, of more than one dose. They indicate that many efficacy and safety data can be obtained from these trials.

Drug Interactions

It is not possible to study all possible or potential drug or other interactions. Those studies that are done should focus on the following:

- Drug-drug interactions should be looked at using those drugs that might be expected to produce safety issues resulting from known metabolic pathways (e.g., certain cytochrome P450 enzymes). Logical choices of test drugs should be made (e.g., for a new cholesterol-lowering treatment, examining the consequences of concomitant use of HMG CoA reductase inhibitors).
- Drug-demography interactions should be sought where gender, age, race, or other demographics might play a role.
- Drug-disease interactions should be examined if necessary.

- Drug-dietary supplement interactions may need to be evaluated (e.g., interactions between an antidepressant and St. John's wort).

The FDA recommends that pharmacokinetic assessments be built into some late-phase clinical trials to see whether unexpected interactions can be picked up.

Drug-drug interactions, in particular, remain a difficult nut to crack. Certain standard studies looking at the key cytochrome P450 enzyme pathways or drugs known to have many interactions (e.g., Coumadin®, anticonvulsants) are straightforward and generally done routinely, as are drug-food and drug-alcohol studies. It is only after marketing that "surprise" interactions are seen (e.g., St. John's wort and human immunodeficiency virus drugs). Sometimes pharmacokinetic interactions are seen (e.g., loratadine and clarithromycin) but have no pharmacodynamic or clinical implications (Carr, Edmonds, Shi, et al., Antimicrob Agents Chemother 1998;42:1176-1180). These types of effects are unpredictable and, once seen, often hard to study. It may not be feasible, safe, or ethical to treat normal subjects with two drugs to see whether the drugs interact. Similarly, it may not be feasible, safe, or ethical to treat a cohort of patients already on a drug (e.g., acquired immunodeficiency syndrome patients, asthmatics) with the new drug to see whether there is an interaction.

Comparative Safety Data

The FDA next comments on safety data and comparators in clinical trials. They note, consistent with their long-standing feelings but not always consistent with European and some US clinical practice views, that "much of the safety data in an application may be derived from placebo-controlled trials and single-arm safety studies, with little or no comparative safety data." Many believe that comparisons against a placebo (both for safety and efficacy) are less useful in the "real world" because physicians do not usually prescribe placebos. They do not care that a drug is better than a placebo but rather want to know whether the drug is better (or worse or the same) as the current treatment used.

Nonetheless, the FDA notes that active controls and/or a placebo arm if possible would be useful in the following circumstances:

- The background rate of AEs is high. Using a single-arm study might show an alarmingly high rate of AEs, which would be of less concern if a placebo arm showed a similar high rate.
- There is a well-established treatment already. A single-arm trial would likely be uninformative and a

placebo control unethical. Thus an active comparator is the usual choice.

- A superiority claim for safety or efficacy is desired. A control then is obviously needed.

Special Circumstances

Certain special circumstances require a tailored approach:

- Chronically used, long-half-life drugs and/or drugs with dose-related toxicities should have studies to determine whether a lower dose or less frequent dose is appropriate.
- If a specific titration schedule is needed, this schedule should be based on specific studies to determine the best titration scheme.
- If certain AEs are not likely to be detected or reported without special attention or tests, studies should include these. As an example, the FDA cites a new drug with central nervous system effects and notes that it should have assessments of cognitive function, motor skills, and mood.
- In pediatric studies, special attention should be paid to effects on growth and neurocognitive development if the drug is used in the very young, to excipients, and to immunization recommendations.
- The sponsor should evaluate whether and when the collection from some or all patients of blood or other bodily tissues or fluids during phase III studies for analysis at a later time should be done. This might be useful for analyzing unusual signals or for retrospective analyses at a later date.

Large Simple Safety Studies

These are usually randomized controlled studies done to assess limited specific safety outcomes in large numbers of patients. Rarely, they may be uncontrolled if the event being assessed is very uncommon. The FDA notes these are usually done as formal phase IV commitments, although they could be done occasionally earlier in development. Another place for a large study is a product developed for preventive use in at-risk subjects who are otherwise healthy and where the benefits may be small.

Medication Errors

Although historically not a part of drug safety or pharmacovigilance, medication errors are now a high FDA priority in risk management. The FDA now wants sponsors to pay close attention before marketing to possible areas of medication error such as packaging, drug name, and labeling. Should medication errors or potential for errors be noted in the premarketing clinical trials, they should be acted on to remove potentials for errors. The FDA recommends drawing from the experience of Good Manufacturing Practice and device development by

- Conducting a failure mode and effects analysis
- Using expert panels
- Using computer-assisted analysis
- Using direct observation during clinical trials
- Using directed interviews of consumers and medical and pharmacy personnel to better understand comprehension
- Using focus groups
- Using simulated prescription and over-the-counter use studies

Assessing Safety during Product Development

During the development of all new small-molecule drugs the following should be addressed as part of the NDA:

- Drug-related QTc prolongation (to exclude arrhythmic potential)
- Drug-drug interactions
- Polymorphic metabolism

These experiments are conducted with "normal" doses in humans and are now known as safety pharmacology, in contrast to animal toxicology, which consists of increasing dosages until some untoward effect occurs:

- Drug-related liver toxicity
- Drug-related nephrotoxicity
- Drug-related bone marrow toxicity

Not all drugs require studies looking at all of these issues. They should be done where scientifically appropriate. The FDA does note, however, "For some issues, such as QTc, specifically conducted preclinical and clinical studies are generally recommended."

Biologic products may require additional testing:

- Immunogenicity: "...both the incidence and consequences of neutralizing antibody formation and the potential for adverse events related to binding antibody formation."
- Transfection of nontarget cells and infection transmissibility to close contacts should be evaluated for gene-based products.
- "For cell-based products, assessment of AEs related to distribution, migration and growth beyond the initial intended administration are important as are AEs related to cell survival and demise."

Data Analysis and Interpretation

The FDA refers the reader to three ICH guidances on preparing NDAs, clinical study reports, and the common technical document. The FDA notes that the later phases of product development are primarily aimed at efficacy, with endpoints identified in advance and with statistical calculations based on these endpoints. In contrast, the safety measures are usually not addressed with any pre-specified level of statistical sensitivity. Thus premarketing safety data are often only exploratory and useful primarily for signal development.

Describing AEs to Identify Signals (Coding)

The FDA recommends use of a single coding system (e.g., MedDRA), with a standardized coding convention and without updates throughout the program. If that is not possible (and it often is not), then care should be taken to handle the groupings and updates appropriately so as not to lose signals and safety data.

Coding Accuracy

Care should be taken with investigators and coders such that the reported verbatim terms are accurately reflected in the MedDRA codes used for these reported AEs. Severity and magnitude should not be exaggerated (e.g., coding acute liver failure when all that occurred was isolated transaminase elevation without elevated bilirubin, coagulopathy, or encephalopathy) or masked (using a nonspecific and "unimportant" term to describe a serious AE). The sponsor may "recharacterize" an AE code when appropriate but with an audit trail and with FDA consultation.

Verbatim terms from investigators should be captured, verified to be accurate, and mapped to the appropriate MedDRA term (e.g., the verbatim term "suicidal ideation" should not be captured as "emotional lability"). The sponsor should ensure that verbatim terms are consistent across studies and individual coders. The FDA also suggests that the sponsor "consider a coded event in conjunction with other coded events in some circumstances" and may define certain entities as "an amalgamation of multiple coding terms." They give as an example "acute liver failure," which could be used if it is based on recognized definitions of this term. The FDA does not, however, come down squarely on one side or the other in the "lumpers" versus "splitters" debate (i.e., combine terms or report them separately). This is an area of continued controversy with various coding conventions proposed.

Coding Analysis

The FDA cautions about how analyses can be altered or obscured by the way coding is done. They urge the sponsor to pay attention and use coding (whether lumping or splitting) to obtain the best signals:

■ Splitting: Using multiple terms may at times be more useful than combinations. They give the ex-

ample that "dyspnea, cough, wheezing and pleuritis" is more sensitive and useful than "pulmonary toxicity" but warn that "constipation" might include and hide cases of "toxic megacolon."

■ Splitting may, however, falsely decrease the incidence of AEs. "Fluid retention" may give a better signal and truer incidence than dividing the AEs into "pedal edema, generalized edema, peripheral edema."

■ Prospective grouping may be useful in clinical programs where appropriate: serotonin syndrome, parkinsonism, and drug withdrawal are useful and "not well characterized by a single term." Other groupings may be done retrospectively, although the FDA should be consulted.

Analyzing Temporal and Other Associations

The FDA next gives a high-level discussion of factors that need to be considered in analyzing signals. They note that simple comparisons of frequency may not be sufficient to analyze a signal and that temporal associations may aid in evaluating causality. This includes duration of exposure to a product, time to onset, and so on. Various statistical methods, including the Kaplan-Meier approach, may be useful for evaluating risks of AEs. The product's pharmacokinetic and pharmacodynamic profiles as well as "an appreciation of physiologic, metabolic and host immune responses may be important in understanding the possible timing of treatment-related AEs." Concomitant medications, the initiation or withdrawal of other therapies, and changes in the preexisting conditions over time should also be considered.

Analyzing Dose Effect

AEs should be analyzed as a function of dose. That is, are there different AE responses at different doses? It may be useful to consider weight or body surface area adjusted doses. Subgroup analysis by dose may also be useful.

The FDA also makes the important point that "the likelihood of observing false positive signals increases with the number of analyses conducted." Consistency across studies should be investigated to help validate such findings.

Data Pooling

The FDA notes that "...data pooling is performed to achieve larger sample sizes and data sets because individual clinical studies are not designed with sufficient sample size to estimate the frequency of low incidence events or to compare differences in rates or relative rates between the test drug (exposed group) and the control (unexposed group)." Further, "pooled analyses can enhance the power to detect an association between product use and an event and provide more reliable estimates of the magnitude of risk over time...and can also provide insight into a positive signal observed in a single study by allowing a broader comparison." The FDA discusses issues for and against use of such pooled data.

The FDA next notes that all placebo-controlled trials should be considered for data pooling. The patient populations should be relatively homogeneous and have similar methods of AE and dropout ascertainment. Phase I trials should generally be excluded. Risks should not just be expressed in event frequency (e.g., AEs per 100 persons) but also in time-event analyses when appropriate.

Rigorous Ascertainment of Reasons for Withdrawals from Studies

The FDA emphasizes that all dropouts must be followed up to fully understand why they did so. Some reasons may be irrelevant and trivial (e.g., moved away) or very important in regard to safety (e.g., had a stroke, was intolerant to adverse reactions). Terms like "withdrew consent," "failed to return," "administratively withdrawn," or "lost to follow-up" are too vague to be useful. These reasons should be followed up for more specific causes, especially if safety issues are involved. Dropouts due to abnormal laboratory tests, vital signs, or electrocardiographic findings may not always be characterized as AEs but should be followed up and accounted for. Follow-up on safety issues should be done until the AE is resolved or stabilized.

Long-Term Follow-Up

In some instances (e.g., the drug has a very long half-life, is deposited in bone or brain, or might cause irreversible AEs such as cancer) patients should be followed to the end of the study or even after the study ends. This may mean follow-up long after the drug treatment ends. This is especially true in long-term treatment and outcome studies. The FDA recommends discussions with the agency for these special cases.

Important Aspects of Data Presentation

Finally, the FDA makes several comments on data presentation in the NDA integrated summary of safety and elsewhere.

- AE rates should be presented from more restrictive (e.g., myocardial infarction) to less restrictive (e.g., myocardial ischemia).

- AEs for the drug that are important and seen for other drugs in the class should be discussed.

- Analyses of pooled data looking at gender, age, extent of exposure, concomitant medical conditions, and concomitant medications should be included.

- Differential discontinuation rates (e.g., placebo-treated patients may drop out of a trial earlier than drug-treated patients) must be accounted for.

- Case report forms submitted for patients who died or discontinued should have relevant hospital records, biopsy reports, and so forth included.

- Narrative summaries of important AEs should be sufficiently detailed to allow the case to be understood and analyzed.

The US Food and Drug Administration's Development and Use of Risk Minimization Action Plans Guidance of March 2005

➡️ **NOTE:** (Unless otherwise noted, the word "drug" or "drug product" should be taken in this book to include "biologics" and "vaccines.")

■ Background

In March 2005, the US Food and Drug Administration (FDA) issued three guidances, which were years in the making, summarizing the agency's views on risk management. These documents are of critical importance in conveying how the FDA (and other health agencies) views risk. Each guidance is examined in detail in Chapter 15, this chapter, and in Chapter 17.

The document Development and Use of Risk Minimization Action Plans can be found at the FDA's website (Web Resource 16-1).

■ The Theory and the Practice

This document advises industry on

■ Initiating and designing plans, called risk minimization action plans (RiskMAPs), to minimize identified product risks

■ Selecting and developing tools to minimize those risks

■ Evaluating RiskMAPs and monitoring tools

■ Communicating with the FDA about RiskMAPs

■ Recommending components of a RiskMAP submission to the FDA

The FDA begins by noting that its approval of a product for marketing means that it is "considered safe if it has an appropriate benefit-risk balance for the intended population and use." Benefits may be cosmetic, symptomatic, or curative; may alter the course of the disease; or may affect mortality. Risks may be at the individual or population level. The FDA notes that the usual product labeling is sufficient in most cases to minimize risk. There are some cases where a RiskMAP might be needed. The FDA "recommends that RiskMAPs be used judiciously to minimize risks without encumbering drug availability or otherwise interfering with the delivery of product benefits to patients." The FDA defines a RiskMAP as a strategic safety program designed to meet specific goals and objectives to minimize known risks while preserving the product's benefits. Outcomes and tools are defined. The FDA references the International Conference on Harmonization E2E document on Pharmacovigilance Planning in designing a RiskMAP.

Goals

The RiskMAP should state its goal(s) in "absolute terms" to achieve maximum risk reduction. Examples include "patients on X drug should not also be prescribed Y drug" or "fetal exposures to Z drug should not occur."

Objectives

The objectives should be pragmatic, specific, and measurable. For the goal stated above of "patients on X drug should not also be prescribed Y drug" or "fetal exposures to Z drug should not occur," the objective could be "lowering physician coprescribing rates and/or pharmacist codispensing rates."

Tools

In this example, possible tools include targeted education and outreach to health care professionals and patients, reminder systems or forms, and limiting access.

When to Develop a RiskMAP

A RiskMAP may be developed anytime during a product's life cycle. It may be done by the company or proposed by the FDA. Several considerations should be kept in mind when developing the RiskMAP:

- The types, magnitude, and frequency of risks and benefits
- The populations at greatest risk and/or those likely to derive the most benefit
- The existence of treatment alternatives and their risks and benefits
- The reversibility of the adverse events observed
- The preventability of the adverse events in question
- The probability of benefit

As examples, the FDA recommends the following:

- All schedule II controlled substances (especially extended-release or high-concentration opiates) for pain control have a RiskMAP aimed at minimizing overdose, abuse, and addiction.
- Teratogens should also have a RiskMAP.
- Drugs requiring specialized health care skills, training, or facilities to manage the therapeutic or adverse effects of a drug.

- Discussion by all the stakeholders at an early point in the process and notes that a public FDA advisory committee meeting may be useful in some cases.

Mechanisms Available to Industry to Minimize Risk

Tools are created to achieve the desired objectives. There are three broad types of tools.

1. *Targeted education and outreach.* These tools include specific targeted programs to health care practitioners and consumers (and possibly others). They should typically be used where the usual risk minimization (e.g., labeling) is not sufficient and where there is also a reminder or performance-linked access system (see below). Occasionally, they may be used alone. Examples include letters, training programs, continuing medical education, "prominent professional or public notifications," patient medication guides and package inserts, direct-to-consumer advertising highlighting the risks in question, and disease management/patient access systems with patient-sponsor interactions.

2. *Reminder systems.* These tools prompt, remind, or double-check health care practitioners and/or patients. Examples include consent forms where patients read directed material and agree to follow its instructions, health care provider training and testing, enrollment of patients, prescribers, and/or pharmacies in special data collection systems to reinforce appropriate product use, limiting the amount of product dispensed in a prescription or forbidding refills, and special packaging and systems to attest that safety measures have been done (e.g., prescription stickers).

3. *Performance-linked access systems.* These tools link product access to laboratory testing of other specific documentation. Because these tools are burdensome, costly, and interrupt the usual flow of patient care, they should be used where significant benefits occur but significant risks also exist, such as irreversible disability or death, and where less burdensome systems are believed to be insufficient. Examples include obligatory actions before making a product available such as a laboratory test or a signed informed consent, enrollment in a special support program, special certification of prescribers, and limited dispensing to only certain pharmacies. The FDA is planning a website to list available tools in use.

The FDA recommends careful selection of the tools to use on a case-by-case basis and gives some general suggestions:

- Use the least burdensome tools possible.
- Identify all the key stakeholders and define the role of each. Seek their input on the feasibility and acceptability of the tools.
- The RiskMAP should be compatible with current technology.
- Make them applicable to inpatient and outpatient use.
- Make them accessible to patients in diverse locales (i.e., nonurban settings).
- Make them consistent with other tools that have been shown to be effective.
- Consider looking not just at direct evidence of a tool's effectiveness but also indirect evidence.
- Avoid tools that will drive patients to inappropriate alternatives ("unintended consequences") such as the use of counterfeit products, Internet sales, or inappropriate alternative treatment.

Mechanisms Available to the FDA to Minimize Risks

The FDA has legal and regulatory powers to minimize risks, including product recalls, warning and untitled letters, import alerts, safety alerts, guidance documents, and regulations and judicial enforcement procedures such as seizures or injunctions.

Assessing the Effectiveness of the Tools and the Plan

It is now recognized that it is not sufficient to only implement a risk management plan without analyzing its effectiveness. To do so, the FDA recommends that "well defined, evidence based and objective performance measures tailored to the particular RiskMAP" be used. Measures that can be used are as follows:

- Direct measurements (e.g., if the goal is to prevent a particular complication from product use, the measurement of the complication rate could be used).
- Surrogate measurements (e.g., emergency room visits). The sensitivity, specificity, and predictive value of such markers need to be established before their use.
- Process measurements (e.g., performance of a monitoring laboratory test, signature on an informed consent).

- Assessments of comprehension, knowledge, attitudes, and behavior changes (e.g., of the prescriber, pharmacist, or patient).

As an example, for a RiskMAP to avoid liver failure due to a product, the measures used, in order of preference, could be (1) rate of liver failure in the user population, (2) hospitalization for severe liver injury, and (3) frequency of liver function monitoring. The FDA notes that if a method is chosen that is not direct, it may be necessary to compensate for the methodologic shortfalls. It cites the weaknesses of certain systems:

- Spontaneous adverse event reporting is biased as an outcome measure because reporting varies due to many factors and represents an unknown and variable fraction of the adverse outcome in question that is actually occurring.
- Population-based evaluation using administrative or claims-based databases (with validation done by examination of the actual medical charts) may not represent the actual population exposed to the drug. In addition, the number of patients actually exposed to the drug may be limited, thus reducing the power to detect the outcome being sought. There are also time lags between the collection of the data, entry into the database, and ability to retrieve and analyze it.
- Active surveillance using sentinel reporting sites is costly and may not detect rare events.
- Surveys of patients or practitioners may be limited by inadequate response rates, poor representativeness, and reporting biases.

Because of these issues, the FDA recommends, where feasible, that two different methods be used for each critical RiskMAP goal. Failing that, quantitative methods using multiple-site sampling or audits should be done. There is a literature and methodology available, such as failure modes and effect analysis, that the FDA recommends considering.

Evaluating Effectiveness of the RiskMAP

The FDA recommends periodic evaluation of the RiskMAP, its tools, and its effectiveness so that ineffective tools can be eliminated and better ones adopted. The sponsor should distinguish between the goals and the tools used. A RiskMAP goal may be achieved even though the tools may be performing poorly or vice versa. In particular, the FDA asks that sponsors evaluate a tool's acceptability and unintended consequences. RiskMAP tools should be evaluated before implementation where possible. Techniques include using tools with a known (published) track record of effectiveness and pretests or pilot tests before full-scale implementation. This might include using a tool in a small phase II trial before use in a large phase III trial. For other tools multiple interviews or focus groups may be useful with targeted education and outreach tools.

FDA Assessment and Publication of RiskMAP Results

If a sponsor makes a RiskMAP submission to the FDA, the submission should include a timetable of when the sponsor will send in periodic evaluation results to the FDA. The submissions should include the data, all the analyses, conclusions regarding effectiveness, and any proposed modifications. The FDA then does its own analysis and discusses the respective evaluations with the sponsor afterward. In high-risk areas, if results are ambiguous, or if there is disagreement, the FDA may call a public advisory committee meeting to evaluate the data.

The FDA maintains a website that describes all publicly available information about RiskMAPs and tools. The FDA also discusses the effectiveness of particular RiskMAP tools.

The FDA recommends that sponsors consider setting up a dialogue with the FDA review division in question to "benefit from the Agency's experience in reviewing previously implemented plans." That division may discuss the RiskMAP with other FDA divisions. The sponsor should share information and analyses regarding the product's risks and benefits; discuss the choice of goals, objectives, and tools; and discuss the evaluation plan, including the specifics of times for evaluation, performance, measures, and analyses. Information should be supplied to the FDA before the meeting. The FDA develops internal policies and manuals for RiskMAPs.

For products not yet marketed, the RiskMAP may be submitted to the New Drug Application for drugs or Biologic License Application for biologics or, if earlier in the product life cycle, to the Investigational New Drug Application. After marketing, the RiskMAP may be submitted as a supplement to the New Drug Application or Biologic License Application.

The guidance concludes with two sections on the format and contents of a RiskMAP submission to the FDA and a RiskMAP progress report. The reader is referred to the guidance for the specifics of these sections.

■ The Practice

This guidance represents the formalization of risk evaluation for products. It is clearly quite high level and short on specifics. Although risk evaluation has been going on for some time, it has been by a less formal, more customized, case-by-case basis. Examples of risk management programs exist to ensure that women avoid pregnancy if taking potentially teratogenic drugs (e.g., ribavirin and interferon alpha, isotretinoin) or agranulocytosis (Clozaril).

Nonetheless, the FDA is putting risk management on a "higher burner." For example, in August 2005 the FDA altered the program in place for isotretinoin:

> "FDA notified healthcare professionals and patients of the approval of a strengthened risk management program, called iPLEDGE, for Accutane and generic isotretinoin. The strengthened program requires registration of wholesalers, prescribers, pharmacies and patients who agree to accept specific responsibilities designed to minimize pregnancy exposures in order to distribute, prescribe, dispense and use Accutane. In addition to approving the iPLEDGE program, FDA has approved changes to the existing warnings, patient information and informed consent document so that patients and prescribers can better identify and manage the risks of psychiatric symptoms and depression before and after prescribing isotretinoin."

See the FDA's website for further information (Web Resource 16-2). It is likely that the risk management efforts of the FDA will change over time as experience grows.

17

The US Food and Drug Administration's Good Pharmacovigilance Practices and Pharmacoepidemiologic Assessment Guidance of March 2005

➡️ **NOTE:** (Unless otherwise noted, the word "drug" or "drug product" should be taken in this book to include "biologics" and "vaccines.")

■ Background

In March 2005, the US Food and Drug Administration (FDA) issued three guidances, which were years in the making, summarizing the agency's views on risk management. These documents are of critical importance in conveying how the FDA (and other health agencies) looks at risk. Each guidance is examined in detail in Chapters 15 and 16 and in this chapter.

The document FDA's Good Pharmacovigilance Practices and Pharmacoepidemiologic Assessment Guidance can be found on the FDA's website (Web Resource 17-1).

■ The Theory and the Practice

In this guidance the FDA discusses pharmacovigilance and how a product is marketed. The agency notes that because it is impossible to identify all safety issues in the clinical studies, pharmacovigilance must be very active after New Drug Application approval. Only after a large number of patients with other comorbid conditions and taking other drugs are exposed to the new product after marketing is a better safety profile known.

The FDA takes a broad definition of pharmacovigilance: "All scientific and data gathering activities relating to the detection, assessment, and understanding of adverse events. This includes the use of pharmacoepidemiologic studies." The FDA also defines "signal" as "a concern about an excess of adverse events compared to what would be expected to be associated with a product's use...(though) even a single well-documented case report can be viewed as a signal... Signals generally indicate the need for further investigation, which may or may not lead to the conclusion that the product caused the event."

Identifying Signals: Good Reporting Practice

The FDA notes that individual case reports submitted to the sponsor or the FDA or cases found in clinical trials or the literature may generate safety signals and that these signals need to be pursued. Sponsors make "reasonable" attempts to get complete information at the initial and at follow-up contacts, especially for serious adverse events

(AEs). The "detective work" should be done by experienced health care professionals. The greatest efforts should be made to obtain follow-up information for serious cases, particularly ones that are not already known to occur with the drug in question. For consumer reports, an attempt should be made to obtain corroborative details from the consumer's health care practitioner and to obtain medical records.

Case reports should contain all of the following elements:

1. Description of the AEs, including time to onset
2. Suspected and concomitant medication details (i.e., dose, lot number, schedule, dates, duration), including over-the-counter medications, dietary supplements, and recently discontinued medications
3. Patient demography (e.g., age, race, sex), baseline medical condition before product therapy, comorbid conditions, use, relevant family history, and risk factors
4. Documentation of the diagnosis and procedures done regarding the AEs
5. Clinical course of the event and outcome (e.g., hospitalization or death)
6. Relevant therapeutic measures and laboratory data at baseline, during, and after therapy
7. Information about response to dechallenge and rechallenge

Medication errors should also be captured in detail.

Developing a Case Series

If a signal is noted from postmarketing spontaneous reports, the sponsor should develop a case series by looking for additional similar cases in its safety and clinical trial databases, the FDA's Adverse Event Reporting System database, published literature, and elsewhere. Formal written case criteria/standards should be developed to ensure that similar cases are chosen for the series. Next, each case in the series should be evaluated with emphasis on the serious unlabeled AEs. Incomplete cases should have follow-up done. Duplicate cases should be removed.

During the evaluation of each case, causality should be evaluated. Note that this causality is not needed for sending expedited 15-day reports to the New Drug Application. Rather the causality is needed for the signal analysis. There are, as the FDA notes, no internationally accepted standards for causality, especially for events with a high background or spontaneous incidence in the population. "FDA does not recommend any specific categorization of causality, but the categories *probable, possible,*

or *unlikely* have been used previously." If different categories are used, the criteria should be clearly spelled out.

The FDA suggests using the following criteria for causality reviews:

1. Occurrence of the AE in the expected time frame (e.g., type 1 allergic reactions occurring within days of therapy; cancers developing after years of therapy)
2. Absence of symptoms related to the event before exposure
3. Evidence of positive dechallenge or positive rechallenge
4. Consistency of the event with the established pharmacological/toxicologic effects of the product (medical and pharmacological plausibility)
5. Consistency of the event with the known effects of other products in the class
6. Existence of other supporting evidence from preclinical, clinical, or pharmacoepidemiologic studies
7. No other alternative explanations for the event

After this review, those cases that are "unconfounded," that is, "clean cases" where no other explanation seems possible, should be evaluated separately.

If, following this exercise, the case series suggests that additional investigation be done, the case series data should be assembled as a chart as follows:

1. The clinical and laboratory manifestations and course of the event
2. Demography (e.g., age, gender, race)
3. Exposure duration
4. Time from initiation of product exposure to the AE
5. Doses used and lot numbers, if available
6. Concomitant medications taken
7. The presence of comorbid conditions, particularly those known to cause the AE
8. The route of administration
9. Changes in event reporting rate over calendar time or product life cycle

Data Mining

The FDA gives a brief description of data mining or the use of statistical or mathematical tools to derive additional information on excess AEs (signals) in a database containing AE reports such as the FDA's Adverse Event Reporting System database. The FDA notes that these techniques are "inherently exploratory and hypothesis generating" and that caution should be used with them due to incomplete data, duplicate reports, underreporting, stimulated reports due to publicity or litigation ("secular effects"), and other biases.

The tools vary but fundamentally do the same type of analysis. This involves generating a numerical value (or score) for a particular AE-drug combination (e.g., liver failure with drug A) and comparing this with the score for all drugs in the database (e.g., liver failure with all drugs). If the score for AE-drug A is greater than that for AE-all drugs, this may represent a signal (AE-drug A divided by AE-all drugs >1.0). The technique can be refined using a threshold higher than 1.0 or making corrections for age, gender, time period, and so on.

Other data mining methods (such as the neural network and proportional reporting ratios) are referenced in the FDA's guidance along with a note that, except when sample sizes are small, the methods generally produce similar results. The FDA notes that the use of data mining techniques is not obligatory but if submitted to the FDA, it should be done in the context of a larger clinical and epidemiologic evaluation.

Safety Signals That May Warrant Further Investigation

Once a signal is identified, a decision must be made by the sponsor and/or the FDA about doing further investigation. Signals that generally do warrant further workup include

1. New unlabeled AEs, especially if serious
2. An apparent increase in the severity of a labeled event
3. Occurrence of serious events thought to be extremely rare in the general population
4. New product-product, product-device, product-food, or product-dietary supplement interactions
5. Identification of a previously unrecognized at-risk population
6. Confusion about a product's name, labeling, packaging, or use
7. Concerns arising from the way a product is used (e.g., AEs seen at higher than labeled doses or in populations not recommended for treatment)
8. Concerns arising from potential inadequacies of a currently implemented risk minimization action plan (RiskMAP) (e.g., reports of serious AEs that appear to reflect failure of a RiskMAP goal)

Reporting Rates Versus Incidence Rates

The FDA next discusses a chronically vexing issue in pharmacovigilance: reporting rate calculations. Clearly, in epidemiology risk assessment it is worth calculating the number of new cases of an event that occur in the exposed population (the incidence rate). In clinical or epidemiologic studies this is doable.

However, for spontaneously reported AEs problems arise in both the numerator (reports of an AE) and in the denominator (population exposed). In regard to the numerator, there is always underreporting by a variable and unknown amount. In regard to the denominator, it is difficult to get accurate estimates of the number of patients exposed to the product and the duration of treatment. In addition, the data may be unreliable because it is often difficult to exclude patients who are not at risk or a product may be used in different populations for different indications.

Given all these limitations, the FDA still believes it is worthwhile to calculate the reporting rate using reported cases divided by estimates of national (i.e., US) exposure of patients or patient-time. Only if this is not available should surrogates be used for exposure such as prescriptions filled or kilograms of product sold.

The FDA then notes that comparisons of reporting rates and their temporal trends may be useful and may be done with caution. Reporting rates can never be considered as incidence rates, however, and should never be compared with them.

It is also useful to obtain estimates of background occurrence rates in the population or in subpopulations (e.g., diabetics, premenopausal women, etc.) from published literature and health statistics from databases or studies. Cautious comparisons of these data with reporting rates may be useful in some situations.

The FDA then comments on the interpretation of reporting rates. Because underreporting is often substantial, if the reporting rate is higher than background expectations, this may be a strong indicator of a high true incidence rate. Conversely, a lower than background reporting rate does not necessarily mean the product is not associated with an increased risk for the AE in question. *Nor does it imply that the drug protects against this AE, as has been claimed by some sponsors!*

Epidemiologic Studies

The FDA encourages sponsors to consider the use of nonrandomized observational studies, particularly if randomized trials are not possible or feasible. Three categories of observational studies are discussed: pharmacoepidemiologic studies, registries, and surveys.

Pharmacoepidemiologic Studies

Several types of epidemiologic studies are possible, including prospective or retrospective cohort studies, case-control studies, nested case-control studies, case-crossover studies, or others. A clinical trial is not feasible in the following situations:

- The AE in question is uncommon (e.g., 1:2,000-3,000), and clinical trials are not practical due to the very large number of patients needed.
- Exposure to the product is chronic.
- Exposure to the product is done in patients with significant comorbid conditions.
- Patients are taking multiple comedications.
- The study is meant to identify risk factors for an AE.

Pharmacoepidemiologic studies, however, have their own set of problems, including confounding (other conditions produce the same outcome or AE), effect modulation (the association between the drug and the AE is altered by another factor, e.g., ethnic background), and other biases. There is no "one size fits all" set of criteria to allow an easy choice of which study type to use. Each situation should be considered individually, with the best choice being the one that minimizes these biases. Sometimes more than one study is needed. Each study should have a detailed description of the methodology used, including

- The population to be studied
- The case definitions to be used
- The data sources to be used (including a rationale for data sources if from outside the United States)
- The projected study size and statistical power calculations
- The methods for data collection, management, and analysis

The choice of the database for the study also entails some careful analysis. Many studies are now done in automated (insurance) claims databases (e.g., health maintenance organizations, Medicaid). The choice of the database should be based on

- Demography of the patients enrolled in the health plans (e.g., age, geographic location)
- Turnover rate of patients in the health plans
- Plan coverage of the medications of interest
- Size and characteristics of the exposed population available for study
- Availability of the outcomes of interest

- Ability to identify conditions of interest using standard medical coding systems (e.g., International Classification of Diseases)
- Access to medical records
- Access to patients for data not captured electronically

The results should be validated by review of some or all the medical records of the patients in the database.

Finally, the FDA recommends discussions between the sponsor and the agency during the development of such trials.

Registries

The FDA defines registries in this context as "an organized system for the collection, storage, retrieval, analysis, and dissemination of information on individual persons exposed to a specific medical intervention who have either a particular disease, a condition (e.g., a risk factor) that predisposes [them] to the occurrence of a health-related event, or prior exposure to substances (or circumstances) known or suspected to cause adverse health effects." When possible, a control or comparison group should be included. They may be used when such data are not available in automated databases or when collection is from multiple sources (e.g., medical doctors, hospitals, pathologists, etc.) over time.

The FDA suggests that all registries have written protocols describing objectives, a literature review, plans for systematic patient recruitment and follow-up, methodology for data collection, management and analysis, and registry termination conditions. Again, the FDA suggests collaboration between the sponsor and agency in the development of the registry.

Surveys

Surveys of patients or health care providers can provide information on signals, knowledge of labeled AEs, actual use of a product, compliance with RiskMAP requirements, and confusion over sound-alike or look-alike products. As with registries, the FDA suggests a written protocol with details on the methodology, including patient or health care professional recruitment and follow-up, projected sample size, and methods of data collection, management, and analysis. Validation should be done against medical or pharmacy records or through interviews with health care providers. Where possible, validated or piloted instruments should be used. And again, discussion between the sponsor and the FDA is encouraged.

Interpreting Signals

After identifying a signal, studying the individual cases in the series, using as needed data mining, reporting rate calculations, a literature review, and possibly other data (e.g., animal studies), the sponsor should consider whether a study should be done to determine whether a safety risk exists.

Whenever in the process the sponsor concludes that there is a potential safety risk, a submission to the FDA should be made of all available safety information and analyses (from preclinical data on). The submission should include

- Spontaneous and published cases with denominator or exposure information
- Background rate for the event in general and specific patient populations, if available
- Relative risks, odds ratios, or other measures of association derived from pharmacoepidemiologic studies
- Biologic effects observed in preclinical studies and pharmacokinetic or pharmacodynamic effects
- Safety findings from controlled clinical trials
- General marketing experience with similar products in the class

The sponsor should make a benefit-risk assessment for the population as a whole and for identified at-risk groups and propose, if appropriate, further studies and/or risk minimization actions. The FDA also makes its own evaluation. These analyses should be done iteratively in an ongoing logical sequence and manner as the data become available.

Items that the sponsor and the FDA should consider in their evaluations include

1. Strength of the association (e.g., relative risk of the AE associated with the product)
2. Temporal relationship of product use and the event
3. Consistency of findings across available data sources
4. Evidence of a dose-response for the effect
5. Biologic plausibility
6. Seriousness of the event relative to the disease being treated
7. Potential to mitigate the risk in the population
8. Feasibility of further study using observational or controlled clinical study designs
9. Degree of benefit the product provides, including availability of other therapies

Developing a Pharmacovigilance Plan

Depending on the situation at hand, the sponsor may wish to develop a pharmacovigilance plan above and beyond the usual postmarketing spontaneous AE collection and analysis. The FDA refers to the guidance on RiskMAPs issued in March 2005. The need for a plan should be based on

1. The likelihood that the AE represents a potential safety risk
2. The frequency with which the AE occurs (e.g., incidence rate, reporting rate, or other measures available)
3. The severity of the event
4. The nature of the population(s) at risk
5. The range of patients for which the product is indicated
6. The method by which the product is dispensed (through pharmacies or performance linked systems only)

In general, RiskMAPs should be developed for products with serious safety risks that have been identified or where at-risk populations have not been adequately studied. Such a plan could include the following:

- Submission of specific serious AEs in an expedited manner beyond routine required reporting (i.e., as 15-day reports).
- Submission of AE report summaries at more frequent prespecified intervals (e.g., quarterly rather than annually).
- Active surveillance to identify AEs that may or may not be reported through passive surveillance. Active surveillance can be (1) *drug based*, identifying AEs in patients taking certain products; (2) *setting based*, identifying AEs in certain health care settings where they are likely to present for treatment (e.g., emergency departments, etc.); or (3) *event based*, identifying AEs that are likely to be associated with medical products (e.g., acute liver failure).
- Additional pharmacoepidemiologic studies.
- Creation of registries or surveys.
- Additional controlled clinical trials.

The sponsor should periodically reevaluate the plan's effectiveness. The FDA will also do so and may choose to bring questions to its Drug Safety Risk Management Advisory Committee or an FDA advisory committee dealing with the specific product.

In practice, companies are now actively setting up risk management departments and staffing them with the appropriate personnel. Data mining tools are now being developed commercially and are being evaluated and set up so that data can be exported from the safety database (if the tool is not an integral part of the database) for analysis. Criteria for RiskMAPs are being developed, and integration of the European Union, Japanese, and US requirements is also being developed because there is not total overlap of the various risk management requirements worldwide. As with other areas in drug safety, this is a developing field.

Epidemiology and Pharmacoepidemiology: What Are They? What Are Their Limitations and Advantages?

➡ **NOTE:** (Unless otherwise noted, the word "drug" or "drug product" should be taken in this book to include "biologics" and "vaccines.")

This chapter is not meant to be an introduction to epidemiology or pharmacoepidemiology. There are many excellent textbooks and references in those fields. Rather this chapter attempts, briefly, to place epidemiology and pharmacoepidemiology in the context of their use in the practical world of drug safety. An excellent website to visit is that of the International Society of Pharmacoepidemiology (Web Resource 18-1).

■ The Theory and the Practice

What is epidemiology? There are several similar definitions:

■ The study of the distribution and determinants of health-related states or events in specified popula-

tions, and the application of this study to the control of health problems. From the Centers for Disease Control and Prevention (Web Resource 18-2).

■ The study of the frequency, distribution, and behavior of a disease within a population (Web Resource 18-3).

■ The study of the incidence, distribution, and control of disease in a population (Web Resource 18-4).

■ The study of a disease that deals with how many people have it, where they are, how many new cases develop, and how to control the disease (Web Resource 18-5).

■ Study of disease incidence and distribution in populations, as well as the relationship between environment and disease (Web Resource 18-6).

■ The study of the incidence, distribution, and determinants of an infection, disease, or other health-related events in a population. Epidemiology can be thought of in terms of who, where, when, what, and why. That is, who has the infection/disease, where are they located geographically and in relation to each other, when is the infection/disease occurring, what is the cause, and why did it occur (Web Resource 18-7).

What is pharmacoepidemiology?

- The study of the utilization and effects of drugs in large numbers of people (Web Resource 18-8).
- The study of the utilization of drugs by populations, good and bad, and the effect of these drugs on those populations, for better or for worse.

For the purposes of this chapter I use epidemiology and pharmacoepidemiology interchangeably.

Of necessity, (pharmaco)epidemiology uses numbers and statistical analyses. It is the study of populations as opposed to the study of individuals. Thus, it is used to answer questions about groups of people rather than about individual patients. It is also used to extrapolate and generalize from individuals to groups and populations. Thus it would answer questions like "Are the women who live on Long Island, New York at greater risk for breast cancer than those who live elsewhere?" or "Is the use of drug X associated with a higher incidence of atrial fibrillation in elderly men?" as opposed to questions like "Does Ms. Jones have breast cancer because she lives on Long Island?" or "Did drug X produce atrial fibrillation in 79-year-old Mr. Jones?"

In the world of drug safety, epidemiology is used to answer questions about adverse events (AEs) in populations after (usually) a signal has been generated based on one or more individual case reports. The purpose is to confirm and quantify the signal or to rule it out. Such studies can rarely answer questions about causality but rather give information on risks and associations.

In this chapter we give a very high level view of the handful of concepts that continually appear in the drug safety and pharmacovigilance literature and for which a passing knowledge (at least) is useful. Pharmacoepidemiology is now an area of much research and interest and will play a larger and larger role in drug safety.

Case Report

A case report is a clinical observation in a patient who received a drug and experienced one or more AEs. The most common formats for presentation of a case report are the MedWatch form and the CIOMS I form, also called an "individual case safety report (ICSR)." Some are published as short reports in medical journals.

Aggregate Reports

Aggregate reports are descriptions of a group of patients exposed to a drug (or sometimes more than one drug, e.g., combination products) and the AEs. There are multiple standard formats, including US New Drug Application periodic reports and Periodic Safety Update Reports, which include CIOMS II line listings.

Randomized Clinical Trial

This is the type of study that most people are familiar with. It is an experimental study, not an observational study, because the investigator, using a protocol, determines who receives what drug treatment; the protocol may differ from the normal practice of medicine. In an observational trial, one merely observes and records what happens in the normal course of medical practice and treatment.

A randomized clinical trial is prospective. It involves two or more groups of patients with a disease receiving different treatments. For example, one group may get drug A and the other group may get drug B or placebo. It may be single blinded (the patient does not know what the treatment is) or double blinded (neither the patient nor the investigator knows what the treatment is). The study may also be randomized to minimize known and unknown biases (factors other than the drugs being tested that may alter or explain the results). These studies are often long and costly. They represent the gold standard of research: the double-blind, randomized, controlled trial. These studies are usually done during phases I, II, and III of drug development and for many reasons (ethical, availability of patients, etc.) may not be feasible after the drug is marketed. The results are usually clear and easily understandable with the calculation of a risk difference between groups. For example, the group receiving drug A had a 4.1% incidence of AEs and the placebo group a 2% incidence of AEs, a difference of 2.1%.

Case-Control Study

This concept is sometimes hard to grasp intuitively. This type of study determines the chance (or "odds" or "probability") of having taken the suspect drug in a group of patients already suffering from an AE and compares that with the chance of having taken the drug in a group of patients who did not have the AE. To put it more simply, take a group of patients who had the AE and another group who did not have the AE and see how many in each group took the drug in question.

Using a large database (e.g., a claims database, a hospital database), patients with the AE (cases) are selected who have experienced the AE in question. Another group that did not experience the AE (control subjects) is also selected. Usually, the investigator attempts to match the two groups as closely as possible (ideally they should be identical) based on demographic characteristics (e.g., age, sex, race, indication treated, concomitant diseases, and medications, etc.) so that the groups are comparable. Both groups should have the same medical profile and opportunity to receive the drug. For example, if a health maintenance organization or hospital database is used, the drug should be on the pharmacy formulary for the entire time period examined in the study. This is a retrospective study because the AE has occurred and the investigator is looking back in time before the AE occurred into the medical history of the patient.

The patients' medical histories are then examined to see which patients in each group used the drug in question. The data are then filled in a 2×2 table as follows:

Took the Drug

Yes	No		
a	b	Yes	Experienced the AE
c	d	No	

$$\text{Odds ratio} = \frac{a/(a + c)/c(\,a+ c)}{b(b + d)/d(b + d)} = ad/bc$$

After the data are filled in, the odds ratio is calculated. For example, the data might show the following:

■ 120 patients experienced the AE
  ▪ 90 took the drug and
  ▪ 30 did not

■ 120 control patients did not experience the AE
  ▪ 50 took the drug and
  ▪ 70 did not

The table would look like the following:

Took the Drug

Yes	No		
90	30	Yes	Experienced the AE
50	70	No	

The odds ratio is calculated by dividing the odds of having the AE in the group that took the drug (90 of 140 patients or 90:50 = 1.8) by the odds in the group that had the AE but did not take the drug (30 of 100 patients or 30:70 = 0.43). The division is 1.8/4.3 = 4.2. Using the formula above

$$\text{Odds ratio} =$$
$$\frac{90/(90 + 50)/50/(90 + 50)}{30/(30 + 70)/70/(30 + 70)} = (90 \times 70)/(50 \times 30) = 4.2$$

A value over 1.0 is suggestive of an association between the drug and the AE. As a rule of thumb, anything over 2.0 is believed to be fairly strong and quite suggestive of an association. In our example, this is a very high value (4.2) and is very suggestive that there is an association between taking the drug and having the AE.

Advantages of case-control studies are that they are useful for studying very rare AEs because the investigator seeks out a database where this AE is found in a large enough number of patients. Obviously, the patients also had to have the opportunity to take the drug if this database is to be used. These studies are fast and relatively inexpensive. However, they are liable to significant bias both in the selection of the patients for the two groups and in the amount and quality of the drug exposure and medical history data.

Cohort Study

A cohort study is the other basic type of epidemiologic study used in pharmacovigilance. This type of study is easier to grasp intuitively. Two groups of patients are chosen from a database. The first group is those who took the drug in question for a certain amount of time and the second group is those who did not (the "cohort") take the drug. The investigator attempts to choose a cohort that is as close demographically to the drug group as possible.

The patients' records are reviewed and the incidence of the AE in question is calculated for each of the groups. These studies are prospective as the investigator picks a point in time and studies the two groups as they move forward in time to see whether they develop the AE. This study may be done on data that have already been collected and stored in a database or it may be done on data that are being collected now and moving forward. The advantage of the cohort over the case-control is the ability to calculate the excess risk, the absolute risk difference. The excess risk is useful in determining the number needed to harm, that is, the number of patients that need be exposed to a drug to produce a specified AE.

Took the Drug

Yes	No		
a	b	Yes	Experienced the AE
c	d	No	

Relative risk = $[a/(a + c)] \div [b/(b + d)]$ or the rate in exposed divided by the rate in the unexposed. Absolute risk = $[a/(a + c)]–b/(b + d)]$ or rate in exposed minus rate in unexposed.

After the data are filled in, the absolute and relative risks are calculated. Using the same example as above:

Took the Drug

Yes	No		
90	30	Yes	Experienced the AE
50	70	No	

Relative risk = [90/(90 + 50)]/30/(30 + 70)] = 0.643/0.300 = 2.14 times more cases of AE, whereas absolute risk = 0.643–0.3 = 0.343.

This tells us that the drug group is more than two times at risk for this AE compared with the cohort group. If the relative risk were 1, the likelihood of getting the AE is the same in the drug and cohort group. If the relative risk is less than 1 (but greater than zero—the value in this calculation is always greater than zero), then the risk of getting the AE in the drug group is less than that in the cohort group.

The absolute risk tells us there were 343 additional cases of AE per 1,000 patients exposed to the drug. Therefore the number needed to harm is about 3; that is, every third patient on the average will develop the AE (something the clinician should keep in mind).

For an excellent discussion of risk ratios and odds ratios, their differences, when they are close to being the same (i.e., when the AEs are very rare) and other complex issues, please see the article by Jon Deeks of The Centre for Statistics in Medicine Oxford at Web Resource 18-9. The entire Bandolier site (Web Resource 18-10) is worth looking at for, as they put it, "Evidence based thinking about health care."

Nested Case-Control Study

This is a type of case-control study that is inside or nested in a cohort study. The nested case-control design uses estimates from a sample of the cohort rather than the whole cohort. It permits the collection of less data than in a full cohort study with an acceptable statistical analysis and saves time and money.

Confidence Interval

Most studies are based on samples, not entire populations. The confidence interval reflects the resulting uncertainty. Based on the sample of the population, a particular result is obtained (e.g., 15% of the users of drug A had serious AEs). Because we did not study the whole population, we cannot be totally sure that the 15% figure is correct and represents the true value for the whole population rather than just for the smaller sample. The confidence interval represents the range of the correct or true value for the whole population. One can calculate various levels of "assurance," 90%, 95%, 99%, 99.9%, and so on, for the confidence interval. Usually, the 95% level is used. The narrower or smaller the distance between the upper and lower values of the confidence interval (called the confidence limits), the better. In general, the more patients in the study, the narrower (better) the confidence interval.

With the arrival of risk management as an integral part of the development and lifespan of all drugs, the fields of pharmacoepidemiology and drug safety are now more tightly linked than ever. Health authorities require epidemiologic safety studies, and companies are more willing to do them. Large databases and the practitioners who know how to do these studies become more and more available and the methodology becomes more refined and automated. Most pharmaceutical companies now have or will soon form risk management/pharmacoepidemiology departments to handle these studies.

19

Product Quality Issues

■ Background

In the last several years, it has been realized that many other issues in addition to adverse events (AEs) play a significant role in drug safety and pharmacovigilance. This has come about because of the realization that a safety issue may be related to the active ingredient (moiety) itself, excipients (see Chapter 5), residues from the manufacturing process, quality control, the container and packaging, storage issues in the pharmacy or home, tampering, and other adventures that occur after the product has left the factory. This chapter summarizes briefly issues that revolve around quality and manufacturing.

Patient or health care professional product complaints can revolve around the following:

- The drug didn't work (lack of efficacy).
- The drug produced an AE (safety issue).
- The drug looked, tasted, or smelled funny or differ-

ent. It was crumbling. There was a powder on the pill and so forth (product manufacturing and/or quality issue).

- The drug was a tablet in the past, but this time it was capsules (quality issue in packaging, dispensing, etc.).
- I want my money back or I am suing.
- Others ("My dog accidentally ate the pills...").

Not infrequently, one sees multiple issues with a single phone call: "The pill was the wrong color and when I took it I developed chest pain and I want my money back or I'll sue." Part of the issue here involves getting the correct people within the pharmaceutical company to act on each of the issues involved: the AE component, the product quality component, and the monetary/legal component. In this chapter we address product quality issues.

■ The Theory

Product quality is regulated under Good Manufacturing Practices. As one can imagine, this is an extensive subject covered in great detail in the Code of Federal Regulations section 21CFR211, Current Good Manufacturing Practice for Finished Pharmaceuticals.

The specific section covering product quality issues is 211.198 Complaint Files. This section obliges the manufacturer to maintain written procedures on the handling of written and oral complaints. The procedures should include provisions for review and investigation by the quality control unit.

The US Food and Drug Administration (FDA) performs inspections (over 22,000 in 2003), and product quality issues are often cited. An example follows from a 2003 warning letter to a pharmaceutical company:

> **"2. Failure to follow established Standard Operating Procedures regarding the handling of written and oral drug product quality complaints [21 CFR 211.198(a)]**
>
> Your firm's QCU failed to follow established written Standard Operating Procedures (SOP) for investigating drug product quality complaints received by your firm. Specifically, your firm's SOP states that it is the responsibility of the support departments (e.g., Quality Assurance, Quality Control, etc.) to complete their part of the complaint investigation "usually within 30 days. Yet, our Investigator observed incomplete complaint investigations lasting as long as 247 and 301 days after receipt of the complaint."

Warning Letter to Koss Pharmaceuticals, December 29, 2003. See the letter at the FDA's website (Web Resource 19-1).

■ The Practice

The responsibility for investigation of product complaints generally falls within the competence of one of the quality units in a company. The drug safety department usually becomes involved when there is a product quality complaint, a medical error, or an AE. That is, even though there was an issue with the manufacturing or quality of the product, the subject took the product and had an AE. Sometimes, of course, the quality issue is only discovered or noted after the use of the product (e.g., the patient had an AE and went back to look at the package and noted the tablets smelled funny and were off color—a quality issue).

Within the pharmaceutical company this is a "double issue" with an evaluation of the AE by the drug safety group and an evaluation of the product complaint by the quality unit concerned. There are several critical operational issues:

- Both units (drug safety and quality control) must be informed that the other unit is involved in the same case if the case was received and triaged elsewhere (e.g., in Medical Affairs or Medical Communications). Each unit follows its procedures and does its evaluation, usually simultaneously.

- The two units must communicate their findings to each other because one or both will likely be required to submit the findings to the FDA. A mechanism must be developed to request the patient who had the complaint to return any unused product to the company for analysis. Some companies do this for all complaints, whereas others set up criteria for such requests for return of product. The quality workup may include review of batch records, testing of the retained sample, and testing of the sample returned by the patient.

- The results of this testing must be conveyed to the drug safety unit for inclusion in the report to the FDA. If this is an expedited report, the quality unit must get the new information to the drug safety unit so that the follow-up to the FDA is done within the required time (15 calendar days). The quality unit must not delay sending the information to the drug safety group. Similarly, relevant clinical follow-up information (e.g., lot numbers) from the drug safety unit should be forwarded to the quality unit on the case.

- The case may have two different identification numbers—one in the drug safety unit and the other in the quality unit. If the computer system(s) cannot handle the two numbers for the same case, then another method of tracking must be developed to ensure that the case does not fall through the cracks. For large companies, the volume of such investigations may be quite high with many data flowing back and forth between the departments. In addition, a third or even fourth department may be involved if the case involves a refund of money to the patient or a possible legal or police action (e.g., a lawsuit or police investigation for tampering).

- AEs and product quality complaints are now considered "two sides of the same coin." That is, if an AE occurs after taking a drug, it is not always evident that the event is due to the active ingredient. It might be due to an excipient or to a problem in manufacturing or storage or shipping. It is now good pharmacovigilance practice for the drug safety group or the pharmacovigilance or risk management group to periodically examine product quality issues on a regular basis to see whether there is a clue or suggestion that quality issues have produced AEs. The methodology for this evaluation has not been well worked out yet and remains one of "global introspection" for the most part. Some of the newer AE databases are now able to capture product quality issues for cases in addition to the usual AE data. The analysis should attempt to see whether there are similar cases (AEs and product complaints) seen with that product's lot or batch number or geographic area. (Mail order pharmacy systems distributing drugs from centralized locations to all parts of the United States now make geographic tracking much harder and less useful. The days when a particular batch of a drug was used in a localized geographic area are disappearing.)

■ Product quality issues that are significant and severe, in particular those that risk patient health or produce serious AEs or suggest tampering, must be acted on immediately. The pharmaceutical company must have a mechanism in place to recognize such issues, investigate them, and bring the information in a timely fashion to the responsible levels of the company and the FDA and other health agencies if the product was shipped outside the United States. If necessary, a product may need to be withdrawn immediately, public announcements made, protocols stopped, and so forth. The company should have a procedure whereby the team that would need to perform these actions is easily mobilizable for action.

■ Many of the AE/product quality issues are often small and noncritical. Examples include the discovery that a part of the packaging (e.g., vials or stoppers) was obtained from a new vendor, looked or acted differently, or late stability testing showed problems. Sometimes it is discovered that a part or procedure was slightly but clearly out of specification. The determination of how far to proceed in terms of analysis and recall of products is often a difficult decision that requires the assistance of multiple departments within the company and the FDA. A formal written procedure must be developed and used.

Examples of some of the more serious issues resulting in recalls can be seen at the FDA's website (Web Resource 19-2). For example, a partial listing of some of the recalls for one week in August 2005 (Web Resource 19-3) include (note that only one of these recalls involved AEs, whereas the rest were product quality problems):

■ Albuterol sulfate inhalation solution: discoloration

■ Anagrelide hydrochloride capsules: dissolution failure

■ ("Name removed") tablets: oversized tablets

■ Adenoscan adenosine injection (there has been an increase in AEs reported for this lot of Adenoscan)

■ Nystatin and triamcinolone acetonide cream: subpotent on 21-month stability

■ Ethynodiol diacetate and ethinyl estradiol (there was an out-of-specification result for total impurities at the 12-month stability test point)

■ ("Name removed") brand acid reducer tablets (Ranitidine USP), 75 mg (mispacked; lot was packaged without a desiccant)

20

Pregnancy, Lactation, and Adverse Events (AEs): AEs in Pregnant Partners of Males Taking a Drug, Pregnancy Registries, and the Swedish Pregnancy Registry

➡ **NOTE:** (Unless otherwise noted, the word "drug" or "drug product" should be taken in this book to include "biologics" and "vaccines.")

■ Background

The testing of pregnant animals is done as part of the usual preclinical development of new drugs, but a drug that is not teratogenic (leading to congenital malformations) in some or all animal species tested may sometimes, unfortunately, be noxious in women. For obvious reasons, clinical testing is almost never done in pregnant women during the development of new drugs unless the drug is developed expressly for use in pregnancy. Thus the safety and efficacy of drugs in pregnant women is largely unknown at the time of marketing, and little additional information is gained from spontaneous reporting of adverse events (AEs).

Some drugs are used and, to some degree, tested in pregnancy, usually in situations where treatment is obligatory for either the mother or unborn child (e.g., hypertension, asthma, rheumatoid arthritis, epilepsy, etc.). The studies are usually not blinded and are prospective or retrospective observational or surveillance studies.

■ The Theory

Table 20-1 lists the US Food and Drug Administration's (FDA's) pregnancy categories.

FDA Guidance for Industry—2002

In August 2002, the FDA issued a guidance for industry on the establishment of pregnancy registries. In this guidance the FDA gives a very specific definition of a birth registry to differentiate it from a teratology registry:

"A pregnancy exposure registry is a prospective observational study that actively collects information on medical product exposure during pregnancy and associated pregnancy outcomes."

This type of registry is not a pregnancy prevention program. The FDA does not recommend a registry for all drugs:

"We recommend that a pregnancy exposure registry be seriously considered when it is likely that

Table 20-1	FDA Pregnancy Categories
Category	**Interpretation**
A	Adequate, well-controlled studies in pregnant women have not shown an increased risk of fetal abnormalities to the fetus in any trimester of pregnancy.
B	Animal studies have revealed no evidence of harm to the fetus; however, there are no adequate and well-controlled studies in pregnant women. OR Animal studies have shown an adverse effect, but adequate and well-controlled studies in pregnant women have failed to demonstrate a risk to the fetus in any trimester.
C	Animal studies have shown an adverse effect, and there are no adequate and well-controlled studies in pregnant women. OR No animal studies have been conducted, and there are no adequate and well-controlled studies in pregnant women.
D	Adequate well-controlled or observational studies in pregnant women have demonstrated a risk to the fetus. However, the benefits of therapy may outweigh the potential risk. For example, the drug may be acceptable if needed in a life-threatening situation or serious disease for which safer drugs cannot be used or are ineffective.
X	Adequate well-controlled or observational studies in animals or pregnant women have demonstrated positive evidence of fetal abnormalities or risks. The use of the product is contraindicated in women who are or may become pregnant.

the medical product will be used during pregnancy as therapy for a new or chronic condition.

"A medical product may also be a good candidate for a pregnancy exposure registry when one of the following conditions exists:

- Inadvertent exposures to the medical product in pregnancy are or are expected to be common such as when products have a high likelihood of use by women of childbearing age.

- The medical product presents special circumstances, such as the potential for infection of mother and fetus by administration of live, attenuated vaccines.

"Pregnancy exposure registries are unlikely to be warranted in the following situations: (1) there is no systemic exposure to the medical product, or (2) the product is not, or rarely, used by women of childbearing age."

A registry can be established at any time during the life of a drug. The sponsor or the FDA may initiate the request. The design of the registry is a function of the objective. It

may be an open-ended surveillance to the specific testing of a hypothesis using standard Good Epidemiologic Practices.

The guidance then goes into detail on the critical elements of a registry, including objectives, exposure, sample size, eligibility requirements, data source and content, fetal anomalies sought, use of an independent data monitoring committee, an investigational review board, and informed consent. The reader is referred to the guidance for these epidemiologic details.

A few points of note:

- "When estimating the number of exposed pregnancies to be enrolled prospectively, it is important to be aware that approximately 62 percent of clinically recognized pregnancies will result in a live birth, 22 percent will end in elective termination, and 16 percent will result in fetal loss (i.e., spontaneous abortions and fetal death/stillbirth" (Ventura, Mosher, Curtin, et al., *Vital Health Stat*, 2000;21:56).

- Birth defects occur "spontaneously" in a fairly high number of women. The March of Dimes Birth Defect Foundation, Fact Sheet 2001, available on its website (Web Resource 20-1), reports the following rates for various pregnancy outcomes and fetal abnormalities:

- Spontaneous abortions/miscarriage (loss before 20 weeks): 1 in 7 known pregnancies
- Low birth weight (<2,500 grams): 1 in 12 live births
- Fetal death/stillbirth (loss after 20 weeks): 1 in 200 known pregnancies
- Any major birth defect: 1 in 25 live births
- Heart and circulation defects: 1 in 115 live births
- Genital and urinary tract defects: 1 in 135 live births
- Nervous system and eye defects: 1 in 235 live births
- Club foot: 1 in 735 live births
- Cleft lip with or without cleft palate: 1 in 930 live births

- The guidance also notes that other types of studies, such as case-control studies, may be useful to evaluate rare adverse birth outcomes and identify whether the drug in question is an associated risk factor. They are useful when long-term follow-up is needed. They can be nested within other existing pregnancy registries. Automated database studies (e.g., health maintenance organizations, Medicaid) may be useful also.

Regulatory Reporting Requirements

Registries are considered solicited information and thus must be reported as if they were clinical trial AEs: The cases must be serious, unexpected, and have a reasonable possibility that the product caused the AE. See 21 CFR 310.305(c)(1), 314.80(c)(2)(iii) and (e), and 600.80(c)(1), (c)(2)(iii) and (e)). Note also that congenital anomalies are considered serious AEs (21 CFR 314.80(a) and 600.80(a)). Registries run independently of sponsors holding New Drug Applications are not subject to postmarketing reporting requirements.

The sponsor must submit an annual status report to the FDA on any registry being run. A registry may be discontinued if

- It has accumulated sufficient data to meet the registry objectives.
- The feasibility of collecting sufficient information diminishes to unacceptable levels due to low exposure, poor enrollment, or loss to follow-up.
- Better methods are developed.

- Termination criteria should be listed in the original protocol.

In conclusion, sponsors who are studying or marketing drugs that may pose a pregnancy/teratology threat must give careful and early consideration to adequate data gathering to determine whether a safety problem exists or if it is already known to exist to quantify and track safety problems. The obvious aim is risk minimization using the various means available.

Lactation

In general, the obvious truism is that no breast-feeding infant should be exposed to products taken by the mother. In practice, it is not always feasible for the mother to stop certain critical drugs. Fortunately, contrary to pregnancy studies, lactation studies are relatively easy to do and are done routinely in the study of new drugs. The FDA issued a guidance in October 2004, "Guidance for Industry, Pharmacokinetics in Pregnancy—Study Design, Data Analysis, and Impact on Dosing and Labeling." See its website for the document (Web Resource 20-2).

As the World Health Organization (WHO) states in its publication, "Breast Feeding and Maternal Medication. Recommendations for Drugs in the 11th WHO Model List of Essential Drugs": "There are very few kinds of treatment during which breastfeeding is absolutely contraindicated. However, there are some drugs which a mother may need to take which sometimes cause side effects in the baby." See its website for the document (Web Resource 20-3). This publication gives specifics for many drugs with specific recommendations such as "compatible with breastfeeding," "avoid if possible," "avoid breastfeeding," and "no data available."

The FDA covers some of these same issues in its Office of Women's Health Information website (Web Resource 20-4). Included is an excellent but now somewhat old (1998) publication on "Breast Milk or Formula: Making the Right Choice for Your Baby" (Web Resource 20-5).

AEs in Pregnant Partners of Males Taking a Drug

This is an area with little information. Reproductive studies in animals are done to determine the effects of new drugs on the testes and sperm. Thus there are often animal data in regard to whether a drug is toxic to the male reproductive system. There are few data, however, on toxicity in the female and the fetus due to transfer of the drug into the female from the male's semen or other body fluids. There are a few examples in the medical literature.

Ribavirin is an antiviral used in combination with interferon-alpha for the treatment of hepatitis C. The FDA approved package insert notes as follows:

"REBETOL® and combination REBETOL/PEG-INTRON® therapy must not be used by women, or male partners of women, who are or may become pregnant during therapy and during the 6 months after stopping therapy. REBETOL® and combination REBETOL/PEG-INTRON® therapy should not be initiated until a report of a negative pregnancy test has been obtained immediately prior to initiation of therapy. Women of childbearing potential and men must use effective contraception (at least two reliable forms) during treatment and during the 6-month post treatment follow-up period. Significant teratogenic and/or embryocidal effects have been demonstrated for ribavirin in all animal species in which adequate studies have been conducted. These effects occurred at doses as low as one twentieth of the recommended human dose of REBETOL®. If pregnancy occurs in a patient or partner of a patient during treatment or during the 6 months after treatment stops, physicians are encouraged to report such cases". Package insert for Rebetol® is available at Web Resource 20-6.

"Ribavirin, including COPEGUS®, may cause birth defects and/or death of the fetus. Extreme care must be taken to avoid pregnancy in female patients and in female partners of male patients. Ribavirin causes hemolytic anemia. The anemia associated with ribavirin therapy may result in a worsening of cardiac disease. Ribavirin is genotoxic and mutagenic and should be considered a potential carcinogen." Package insert for Copegus® (Web Resource 20-7).

The area of female exposure to drugs or teratogenic effects from male partners taking the drugs requires significant additional study. However, the methodology for such work is and will remain exceedingly difficult.

■ The Practice

From a practical point of view the critical issue for health care practitioners, consumers, and health authorities is to determine what drugs may be safely taken before and during pregnancy (including the weeks after conception and before diagnosis of the pregnancy) and lactation.

An excellent website is perinatology.com (Web Resource 20-8). This site has multiple links as well as information on specific drugs, their effects in the various trimesters (if known), lactation information, neonatal AEs, and a literature search.

A major center in the world for information on pregnancy and drugs, called Motherisk, is located at the Hospital for Sick Children in Toronto, Canada. See its excellent website (Web Resource 20-9). Its goal, as noted on its website (Web Resource 20-10), is as follows:

"The Motherisk Program at The Hospital for Sick Children in Toronto, is a clinical, research and teaching program dedicated to antenatal drug, chemical, and disease risk counseling. It is affiliated with the University of Toronto. Created in 1985, Motherisk provides evidence-based information and guidance about the safety or risk to the developing fetus or infant, of maternal exposure to drugs, chemicals, diseases, radiation and environmental agents."

Further, its web page (Web Resource 20-11), devoted to drugs, includes the following:

"Pregnancy, whether planned or a pleasant surprise, brings with it important concerns about prescription and over the counter drugs. Not every medication poses a risk to your unborn baby. However, some do. If you are already pregnant, Motherisk's published research can help you and your doctor make informed decisions about possible drug therapy. Since 1985, Motherisk has reviewed data from around the world, conducting controlled, prospective studies to determine the potential risks of therapeutic drugs during pregnancy. It is now clear that there are many drugs that are safe for use in pregnancy."

They list several classes of drugs with references, including anticonvulsants, antihistamines, antiinfectives, antiinflammatories, antirheumatics, psychotropics, cardiovascular agents, chemotherapeutic agents, contraceptives, gastrointestinal agents, herbal products, nausea/vomiting and treatment, radiation, recreational/social drugs, vitamin A, and congeners. The reader is referred to this website for the specific references and studies.

Note, however, that this information represents the opinion of Motherisk and is not necessarily the same as that of the approved drug labeling in the United States or elsewhere. It should not be taken as an approval, guarantee, or clearance that a particular drug is safe to use in a pregnant woman. Others may disagree about the safe use of these drugs in pregnancy. This question should always be one between the woman and her physician.

Given the scarcity of information, it is now recognized that tracking the pregnancy and its outcome in women who have taken products either accidentally (not knowing they were pregnant) or knowingly is a very important way to understand the potential toxicity (and efficacy) of drug products.

- An umbrella organization for the teratology agencies is The Organization of Teratology Information Services covering the United States, Canada, the United Kingdom, and Israel. See its website at (Web Resource 20-12). This organization serves as a clearinghouse for information and research on drug therapies. It often maintains (retrospective) teratology registries of reported birth defects from hospitals in its catchment area. A European counterpart is The European Network of Teratology Information Services at Web Resource 20-13. There are also various teratology and mutagenicity societies around the world in the pharmaceutical and chemical industries, among others. Eurocat is a European network of population-based registries for the epidemiologic surveillance of congenital anomalies covering 43 registries in 20 countries and 29% of the European birth population. See its website (Web Resource 20-14).

One center of particular interest is the Swedish Medical Birth Registry at Web Resource 20-15, which is a part of the Centre for Epidemiology at the National Board of Health and Welfare in Sweden. What makes this center of unique interest is that its aim is to collect prospective gestation and pregnancy data on all births in Sweden— between 85,000 and 120,000 per year. Data collected include information on previous gestation, smoking habits, medication, family situation, hospital, length of gestation, type of delivery, diagnoses of mother and child, operations, type of analgesia, sex, weight, length, size of head, birth conditions, place of residence, nationality, as well as outcome, delivery, and infant information.

To this end, many health agencies around the world now urge or require the tracking of all known pregnancies by pharmaceutical companies, hospitals, and so on.

Finally, the extraordinary and tragic situation with diethylstilbestrol (DES) deserves mention. This was a drug taken by pregnant women to prevent miscarriages. A major AE (vaginal carcinoma) was found to be produced many years later by DES in the daughters of the women who took the DES (see Chapter 6 for further information). The possibility that ingestion of a drug during pregnancy could produce an AE years later in the patient or even the offspring is a challenge to medical research that does not seem solvable with the state of the art as it exists today.

■ FAQs

Q: What about the more complex areas of drug-drug interactions or drug-food or drug-alcohol interactions in the pregnant and lactating woman?

A: This is really an unknown area. Because gold standard, prospective, blinded studies are rare to impossible with pregnant women, data are difficult to obtain even in the "simpler" situations of a single drug taken by a pregnant woman. The complexities of interactions, particularly with agents that are known to be toxic (e.g., alcohol), are not able to be studied adequately (if at all) at this time. The critical issue is the inability to test hypotheses other than those suggested by epidemiologic studies. That is the state of the art today.

Q: Is there not a paradox of sorts here? If a pregnancy registry is done for a drug that is known or strongly suspected to be harmful to the mother and/or fetus, doesn't the success of the registry in answering whatever question is asked indicate the failure of the warning and risk management program?

A: Indeed, a successful risk management program to avoid pregnancies with a known teratogen will make the registry unnecessary and undoable. It is one of the tragedies in medicine today that women who are pregnant knowingly or unknowingly do take drugs that are clearly known to be teratogens. Much more attention is now being paid to risk management programs to prevent pregnancies in women taking these drugs.

21

Children, the Elderly, and Other Special Groups

➡ **NOTE:** (Unless otherwise noted, the word "drug" or "drug product" should be taken in this book to include "biologics" and "vaccines.")

■ Background

Similar to the testing of new drugs in pregnant women, the testing of drugs in special groups poses issues. Special groups include children, neonates, and the elderly as well as other groups with specific disease states, genetic conditions, and, controversially, various ethnic, racial, or religious backgrounds. The question here is whether the presence of the "special" condition alters the effects of the drug and produces more or different adverse events (AEs).

■ The Theory

Children

Children are a special group because they are not simply "small adults" but rather may be (depending on age and

other factors) biologic beings who absorb, distribute, metabolize, and excrete drugs differently from adults. A good article summarizing these points and presenting the US Food and Drug Administration's (FDA's) position on testing drugs in children first appeared in the early 1990s and is still germane and worth reading: "Why FDA Is Encouraging Drug Testing in Children" can be found at Web Resource 21-1.

This was followed by a series of initiatives by the federal government to encourage the testing of drugs in children.

In December 1998 the FDA issued a final rule entitled "Regulations Requiring Manufacturers to Assess the Safety and Effectiveness of New Drugs and Biological Products in Pediatric Patients," which is available at Web Resource 21-2. This rule required that every new product contain a pediatric assessment or a deferral or waiver of this assessment. It also allowed the FDA to require pediatric studies and required a pediatric section in New Drug Application periodic reports.

In September 1999 the FDA issued a Guidance for Industry entitled "Qualifying for Pediatric Exclusivity Under Section 505A of the Food, Drug and Cosmetic Act," which is available at Web Resource 21-3. This guidance allowed the FDA to request, before approval of a drug, that pediatric clinical trials be done. As an industry incentive to do this, a 6-month additional period of "exclusivity" (patent protection) could be granted. This was followed up by additional FDA actions, including a draft guidance in 2000 on pediatric oncology studies, which can be found at Web Resource 21-4.

Additional guidances and documents have been issued by the FDA since then, including the International Conference on Harmonization (ICH) E11 "Guidance on Clinical Investigation of Medicinal Products in the Pediatric Population," which can be found at Web Resource 21-5. This guidance notes in regard to safety that because children differ from adults in having still developing body systems, "long term studies or surveillance data, either while patients are on chronic therapy or during the post-therapy period, may be needed to determine possible effects on skeletal, behavioral, cognitive, sexual and immune maturation and development...Normally the pediatric (safety) database is limited at the time of approval. Therefore, post-marketing surveillance is particularly important. In some cases, long term follow-up studies may provide additional safety and/or efficacy information for subgroups within the pediatric population or additional information for the entire pediatric population."

The guidance also addresses the question of the definition of a "child," noting the following possible categories and describing the issues in safety and efficacy of each:

- Preterm newborn infants
- Term newborn infants (0-27 days)
- Infants and toddlers (28 days to 23 months)
- Children (2-11 years)
- Adolescents (12-16 or 18 years depending on region)

Other initiatives continue. For example, in 2003 the FDA allocated money for the testing of 12 commonly used drugs in children: azithromycin, baclofen, bumetanide, dobutamine, dopamine, furosemide, heparin, lithium, lorazepam, rifampin, sodium nitroprusside, and spironolactone. See Web Resource 21-6 for further details. The FDA also maintains a pediatric advisory committee. (For an excellent review see Stephenson, *Br J Clin Pharmacol* 2005;59(6):670-673.)

The Elderly

The elderly represent a special group in pharmacology for several reasons. There are certain diseases that are seen only or primarily in the elderly (e.g., Alzheimer's disease or type II diabetes, known previously as "adult-onset diabetes"). The elderly tend to have more diseases than the young, especially those that are related to chronic conditions (osteoarthritis, hyperlipidemia) or habits (smoking, alcohol use); as a consequence, the elderly consume more drugs and for longer durations. Hence, the risk of drug-drug interactions may increase, particularly if there is a decrease in renal and/or hepatic function. Finally, pharmacokinetics and pharmacodynamics may also be altered in the elderly, producing different effects from those that would occur in younger patients. These subjects (with attention to cardiac and central nervous system drugs, which produce frequent AEs in the elderly) are discussed in detail in the excellent chapter by Una Martin and Charles George entitled "Drugs and the Elderly" (In Ron Mann and Elizabeth Andrews, eds. *Pharmacovigilance*. John Wiley and Sons, Chichester, UK: 2002).

It is also worth keeping in mind that swallowing disorders and dysfunction are often worse in the elderly than in the young. A tablet or other oral preparation that is very large, very sticky (having a hydroxycellulose outer layer), or oddly shaped may be difficult to swallow and could even get stuck or cause obstruction in the pharynx or esophagus.

The ICH and FDA Guideline

The ICH guideline E7 entitled "Studies in Support of Special Populations: Geriatrics" of 1993 was published by the FDA in August 1994. It is directed primarily at drugs expected to have significant use in diseases of the elderly (e.g., Alzheimer disease) or for drugs that are used in large numbers by the elderly (e.g., antihypertensives). The guideline takes an arbitrary definition of geriatric as 65 years or over but recommends seeking out patients 75 years and over for studies. In general, there should be no upper age limit. Nor should the elderly with concomitant diseases specifically be excluded because these are frequently the patients that most need to be studied.

The guideline recommends that geriatric patients be included in phase III and, at the sponsor's option, phase II studies in "meaningful numbers." For diseases "not unique to but present in the elderly," a minimum of 100 patients studied is recommended. For studies of diseases of the elderly, it is obviously expected that most of the patients studied will be elderly.

Pharmacokinetic studies should be done to determine whether the drug is handled differently in the elderly compared with younger patients. Studies in patients with renal and/or hepatic insufficiency should be done, although often studies done in the young suffice and separate studies in the elderly may not be needed. Pharmacodynamic dose-response studies usually do not have to be done except for sedative/hypnotic agents and other psychoactive drugs or where phase II/III studies suggest age-associated issues. Drug-drug interaction studies should be done when appropriate and do not necessarily have to be limited to the elderly.

FDA Guideline and Rule

In 1997 the FDA (62 FR 45313) established the "Geriatric Use" section in drug labeling. In October 2001 the FDA issued a guidance on this rule (Web Resource 21-7). It reviews the requirements for geriatric information in the various sections of approved labeling such as the INDICATIONS AND USAGE and CLINICAL PHARMACOLOGY, WARNINGS, PRECAUTIONS sections. In regard to safety specifically, the FDA states that the labeling should include the following:

> "A statement describing a specific hazard with use of the drug in the elderly that references appropriate sections (e.g., CONTRAINDICATIONS, WARNINGS, PRECAUTIONS) in the labeling for more detailed discussion."

The FDA also issued a document in December 2001 aimed at consumers entitled "Medications and Older Adults," available at Web Resource 21-8, which summarizes some of the issues and the labeling initiatives noted above. Reporting requirements for AEs that occur in the elderly are the same as those for other age groups.

■ The Practice

Children

In practice, children are given drugs approved only for adults. Often the practitioner is quite in the dark about dosage, treatment duration, AEs, and so on because children have not been studied. In fact, the pediatrician is almost forced to treat children as "small adults." This lamentable situation is due to the medical and ethical (especially informed consent) difficulties in studying children, particularly where adequate therapies currently exist.

Clearly, the FDA initiatives have produced much more interest and study regarding the safety of drugs in children in spite of the obstacles. However, the safety profiles of drugs in children generally remain less well characterized for any particular drug (unless it is used only in children) than for adults. Drugs are commonly used in children that are approved only for adults or where no mention is made of use in children in the official labeling. In some cases the AE pattern seen in children and adolescents is different from that seen in adults. In addition, occasionally drugs are used in children even where contraindicated (Wilton, Lynda, Pearce, et al., *Pharmacoepidemiol Drug Safe* 1999;8[Suppl 1]:S37-S45).

As expected, controversies continue. A recent one involved the use of selective serotonin reuptake inhibitors in children and the risk of suicide.

As an interim measure, until better methods of study of drugs in children are developed, it is worth encouraging health care professionals to report AEs in children using the spontaneous reporting systems that currently exist for marketed drugs.

The Elderly

The elderly present a different picture from that seen with children. There are generally more data available about drugs in the elderly and about conditions more commonly seen in the elderly, such as renal or hepatic insufficiency, diabetes, and alcohol use. It is, in general, easier to study drugs in the elderly than in children, where the issues of informed consent often do not exist. Thus if there are not actual data from studies in the elderly, there are often data on these conditions that allow the health care professional to alter doses, change duration of therapy, order special tests, and so on to suit the elder patient in question. Drug-drug interactions pose a particular risk in the elderly, and much has been written about this (Bressler, Bahl, *Mayo Clin Proc* 2003;78:1564-1577; see Chapter 22).

Other Special Groups

It is now generally recognized that there is significant biodiversity among humans. There are probably many reasons for this. One major cause relates to drug metabolism pathways. The cytochrome P450 system, which plays a major role in drug metabolism, is well known to exhibit enormous diversity (genetic polymorphism), producing major differences in metabolism of drugs from individual to individual (Evans, Relling, *Science* 1999;286:487-491). Because of the differences in how drugs are absorbed, metabolized, distributed, and excreted by groups and by individuals, a more rational and tailored use of drugs will allow the maximization of effectiveness and the minimization of AEs.

Two further examples of special groups (women and African-Americans) follow. In practice, one can create scores of special groups. How pharmacology and medicine will evolve and characterize these differences in the upcoming years is a fascinating and unanswered issue.

Women

Women have, in general, a smaller proportion of body water and a greater proportion of body fat than men. Men and women may metabolize drugs differently. For example, men have more alcohol dehydrogenase than women and thus metabolize the same amount of alcohol more rapidly (Frezza, di Padova, Pozzato, et al., *N Engl J Med* 1990;322:95-99). Women also handle cardiac drugs differently from men in many instances (Jochmann, Stangl, Garbe, et al., *Eur Heart J* 2005;26:1585-1595).

African-Americans

It is well known that different groups in the United States have significant differences in their general health. For example, a review by the Centers for Disease Control and Prevention (*MMWR* 2005;54[01]:1-3) noted that "For many health conditions, non-Hispanic blacks bear a disproportionate burden of disease, injury, death, and disability."

Similarly, African-Americans may respond less well to certain drugs, such as antihypertensives (Levy, ed., *Ethnic & racial differences in response to medicines: preserving individualized therapy in managed pharmaceutical programs*. Reston, VA: National Pharmaceutical Council, 1993), or may have more AEs, such as angioedema associated with angiotensin-converting enzyme inhibitors (Kalow, *Trends Pharmacol Sci* 1991;12[3]:102-107). From these and other data it is clear that additional studies of the effects of drugs in various ethnic or racial groups are desirable. See an excellent commentary on the need for greater diversity in clinical trials by Prof. Kenneth Davis of the University of Cincinnati in "African-American Health. Clinical Trial Diversity: The Need and the Challenge," at Web Resource 21-9.

Drug Interactions and Polypharmacy

→ **NOTE:** (Unless otherwise noted, the word "drug" or "drug product" should be taken in this book to include "biologics" and "vaccines.")

■ Background

Analyzing adverse events (AEs) and ascribing the causality to a particular drug can be quite difficult. This difficulty, however, is magnified when additional drugs are also being taken by the patient. This is sometimes known as "polypharmacy." It is generally believed that the more drugs taken, the greater the risk of AEs and the greater the risk of drug-drug interactions.

In such cases, it may not be possible to ascribe the AE to one particular drug. In most situations of regulatory reporting, the reporter is generally required to specify one or more "suspect drugs" and, if present, one or more "concomitant drugs." The former are presumed to have a suspected causative role in the AE and the latter not.

Further complicating matters are drug interactions, a situation that occurs when two (or more) drugs are taken that influence each other. That is, the pharmacokinetics (e.g., blood levels) and/or pharmacodynamics (effects in the body) of one or all of the drugs may be altered.

For example, the coadministration of desloratadine (Clarinex®) and erythromycin, ketoconazole, azithromycin, or fluoxetine in pharmacology studies produced increased plasma concentrations (Cmax and AUC0-24h) of desloratadine and its major metabolite but did not produce clinically relevant changes in the safety profile (*Physicians' Desk Reference*, 2005, p. 3021). This is an example of a drug-drug interaction producing changes in pharmacokinetics (the plasma levels) but not in the pharmacodynamics (no clinical safety untoward effects).

A patient may suffer from a pharmacodynamic interaction when taking several products sharing the same adverse reaction. For example, when simultaneously taking aspirin and Plavix® (both reduce the clotting mechanism) plus a nonsteroidal antiinflammatory drug like Feldene® and, unknowingly, another nonsteroidal antiinflammatory drug like ibuprofen (both weaken the gastric lining and promote bleeding), the patient is at great risk of gastrointestinal bleeding.

At the other end of the spectrum is a drug like Coumadin® (warfarin), which can be life-saving but which has over 55 potential drug interactions listed by drug class and over 100 by specific drug name in the US labeling. The interactions may produce elevations or decreases in the prothrombin time/International Normalized Ratio. In some cases the same drug with Coumadin® may produce an elevation in these levels in one patient and a decrease in another patient (*Physicians' Desk Reference*, 2005, p. 1041). These changes have the potential to produce significant clinical effects by putting the patient at risk for hemorrhage or clotting.

It is impossible, in the course of testing new drugs, to run drug-drug interaction studies against all drugs or even all classes of drugs. At best, sponsors run selected interaction studies against

- The most commonly used drugs that the exposed patients would be likely to take due to their age, diseases, sex, and so on.
- Drugs that might be expected to produce interactions based on pharmacology data (e.g., cytochrome P450 metabolism) or based on historical data from similar drugs in the class.

These studies tend to be done on healthy patients in short-term clinical pharmacology trials. Drugs that are suspected of producing interactions but are significantly toxic by themselves (e.g., cancer drugs) generally cannot be studied in this manner because of ethical considerations. It is hoped that one day pharmacogenetics may provide better means of answering drug-drug interaction questions.

The field of drug-drug interactions is complex. For further information see the excellent section in *Stephens' Detection of New Adverse Drug Reactions*, 5th edition, edited by John Talbot and Patrick Waller (Wiley, 2004). Also see the US Food and Drug Administration's consumer leaflet on drug-drug interactions at Web Resource 22-1. Textbooks on drug interactions are also available.

It is also believed that certain patients who are either debilitated or suffer from certain diseases (e.g., autoimmune disorders, cardiovascular disease, gastro-intestinal disease, infection, psychiatric disorders, respiratory disorders, seizure disorders, and others) may be at greater risk for drug interactions and that the more severe the underlying disease, the greater the risk (Brown, *An Overview of Drug Interactions,* in the US Pharmacist at Web Resource 22-2). It should also be noted that there are possible drug-food (e.g., grapefruit juice), drug-nutrient, drug-disease, drug-herbal, and drug-alcohol interactions.

■ The Practice

In reality, drug-drug interactions represent a major problem in medicine today. We may consider some of these to be "medication errors" because known drug interactions where there are significant clinical risks of either lack of efficacy or AEs should not occur. These drugs should not be prescribed or taken together. However, the use of bad drug combinations is common.

In a study of elderly Danish patients, among those less than 70 years, 67.9% used no drugs, 16.5% used one drug, and 15.6% used two or more prescription drugs. The corresponding prevalences for the people over 70 years of age were 35.7%, 15.9%, and 48.4%. The 26,337 elderly patients with at least two drugs used 21,293 different combinations. Of the elderly patients who had purchased two or more drugs, 4.4% had combinations of drugs carrying a risk of severe interactions (Rosholm, Bjerrum, Hallas, et al., *Dan Med Bull* 1998;45[2]:210-213).

In a database study of 1,600 elderly patients in six European countries, the subjects used on average 7 drugs per person; 46% had at least one drug combination possibly leading to a drug-drug interaction. On average, there were 0.83 potential drug-drug interactions per person. Almost 10% of the potential interactions were classified "to be avoided" according to the Swedish interaction classification system, but nearly one-third of them were to be avoided only for predisposed patients. The risk of a subtherapeutic effect as a result of a potential drug-drug interaction was as common as the risk of adverse reactions. Furthermore, differences in the frequency and type of potential interactions were found among the countries (Bjorkman, Fastbom, Schmidt, et al., *Ann Pharmacother* 2002;36:1675-1681). For an excellent review of drug therapy in the elderly, see Bressler and Bahl (*Mayo Clin Proc* 2003;78:1564-1577).

There is a growing recognition that the mechanism for communicating medical information (in this case drug interaction information) is not adequate and is not achieving its goals. A good summary of the situation is found in *JAMA* (*JAMA* 2000;284:3047-3049). In this article, Dr. Woosley notes that the current system of changing the US labeling (package insert) for a drug has not been sufficient to prevent the incorrect or harmful use of various drugs. He notes that cisapride, a gastrointestinal drug, produced in some patients life-threatening ventricular arrhythmias. After a labeling change contraindicating its use in certain situations, the FDA found that "patients with the contraindications continued to receive the drug at nearly the same rate after the warnings were issued as before they were issued."

Interestingly, in the United States, the responsibility and liability for drug interaction issues seem to be falling more on the pharmacist than on the prescribing physician for the following reasons (as cited in Brown, *An Overview of Drug Interactions,* in the US Pharmacist at Web Resource 22-3):

1. Colleges of pharmacy in the United States include courses in their entry level degree program designed to instruct students on aspects of drug interactions, including detection, incidence and significance, types of drug interactions, mechanisms by which interactions occur, and the role of the pharmacist in monitoring drug therapy to either avoid and/or resolve drug interactions.

2. Most pharmacies in the U.S. utilize sophisticated computer software to help pharmacists manage the pharmacy's business operation, and to screen patient medication profiles for drug-drug interactions when processing new and refill prescriptions.

3. The profession of pharmacy through its professional organizations such as the American Pharmaceutical Association, the American Society of Health-Systems Pharmacists, and the American Society of Consultant Pharmacists has publicly proclaimed that the role of the pharmacist in "pharmaceutical care as a practice standard" is to maximize patient outcomes.

4. OBRA-90 legislation charged pharmacists with the responsibility to minimize adverse reactions, which includes drug-drug interactions.

5. The Federal Department of Health and Human Services requires pharmacists who serve the needs of patients in long-term care facilities as consultant pharmacists to review the drug regimen of patients and report any irregularities, including drug interactions, to the facility's medical director.

6. The Joint Commission on Accreditation of Healthcare Organizations (JCAHO) requires that hospitalized patients be educated and counseled on potential food-drug interactions by the pharmacist, dietitian, nurse and physician. The pharmaceutical care component of the JCAHO standard specifies that pharmacists are responsible for identifying drug-drug interactions as well as drug-food interactions.

7. Recent studies suggest a lack of knowledge among physicians about drug interactions, specifically drug-food interactions. These studies also report that fifth-year pharmacy students scored significantly higher than family medicine residents (in their fifth or sixth year of training) in 12 of 14 items on a standardized drug interaction questionnaire.

In the world of drug safety, it behooves the health care professionals, sponsors, and health agencies to be aware of polypharmacy and to consider a possible drug interaction even if the reporter has not mentioned it as an AE or even as a suspicion. Certain AEs that are known to occur in the drug interaction setting (e.g., torsades de pointes, hemorrhage in patients on anticoagulants, seizures, ingestion of grapefruit juice, etc.) should raise the level of suspicion in the medical reviewers. It may be worthwhile to track suspected drug interactions on a potential "signal list" for continued review.

Conversely, the occurrence of an AE when two or more drugs are being taken does not necessarily imply a drug interaction. Ideally, drug blood level abnormalities (or other markers suggestive of an interaction) should be obtained to add evidence to the suspicion of a drug interaction in a specific patient. In a more general sense, a clinical study or a demonstration of metabolism issues (e.g., use of the same cytochrome P450 pathway) is needed to confirm a drug interaction. As noted above, it is difficult, expensive, and sometimes not ethical to perform such studies, and indirect evidence or a high level of suspicion must be relied on to make a determination of a drug interaction.

Drug Labeling and Warnings, the *Physicians' Desk Reference* and Equivalents, and Differences from Country to Country, Prescription vs. OTC Drug Labeling

➡ **NOTE:** (Unless otherwise noted, the word "drug" or "drug product" should be taken in this book to include "biologics" and "vaccines.")

■ Background and Theory

"Labeling" is divided for pharmacovigilance purposes into two different documents. For drugs that are not yet on the market (approved for sale) the labeling used for adverse event (AE) reporting is considered to be the official "Investigator Brochure" as prepared by the sponsor that contains a summary of the known information about the drug, including its chemistry, pharmacology, toxicology, clinical studies, and AEs. It is usually updated yearly. It is this document that is used in the preparation of 7- and 15-day expedited (alert) reports to the US Food and Drug Administration (FDA) and for investigational new drug annual reports. After a New Drug Application (NDA) is approved and the drug is marketed, the labeling that is used for regulatory reporting of AEs now changes to that document prepared by the sponsor and submitted to, negotiated with, and approved by the FDA.

"Labeling" is a general term encompassing many things about a drug. The requirements for labeling are summarized in 21CFR1. The official definition of labeling for a marketed product is 21CFR1.3(a) (see Web Resource 23-1):

(a) Labeling includes all written, printed, or graphic matter accompanying an article at any time while such article is in interstate commerce or held for sale after shipment or delivery in interstate commerce.

(b) Label means any display of written, printed, or graphic matter on the immediate container of any article, or any such matter affixed to any consumer commodity or affixed to or appearing upon a package containing any consumer commodity.

Thus, it includes the FDA-approved written material describing a drug such as the "package insert" and the packaging and box that a drug is shipped or sold in. Synonyms for labeling include "package insert," "professional labeling," "direction circular," and "package circular." It also includes the FDA-approved patient labeling where this exists (see Web Resource 23-2):

The basic components of labeling in the US for prescription drugs include: Boxed warning (if applicable), Indications and usage, Dosage and administration, How supplied, Contraindications, Warnings, General precautions, Drug interactions, Drug/laboratory test interactions, Laboratory tests, Information for patients, Teratogenic effects, Nonteratogenic effects, Labor and delivery, Nursing mothers, Pediatric use. Geriatric use, Carcinogenesis, mutagenesis, impairment of fertility, Adverse reactions, Controlled Substance (if applicable), Abuse, Dependence, Overdosage, Description, Clinical pharmacology, Animal pharmacology/toxicology, Clinical studies and References.

It is generally recognized that drug labeling in the United States is inconsistent, difficult to read, difficult to access, nonstandardized, and difficult to computerize in its present form. This forces patients and health care practitioners to use publications and websites that "digest" this information and present it in a more user-friendly format.

The FDA has undertaken a major review of labeling in the United States, and this has produced major initiatives over the last several years, culminating in a major new labeling requirement issued as a final rule in early 2006.

The first initiative was the development of structured product labeling (SPL) in which all labeling has three basic parts:

1. The header with general information about the label and product
2. The sections with blocks of text (e.g., indications, contraindications, warnings, etc.)
3. The data elements with product-specific information (e.g., active ingredient, dosage form, how supplied, etc.)

In 2003 the FDA introduced the new requirements for SPL in which prescription and over-the-counter (OTC) drug labeling must be filed with the FDA using an XML-based format standard. See Web Resource 23-3 for the final rule. This is an internationally accepted standard and allows for easy accessibility and transfer to other databases. Its use became obligatory as of October 2005. All labeling is stored in a database known as "DailyMed" in the National Library of Medicine. See the FDA presentation at Web Resource 23-4. In addition, International Conference on Harmonization and European Union (EU) initiatives are also underway to develop SPL in other regions.

The most recent initiative promises to have a more far-reaching effect. It represents four guidances for industry released in January 2006. The actual rule and obligation went into effect June 30, 2006:

1. "Guidance for Industry: Adverse Reactions Section of Labeling for Human Prescription Drug and Biological Products—Content and Format" (Web Resource 23-5)
2. "Guidance for Industry: Clinical Studies Section of Labeling for Human Prescription Drug and Biological Products—Content and Format" (Web Resource 23-6)
3. "Guidance for Industry: Labeling for Human Prescription Drug and Biological Products—Implementing the New Content and Format Requirements" (Web Resource 23-7)
4. "Guidance for Industry: Warnings and Precautions, Contraindications, and Boxed Warning Sections of Labeling for Human Prescription Drug and Biological Products—Content and Format" (Web Resource 23-8)

See also the Q&A accompanying the guidances (Web Resource 23-9).

A brief summary of the guidances follows:

FDA has enacted these to manage the risks of drugs and to reduce medical errors. The new rules do not apply to OTC products or to patient information. The first major change is that there will now be a "Highlights" section. This section, which should run about ½ page in length, will include the most commonly used information in the label:

- The date of the approval of the original product.
- A summary of any black box warning.
- Recent major changes made within the last year regarding black boxes, indications and usage, dosage and administration, contraindications, and warnings and precautions.
- Adverse reactions: most frequent adverse reactions that are important for reasons other than frequency.
- AE reporting contact information for both the FDA and the manufacturer.
- Drug interactions.
- Use in specific populations.

There are also format and reordering changes in the labeling in addition to the Highlights section. Risk information is consolidated with the AE section after the Warnings and Precautions section. Some information formerly in the Precautions section (use in specific populations, drug interactions, and patient counseling information) is now in other sections. In addition, bold type is used in some sections as well as more white space and minimum font sizes to make reading easier.

This new rule applies to drugs approved after the rule went into effect as well as drugs approved in the 5 years before the effective date of the rule and older drugs for which there is a major change in the prescribing information. Manufacturers may apply this to older drugs too if they wish. Companies have between 3 and 7 years to implement this for the older drugs depending on when (in the last 5 years) the drug was approved.

Many drug labels and patient information for specific drugs can be found at the FDA website (Web Resource 23-10). In addition, most pharmaceutical companies have posted their product labeling on its websites. If the drug is sold in multiple countries, the local website for each company usually posts the local labeling.

In the United States, many, but not all, drug labels for prescription drugs are printed in the reference book known as the *Physicians' Desk Reference* (PDR), published yearly by Thomson. It is about 3,000 pages long and has photos of many of the products as well as the product information. There are other editions for OTC products, veterinary products, and so on. An electronic version is available free to medical professionals at Web Resource 23-11. Other countries have the equivalent publications with drug labeling. In Canada, the equivalent of the PDR is called the *Compendium of Pharmaceuticals and Specialties*. In France it is called the "Vidal" (this website is in French [Web Resource 23-12]) and in Germany the "Rote Liste" (this website is in German [Web Resource 23-13]).

Most countries of the world have registration and approval systems similar to that of the United States. In these countries, labeling is approved based on information submitted to that health authority. The approvals may vary significantly from country to country based on different data submitted, different indications requested, different formulations, different patient populations treated, and local customs. Thus the labeling in other countries may be quite different from that of the United States. In addition, in non-English-speaking countries the labeling is, of course, in the local language.

In the EU the approved labeling is known as the Summary of Product Characteristics (SPC or SmPC). The EU situation is complex with labeling being the same or similar for some products (often newer products) if the product was approved centrally or if the label was harmonized at the EU level. Many other products, however, have labels that differ from country to country.

There is a curious use of terminology by some people. In the United States, the generic term "labeling" (sometimes called the "package insert") is used to refer to the official FDA-approved US product information. The world "labeling" is also used in the United States for the SPC when referring to European labeling. Some in the EU, conversely, use the term SPC (or SmPC) when they are referring to their own official labeling or to the US labeling. Thus one might hear a reference to the US SPC—a concept that does not really exist in the United States. This refers, in practice, to the US official labeling.

In terms of pharmacovigilance the sections of labeling that are of most interest include the AEs, warnings, drug interactions, precautions, and pregnancy information. In particular, the labeling is used to determine whether a particular AE that is reported for that product is "labeled" or "expected" (see Chapter 37). In general, if an AE is labeled or expected, it does not have to be reported to the FDA as an expedited report. It is also used to determine in which section this AE report is listed in the NDA periodic report.

Changes, additions, removals, and alterations to product labeling must be approved by the FDA for US labeling, with the exception of emergency safety changes, which make the labeling more restrictive to protect the public health. These may be made by the sponsor immediately and are reported to the FDA right afterward.

Note that drug labels do not always use *Medical Dictionary for Regulatory Activities* (MedDRA) terms for AEs. Many of the drugs are quite old and date back several years to pre-MedDRA days. Thus the terms used are either COSTART or WHO-ART or even other terms that are not standardized. This can clearly produce issues when one attempts to determine whether a term (e.g., a MedDRA term) is considered labeled if a similar but not quite exactly matching term is in the label. It is the goal of all parties to move all labels to MedDRA, but this is not likely to happen in the near future, particularly for older products. Newer product labels are written using MedDRA.

■ OTC Products

The labeling for OTC products in the United States is different from that for prescription products. OTC drugs have labeling that is derived from the "monographs" (the CFR sections dealing with these products and specifying which products may be sold without an NDA or Abbreviated New Drug Application [ANDA]). OTC drugs are used by patients and consumers without a health care intermediary (physician, pharmacist, nurse) to explain the product, its use, its adverse events, etc. The labeling is what is written on the package (box) in the section marked "Drug Facts." This is a lay version of a package insert but is often very skimpy in terms of AEs. Sometimes none are listed at all. This is often most surprising in light of the fact that certain products that had extensive lists of AEs (e.g., loratadine, nonsteroidal anti-inflammatory drugs) in the package insert when they were prescription drugs now have minimal safety information in the OTC "Drug Facts." Some OTC products may be sold under an NDA or ANDA and these products may have a more classic package insert. Similarly for food supplements there is a label marked "Supplement Facts." Many companies that sell OTC products sell supplements, drugs, devices, and sometimes even cosmetics, making for very complicated AE collection and reporting.

This labeling situation complicates AE reporting to the FDA. The federal regulations (21CFR310.305) require the reporting of serious AEs that are unexpected for drugs without NDAs. For OTC products with "Drug Facts" labeling with no AEs or lay terms for medical conditions, the criteria for reporting to FDA are sometimes unclear. Many companies have chosen to simply report all serious AEs received for their OTC products rather than risk underreporting to the FDA. It is likely that Congress will change the requirements for reporting within the next year or two. One current proposal will require all serious AEs to be reported to the FDA for OTC products.

In many other countries, for example the EU, OTC products must have Marketing Authorizations (the approximate equivalent of a US NDA) and thus the usual AE reporting requirements are required as for prescription products.

■ The Practice

The pharmacovigilance worker in a company or health agency should be sure that he or she is always sent updated labeling by the group in charge of preparing them. Though obvious, this is not always routine. The labeling is usually prepared by groups other than those who deal with pharmacovigilance, and the preparers may not always remember to distribute the new labeling to drug safety and other groups that need it.

For pharmacovigilance professionals, knowledge of the labeling for the drugs for which they are responsible is absolutely necessary. For drugs with many AEs, it is generally a good idea to prepare a separate table either on paper or in a spreadsheet as a reference, listing the AEs to aid when determining labeledness (expectedness). These AEs may, in fact, appear in multiple sections and at varying levels of specificity. They should be harvested and grouped appropriately so that a ready reference (known as a "cheat sheet") can be consulted when evaluating and coding AEs. It may be useful to list the corresponding MedDRA terms and level (verbatim, preferred term, lower level term) on the list.

It should be kept in mind that many drugs have multiple labeling documents if there are different preparations (e.g., different labeling for intravenous and oral preparations of the same active ingredient). The AEs in the two labels may differ because some will be route specific (e.g., injection site reactions or those related to a first pass effect after oral intake, etc.).

The advent of the Internet has allowed people to compare labels from one country with another, and the differences become readily noticeable. This will most likely lead to more harmonization in the future.

24

Regulations, Directives, Guidances, Law, and Practice in the European Union and United States: What Is Written Down and What Is Traditional Practice

→ **NOTE:** (Unless otherwise noted, the word "drug" or "drug product" should be taken in this book to include "biologics" and "vaccines.")

■ Background and Theory

Pharmacovigilance is governed by a large body of requirements. Some are written and rigid. Others are written and far less rigid, others are not requirements but only guidances, and still others are unwritten customs and practices. Obviously, laws and regulations vary from country to country. The sections below summarize briefly the obligations in the United States and the European Union (EU).

United States

Legal requirements for drug safety come from multiple areas. There are laws, regulations, and guidances issued by the US federal government. These are the predominant formal requirements governing drug safety. In the United States a "law" is a written statute, requirement, ordinance, and so forth that has been passed by a legislature and then signed into law (where required) by the

executive. That is, a federal law is one that is passed by the Congress in Washington, DC and signed by the President. Laws may be created at multiple levels of government (federal, state, and local).

The law governing investigational drugs ("New Drugs") is found in Section 505(i) [21 U.S.C. 355], and the law governing marketed drugs is found in Section 505(k) of the Food Drug and Cosmetic Act (Web Resource 24-1).

In addition to laws, the US Food and Drug Administration (FDA) is empowered to create regulations. Regulations are rules issued by government authorities under the power of laws. Regulations thus have the force of law. To create a regulation, the FDA publishes the proposed version of the new or amended regulation in the *Federal Register* (Web Resource 24-2). A period is defined during which time the public may send written comments on the proposal to the FDA. After review, a final regulation is published in the *Federal Register* and in the Code of Federal Regulations (Web Resource 24-3). A long period may elapse between first publishing the draft and the final regulation; also, the draft regulation may be withdrawn.

Finally, the FDA issues guidances that contain the FDA's preferences on laws and regulations. As the FDA states on its Center for Drug Evaluation and Research Guidance Website (Web Resource 24-4): "Guidance documents represent the Agency's current thinking on a particular subject. They do not create or confer any rights for or on any person and do not operate to bind FDA or the public. An alternative approach may be used if such approach satisfies the requirements of the applicable statute, regulations, or both." It is generally held in practice in the industry to be a wise course of action to follow FDA guidances.

Many of the applicable pharmacovigilance regulations and guidances can be found at Web Resource 24-5. A more complete listing of FDA guidances can be found at Web Resource 24-6.

European Union

The EU situation is very different from that in the United States, in particular because the EU is composed of 25 separate member states (countries) that are different from the 50 US states. The EU member states are sovereign countries; the US states are not. The website covering EU legislation can be found at Web Resource 24-7.

EU "primary legislation" derives from treaties and agreements among the member states. This includes the Single European Act (1987), the Maastricht Treaty (1992), and the Treaty of Amsterdam (1997). "Secondary legislation" derives from the treaties. There are several types. The ones that touch most on pharmacovigilance are as follows:

- Regulations: Directly applicable and binding in all EU member states without the need for any additional national implementation legislation. That is, the regulation as it is published is, word for word, the law in each of the member states. Note that this is different from the use of the word "regulation" in the United States.
- Directives: This legislation binds member states to the objectives of the legislation within a certain time period but allows each member state to create its own form of national law to so achieve it. That is, each member state may modify the wording and requirements of the directive as long as the objectives of the directive are met.
- Recommendations and opinions: nonbinding and similar to FDA guidances.

The EU legislation and guidance documents can be found at Web Resource 24-8.

The EU situation is, in many ways, far more complex than that in the United States for drug safety. In the United States the requirements for drug safety come primarily from the FDA. In practice, there are few state and local requirements that apply to pharmacovigilance for companies. There are, at rare times, requirements imposed by other governmental entities for registries or other safety obligations. In contrast, the EU has the supranational body of directives, regulations, and such as well as legal requirements in each member state, which may differ from or add onto the EU level requirements. EU documents are generally available in all EU languages. Member state documents are published in the language of the member state but are not consistently published in other languages.

Any company dealing in the EU must obtain expertise at the European and member state level to stay in compliance with all safety obligations. In practice, this usually means the creation of affiliates or subsidiaries or the hiring of local companies or agents in the European countries where the drug is sold or studied.

In particular, the EU requires the presence of a "Qualified Person" (Directive 2001/83/EC and Volume 9). This person must be physically in one of the EU member states and is responsible for pharmacovigilance. The person is responsible for "the establishment and maintenance of a system which ensures that information about all suspected adverse reactions which are reported to the personnel of the company, and to medical representatives, is collected and collated in order to be accessible at least at one point in the Community" (i.e., the EU) as well as preparing reports and responding to questions on safety matters, including the risk-benefit analyses of the products. See the directive (articles 103 and 104 in particular) at Web Resource 24-9.

■ The Practice

In practice, the laws and regulations often leave areas of ambiguity. No law or regulation is ever able to predict or account for every conceivable circumstance that may arise. Where feasible, a guidance is issued to clarify issues. However, it is a complex, time-consuming, and difficult bureaucratic process to create laws, guidances, and regulations, and there is always a time lag between the need for a clarification and the publication of such.

For example, the definition of serious (see Chapter 1) would seem fairly clear: "Any adverse drug experience occurring at any dose that results in...death, a life-threatening adverse drug experience, inpatient hospitalization or prolongation of existing hospitalization, a persistent or significant disability/incapacity or congenital anomaly/birth defect. Important medical events that may not result in death, be life-threatening, or require hospitalization may be considered a serious adverse drug experience when, based upon appropriate medical judgment, they may jeopardize the patient or subject and may require medical or surgical intervention to prevent one of the outcome listed in this definition."

In fact, areas are unclear, and there is a long series of dialogues, publications, and meetings to address such ambiguities as follows:

- Is staying in a hospital emergency room overnight considered inpatient hospitalization (and thus a serious adverse event)? The consensus: No.

- Is a preplanned inpatient hospitalization that occurs after an adverse event but perhaps for a totally separate condition considered inpatient hospitalization (and thus a serious adverse event)? The consensus: No.

- What is an "important medical event"? Is thrombocytopenia if the count is 5,000? Yes. 50,000?

Probably yes. 350,000 (where the normal is up to 400,000)? Probably no.

Thus in circumstances where there is no clear answer, the best approach is to take the most conservative course of action and "overcall": If the question is between serious and nonserious, prefer serious; if the question is between reporting and not reporting a case to the FDA, prefer reporting. Calls to the agencies are possible to ask such questions, but it is not always possible to reach the right person to have a policy question answered. In such cases, try to get a written confirmation. If that is not possible, write detailed minutes of the telephone call and file them with the case. For cases being submitted to multiple health authorities around the world, it is not practical to call each authority to get an answer, and it is possible the answers will be contradictory. Again, the best course of action is the most conservative course.

Council for International Organizations of Medical Sciences (CIOMS) and CIOMS Reports

➡ **NOTE:** (Unless otherwise noted, the word "drug" or "drug product" should be taken in this book to include "biologics" and "vaccines.")

This chapter summarizes what the Council for International Organizations of Medical Sciences (CIOMS) is and the six reports issued by working groups created by CIOMS. These reports have been crucial for the International Conference on Harmonization (ICH) and the development of safety regulations in North America, Europe, Japan, and elsewhere. They are worth taking the time to review. Keep in mind that not all proposals from the CIOMS reports were adopted, and those that were adopted were not necessarily adopted directly and without change by ICH and national regulatory authorities.

■ CIOMS

From the CIOMS website (Web Resource 25-1): "CIOMS is an international, non-governmental, non-profit or-

ganization established jointly by WHO (World Health Organization) and United Nations Educational, Scientific and Cultural Organization (UNESCO) (Web Resource 25-2) in 1949. The membership of CIOMS as of 2003 includes 48 international member organizations, representing many of the biomedical disciplines, and 18 national members mainly representing national academies of sciences and medical research councils. The main objectives of CIOMS are:

- To facilitate and promote international activities in the field of biomedical sciences, especially when the participation of several international associations and national institutions is deemed necessary.
- To maintain collaborative relations with the United Nations and its specialized agencies, in particular with WHO and UNESCO.
- To serve the scientific interests of the international biomedical community in general.

CIOMS has several long-term programs, including one on drug development and use. Starting in the early 1980s, working groups composed of experts from industry and governments have been examining key issues in drug safety. They have issued six reports, several of which have served as seminal documents for procedures and regulations that ICH, the US Food and Drug Administration (FDA), the European Union, Japan, and other drug safety authorities have issued. The key documents are summarized below.

CIOMS I (1990): International Reporting of Adverse Drug Reactions

The goal of this working group was "to develop an internationally acceptable reporting method whereby manufacturers could report post-marketing adverse drug reactions rapidly, efficiently and effectively to regulators." It noted the fact that postmarketing surveillance is necessary because premarketing studies in animals and humans have "inherent limitations." It noted the need for standardization internationally.

The report established several conventions that have largely been adopted, including the following:

- The concept and format of a report ("a CIOMS I report") from the manufacturer receiving the event to the regulators.
- "Reactions" are different from "events." "Reactions" are reports of clinical occurrences that have been judged by a physician or health care worker as having a "reasonable possibility" that the report has been caused by a drug. "Events" have not had a causality evaluation made and, thus, may or may not be related to or associated with the drug.
- Causality is discussed. No particular method of assessing causality is recommended. The report does recommend that manufacturers not separate out those spontaneous reports that they receive into those that seem to be drug related and those not seemingly drug related. The physician, by making the report to the manufacturer, is indicating that there is some level of causality possible in the report. This is a "suspected reaction." This has become a fundamental concept in most spontaneous reporting systems around the world wherein all spontaneous reports from physicians (now extended to all health care providers and in some countries, such as the United States and Canada, to consumers) are to be considered possibly related to the drug; that is they are "reactions" not "events."
- Because labels for marketed drugs differ from country to country, it is recommended that all reactions be collected at one point and then submitted to local authorities on a country-by-country

basis based on whether the reactions are labeled locally or not.

- The report discusses the four minimum requirements for a valid report: an identifiable source (reporter), a patient (even if not precisely identified by name), a suspect drug, and a suspect reaction.
- The report recommended that all reports be sent in as soon as received and no later than 15 working days after receipt to create a common worldwide deadline. This concept has been adopted, but the 15 working days has been changed to 15 calendar days due to differences in the designation of "working days" and nonworking days (holidays) around the world. The reporting clock starts the date the report is first received by anyone anywhere in the company.
- The CIOMS I form was created. It is essentially the same form as used now. This form is to be used for reporting to regulatory authorities.
- Reporting of reactions is to be in the English language.

CIOMS II (1992): International Reporting of Periodic Drug-Safety Update Summaries

This working group proposed a standard for Periodic Safety Update Reports (PSURs) of reactions received by manufacturers on marketed drugs. This standard, with modifications from the ICH and other organizations, has been widely adopted. The document defined several key terms:

- CIOMS Reportable Cases or Reports: "serious, medically substantiated, unlabeled ADRs with the 4 elements (reporter, patient, reaction, suspect drug)."
- Core Data Sheet (CDS): A document prepared by the manufacturer containing all relevant safety information, including adverse drug reactions (ADRs). This is the reference for "labeled" and "unlabeled." Note that this concept, which has been widely accepted, has since gotten more complex and one must distinguish labeling from listing (e.g., unlabeled and unlisted).
- International Birth Date (IBD): The date that the first regulatory authority anywhere in the world has approved a drug for marketing.
- Data Lock-Point (Cut-Off Date): The closing date for information to be included in a particular safety update.
- Serious: Fatal, life-threatening, involves or prolongs inpatient hospitalization.

The sections of the PSUR include the following:

Scope
1. Subject drugs for review
2. Frequency of review and reporting

Content
1. Introduction
2. CDS
3. Drug's licensing (i.e., marketing approval) status
4. Review of regulatory actions taken for safety, if any
5. Patient exposure
6. Individual case histories (including a "CIOMS line listing")
7. Studies
8. Overall safety evaluation
9. Important data received after the data lock-point

Other fundamental concepts were established:

- Reports should be semiannual and not cumulative (unless cumulative information is needed to put a safety issue into context).
- The same report goes to all regulatory authorities on the same date irrespective of the local (national) approval date of the drug.
- Reactions reported should be from studies (published and unpublished), spontaneous reports, published case reports, cases received from regulatory authorities, and other manufacturers. Duplicate reports should be eliminated.
- The manufacturer should do a "concise critical analysis and opinion in English by a person responsible for monitoring and assessing drug safety."

A sample simulated PSUR is included based on a fake drug "Qweasytrol."

CIOMS III (1995 and 1998/1999): Guidelines for Preparing Core Clinical Safety Information on Drugs (1995), Including New Proposals for Investigator's Brochures (1998/1999)

The CIOMS III guideline is now out of print but did establish and extend several fundamental concepts that are now in use in much of the world. The idea of the CDS introduced in CIOMS II was extended to the core safety information (CSI). The CDS contains all of the key core data (not just safety data) on a drug. The CSI contains (only) core safety information and is a subset of the CDS. Several fundamental concepts were introduced:

- The CSI is the core safety information that should appear in all countries' labeling for that drug. Additional information could be added at the national level, but the core information should be included in all countries' labels. The CSI (and national labels) are guides for health care professionals and contain the most relevant information needed for the drug's use.
- Marketing considerations should not play a role in the preparation of the CSI.
- The CSI was proposed primarily as a medical document and not as a legal or regulatory document.
- Every drug should have a CSI prepared and updated by the manufacturer.
- Adverse events (AEs) due to excipients should be included.
- AEs that have no well-established relationship to therapy should not be included.
- The CSI should include important information that physicians are not generally expected to know.
- As soon as relevant safety information becomes sufficiently well established, it should be included. The specific time when it is included occurs when the safety information crosses the "threshold for inclusion," which is defined as the time when "it is judged that it will influence physicians' decisions on therapy."
- Thirty-nine factors were proposed that can be ranked and weighed for an AE for a particular drug to see whether the information has crossed the threshold. An extensive discussion on the threshold is given:
  - The threshold should be lower if the condition being treated is relatively trivial, the drug is used to prevent rather than to treat disease, or the drug is widely used or if the ADR is irreversible.
  - Hypersensitivity reactions should be noted early.
  - Substantial evidence is required to remove or downgrade safety information.
- Ten general principles were proposed:
  1. In general, statements that an adverse reaction does not occur or has not yet been reported should not be made.
  2. As a general rule, clinical descriptions of specific cases should not be part of the CSI.
  3. If the mechanism is known, it should be stated, but speculation about the mechanism should be avoided.

4. As a general rule, secondary effects or sequelae should not be listed.

5. In general, a description of events expected as a result of progression of the underlying treated disease should not be included in the CSI.

6. Unlicensed or "off-label" use should be mentioned only in the context of a medically important safety problem.

7. The wording used in the CSI to describe adverse reactions should be chosen carefully and responsibly to maximize the prescriber's understanding. For example, if the ADR is part of a syndrome, this should be made clear.

8. The terms used should be specific and medically informative.

9. The use of modifiers or adjectives should be avoided unless they add useful important information.

10. A special attribute (e.g., sex, race) known to be associated with an increased risk should be specified.

- Where possible, frequencies should be provided, although it is admitted that this is very difficult with spontaneous safety data. A proposed classification is
  - Very common: ≥1/10 (≥10%)
  - Common (frequent): ≥1/100 and <1/10 (≥1% and <10%)
  - Uncommon (infrequent): ≥1/1,000 and <1/100 (≥0.1% and <1%)
  - Rare: ≥1/10,000 and <1/1000 (≥0.01% and <0.1%)
  - Very rare: <1/10,000 (<0.01%)

Many of these recommendations have been adopted in one form or another around the world, though not in their totality. The revised edition (1998/1999) of this document appeared as CIOMS V (see below).

CIOMS IV (1998): Benefit-Risk Balance for Marketed Drugs: Evaluating Safety Signals

From the preface of the report: "CIOMS IV is to some extent an extension of CIOMS II and III. It examines the theoretical and practical aspects of how to determine whether a potentially major, new safety signal signifies a shift, calling for significant action in the established relationship between benefits and risks; it also provides guidance for deciding what options for action should be considered and on the process of decision-making should such action be required."

The report looks at the general concepts of benefit-risk analysis and discusses the factors influencing as-

sessment, including stakeholders and constituencies, the nature of the problem (risk), the indication for drug use and the population under treatment, constraints of time, data and resources, and economic issues. It recommends a standard format and content for a benefit-risk report:

- Introduction
  - Brief specification/description of the drug and where marketed
  - Indications for use, by country, if there are differences
  - Identification of one or more alternative therapies or modalities, including surgery
  - A very brief description of the suspected or established major safety problem
- Benefit evaluation
  - Epidemiology and natural history of the target disease(s)
  - Purpose of treatment (cure, prophylaxis, etc.)
  - Summary of efficacy and general toleration data compared with
    - Other medical treatments
    - Surgical treatment or other interventions
    - No treatment
- Risk evaluation
  - Background
  - Weight of evidence for the suspected risk (incidence, etc.)
  - Detailed presentations and analyses of data on the new suspected risk
  - Probable and possible explanations
  - Preventability, predictability, and reversibility of the new risk
  - The issue as it relates to alternative therapies and no therapy
  - Review of the complete safety of the drug, using diagrammatic representations when possible (risk profiles); when appropriate, focus on selected subsets of serious AEs (e.g., the three most common and three most medically serious adverse reactions)
  - Provide similar profiles for alternate drugs
  - When possible, estimate the excess incidence of any adverse reactions known to be common to the alternatives
  - When there are significant adverse reactions that are not common to the drugs compared, highlight important differences between the drugs

- Benefit-risk evaluation
  - Summarize the benefits as related to the seriousness of the target disease and the purpose and effectiveness of treatment
  - Summarize the dominant risks (seriousness/severity, duration, incidence)
  - Summarize the benefit-risk relationship, quantitatively and diagrammatically if possible, taking into account the alternative therapies or no treatment
  - Provide a summary assessment and conclusion
- Options analysis
  - List all appropriate options for action
  - Describe the pros and cons and likely consequences (impact analysis) of each option under consideration, taking alternative therapies into account
  - If relevant, outline plans or suggestions for a study that could provide timely and important additional information
  - If feasible, indicate the quality and quantity of any future evidence that would signal the need for a reevaluation of the benefit-risk relationship
  - Suggest how the consequences of the recommended action should be monitored and assessed

Several examples of benefit-risk analyses are given (quinine and allergic hematologic events, felbamate and blood dyscrasias, dipyrone and agranulocytosis, temafloxacin and renal impairment and hypoglycemia, remoxipride and blood dyscrasias, clozapine and agranulocytosis, sparfloxacin and phototoxicity).

No example of a real benefit-risk report is given using this format. This type of report seems eminently possible in situations where the risk is small and there is no urgent or immediate action needed to protect the public health. However, in situations where immediate action is needed, usually in multiple markets around the world, the preparation of such a report is probably not feasible.

Several other guidelines and documents on benefit-risk analysis have been published since this CIOMS IV report by the FDA, European Medicines Evaluation Agency, ICH, and others (see Chapters 15-17). Most of these documents use similar conceptual frameworks for benefit-risk analyses but do not follow or propose the rigid CIOMS IV format. Clearly, however, this document served as a stimulus to a much closer and intense examination of benefit-risk analyses around the world. The document is worth reading, in particular for the specific case studies noted above.

CIOMS V (2001): Current Challenges in Pharmacovigilance: Pragmatic Approaches

The CIOMS V report is a 380-page document that covers a wide variety of current issues in drug safety. A summary of some of the proposals follows. Note that not all these recommendations are universally accepted or required.

The sources of individual case reports are recommended as follows:

- Traditionally, the primary source of safety information on marketed drugs was spontaneous reports, with occasional literature reports also appearing. New types of reports are now appearing, including Internet reports, solicited reports from patient support programs, surveys, epidemiologic studies, disease registries, regulatory and other databases, and licensor and licensee interactions. Consumer reports were often not analyzed unless medical validation was obtained.

The CIOMS V report makes various recommendations, some of which are noted below:

- Consumer reports
  - Consumer reports should be scrutinized and should receive appropriate attention.
  - The quality of a report is more important than its source.
  - Spontaneous reports are always considered to have an implied causal relationship to the drug.
  - Respect privacy and the laws and regulations governing it.
  - If a report is received from a third party, that party should be asked to encourage the consumer to report the information to his or her physician or to authorize the sponsor/authority to contact the physician directly.
  - All efforts should be made to obtain medical confirmation of serious unexpected consumer reports. The regulators may be in a better position to get this information if companies have been unsuccessful.
  - If an event is considered not to be drug related, it should be retained in the company database but not reported.
  - Even in the absence of medical confirmation, any ADR with significant implications for the medicine's benefit-risk relationship should be submitted on an expedited and/or periodic basis.

- Consumer reports should be included in PSURs in an appendix or as a statement indicating they have been reviewed and do or do not suggest new findings.
- Literature
  - Cases may appear in letters to the editor.
  - There may be a long lag time between the first detection of a signal by a researcher and his or her publication of it.
  - Publications may be a source of false information and signals.
  - Companies should search at least two internationally recognized literature databases using the International Normalized Nomenclature name at least monthly.
  - Broadcast and lay media should not ordinarily be monitored. If such information is made available to the company, it should be followed up.
  - Judgment should be used in regard to follow-up with the strongest efforts made for serious unexpected ADRs.
  - If the product source or brand is not specified, a company should assume it was its product. The company should indicate in any report made that the specific brand was not identified if this is the case.
  - If there is a contractual agreement between two or more companies (e.g., for comarketing), the contract should specify the responsibility for literature searches and reporting.
  - English should be the standard language for literature report translations.
  - Regulators should accept translation of an abstract or pertinent sections of a publication.
  - References cited in a publication on apparently unexpected/unlisted and serious reactions should be checked against the company's existing database of literature reports. Articles not previously reported should be retrieved and reviewed as usual. Routine tracking down of all such sources is unrealistic unless faced with a major safety issue.
  - The clock starts when a case is recognized to be a valid case (reporter, patient, drug, event).
- The Internet
  - Protection of privacy is particularly important regarding Internet cases.
  - A blank ADR form should be provided on a website to facilitate reporting.
- A procedure should be in place to ensure daily screening of a company's or regulator's website(s) to identify potential case reports.
- Companies and regulators do not need to routinely surf the net beyond their own sites other than to actively monitor relevant special home pages (e.g., disease groups) if there is a significant safety issue.
- The message should be consistent around the world because the Internet does not respect geographic (or linguistic) boundaries.
- Solicited reports
  - Solicited ADR reports arising in the course of interaction with patients should be regarded as distinct from spontaneous unsolicited reports.
  - They should be processed separately and so identified in expedited and periodic reporting.
  - To satisfy postmarketing regulations, solicited reports should be handled in the same way as study reports: Causality assessments are needed. Serious unexpected ADRs should be reported on an expedited basis.
  - Serious expected and nonserious solicited reports should be kept in the safety database and reported to regulators on request.
  - Signals may arise from solicited reports so they should be reviewed on an ongoing basis.
- Aspects of clinical trial reports
  - Generally, safety information reported expeditiously to regulatory authorities should be reported to all phase I, II, and III investigators who are conducting research with any form of the product and for any indication.
  - It is less important to notify phase IV investigators; they will ordinarily use the available up-to-date local official data sheet as part of the investigator's brochure.
  - Quality of life studies should be handled like clinical trial data.
- Epidemiology: observational studies and use of secondary databases
  - Structured epidemiologic studies should have the same reporting rules for suspected ADR cases as clinical trials.
  - For epidemiologic studies, unless there is specific attribution in an individual case, its expedited reporting is generally not appropriate.
  - If relevant, studies should be summarized in PSURs.

- Promptly notify regulators (within 15 days) if a study result shows an important safety issue (e.g., a greater risk of a known serious ADR for one drug versus another).

- For manufacturers, expedited reports from comparator drug data should be forwarded to the relevant manufacturer(s) for their regulatory reporting as appropriate.

- Disease-specific registries and regulatory ADR databases

  - A registry is not a study. Cases should be treated as solicited reports (causality assessment required).

  - Although there are numerous ADR databases created by regulatory authorities, it is unnecessary to attempt to routinely collect them for regular review. If a company is in possession of data from a regulatory database, it should review those data promptly for any required expedited reporting. Careful screening should be done to avoid duplicates.

  - It is advisable to mention in the PSUR that the databases have been examined even if no relevant cases have been found.

- Licenser-licensee interactions

  - When companies codevelop, comarket, or co-promote products, it is critical that explicit contractual agreements specify processes for exchange of safety information, including timelines and regulatory reporting responsibilities.

  - The time frame for expedited regulatory reporting should normally be no longer than 15 calendar days from the first receipt of a valid case by any of the partners.

  - The original recipient of a suspected ADR should ideally conduct any necessary follow-up; any subsequent follow-up information sent to the regulators should be submitted by the same company that reported the case originally.

- Clinical case evaluation

  - The company or regulatory authority staff can propose alternate clinical terms and interpretations of the case from those of the reporter, but unless the original reporter alters his or her original description in writing, the original terms must also be reported.

  - When a case is reported by a consumer, his or her clinical description should be retained even if confirmatory or additional information from a health care professional is obtained.

- There is an important distinction between a suspected ADR and an "incidental" event. An incidental event is one that occurs in reasonable clinical temporal association with the use of the drug product but is not the intended subject of the spontaneous report (it did not prompt the contact with the company or regulator). There is also no implicit or explicit expression of possible drug causality by the reporter or the company's safety review staff. They should be included as part of the medical history and not be the subject of expedited reporting. Incidental events should be captured in the company database.

- Assessing patient and reporter identities

  - When cases do not meet the minimum criteria (patient, reporter, event, drug) even after follow-up, the case should be kept in the database as an "incomplete case."

  - The regulatory reporting clock starts in the European Union at the first contact with a health care professional, but in the United States and Canada it starts when the case is initially reported to the company, even by a consumer.

  - One or more automatically qualify a patient as identifiable: age, age category (e.g., teenager), sex, initials, date of birth, name, or patient number.

  - Even in the absence of such qualifying descriptors, a report referring to a definite number of patients should be regarded as a case as long as the other criteria for validity are met. For example "Two patients experienced..." but **not** "A few patients experienced...."

  - For serious, unexpected, suspected reactions, the threshold for reporting in the absence of confirmatory identity should be lowered.

- Criteria for seriousness

  - Hospitalization refers to admission as an inpatient and not to an examination and/or treatment as an outpatient.

  - All congenital anomalies and birth defects, without regard to their nature or severity, should be considered serious.

  - There is a lack of objective standards for "life threatening" and "medical judgment" as seriousness criteria; both require individual professional evaluation that invariably introduces a lack of reproducibility.

■ Within a company the tools, lists, and decision-making processes should be harmonized globally.

■ Criteria for expectedness

■ The terminology associated with expectedness depends on which reference safety document is being used and for what purpose:

• "Listed" or "unlisted" refers to the ADRs contained in the CSI for a marketed product or within the development CSI (DCSI) in the investigator's brochure.

• "Labeled" or "unlabeled" refers to the ADRs contained in official product safety information for marketed products (e.g., summary of product characteristics in the European Union or the package insert in the United States).

■ Determining whether a reported reaction is expected or not is a two-step process: first, is the reaction term already included in the CSI? Second, is the ADR different regarding its nature, severity, specificity, or outcome?

■ Expectedness should be strictly based on inclusion of a drug associated experience in the ADR section of the CSI. Special types of reactions, such as those occurring under conditions of overdose, drug interaction, or pregnancy, should also be included in this section.

■ Disorders mentioned in "contraindications" or "precautions" as reasons for not treating with the drug are not expected ADRs unless they also appear in the ADR section.

■ If an ADR has been reported only in association with an overdose, it should be considered unexpected if it occurs at a normal dose.

■ For a marketed drug CSI, events cited in data from clinical trials are not considered expected unless they are included in the ADR section.

■ For expedited reporting on marketed drugs, local approved product information is the reference document for expectedness (labeledness).

■ For periodic reporting (PSUR), the CSI is the reference document for expectedness (listedness).

■ Disclaimer statements for causality (e.g., "X has been reported but the relationship with the drug has not been established") are discouraged; however, even if used, the reaction X is still unexpected.

■ Class labeling does not count as "expected" unless the event in question is included in the ADR section.

■ Lack of expected efficacy is not relevant to whether an AE is expected or not.

■ If the treatment exacerbates the target indication, it would be unexpected unless already detailed in the CSI.

■ Unless the CSI specifies a fatal outcome for an ADR, the case is unexpected as long as there was an association between the reaction and the fatality.

■ Case follow-up approaches

■ Highest priority for follow-up are cases that are serious and unexpected followed by serious, expected and nonserious, unexpected.

■ Cases "of special interest" (e.g., ADRs under active surveillance at the request of the regulators) also deserve high priority as well as any cases that might lead to a labeling change.

■ For any cases with legal implications, the company's legal department should be involved.

■ When the case is serious and if the ADR has not resolved at the time of the initial report, it is important to continue follow-up until the outcome has been established or the condition stabilized. How long to follow up such cases requires judgment.

■ It is recommended that collaboration with other companies be done if more than one company's drug is suspected as a causal agent in a case.

■ Follow-up for unexpected deaths and life-threatening cases should be done within 24 hours.

■ If a reporter fails to respond to the first follow-up attempt, reminder letters should be sent as follows:

• A single follow-up letter for any nonserious expected case.

• For all other cases, a second follow-up letter should be sent no later than 4 weeks after the first letter.

• In general, when the reporter fails to respond or is incompletely cooperative, the two follow-up letters should reflect sufficient due diligence.

■ Role of narratives

■ A company case narrative is different from the reporter's clinical description of a case, though the reporter's comments should be an integral part of the company narrative. The reporter's verbatim words should be included for the adverse reactions.

- Alternate causes to that given by the reporter should be described and identified as a company opinion.
- The same evaluation should be supplied to all regulators.
- Narratives should be prepared for all serious (expected and unexpected) and nonserious unexpected cases but not for nonserious expected cases.
- Narratives should be written in the third person past tense. All relevant information should be in a logical time sequence.
- In general, abbreviations (except laboratory parameters and units) and acronyms should not be used.
- Time to onset of an event from the start of treatment should be given in the most appropriate time units (e.g., hours), but actual dates can be used if helpful to the reader.
- If detailed supplementary records are important to a case (e.g., autopsy report), their availability should be mentioned in the narrative.
- Information may be supplied by more than one person (e.g., initial reporter and supplementary information from a specialist); all sources should be specified.
- When there is conflicting information provided from different sources, this should be mentioned and the sources identified.
- If it is suspected that an ADR resulted from misprescribing (e.g., wrong drug or wrong dose) or other medication error, judgmental comments should not be included in the narrative due to legal implications. Only the facts should be stated (e.g., "four times the normal dose was administered," "the prescription was misread and a contraindicated drug for this patient was given").
- The narrative should have eight sections that serve as a comprehensive stand-alone "medical story":
  - Source of the report and patient demography
  - Medical and drug history
  - Suspect drug(s), timing and conditions surrounding the onset of the reaction(s)
  - The progression of the event(s) and their outcome in the patient
  - If the outcome is fatal, the relevant details
  - Rechallenge information, if applicable
  - The original reporter's clinical assessment
  - The narrative preparer's medical evaluation and comment
- PSURs: content modification
  - For reports covering long time periods (e.g., 5 years), it is more practical to use the CSI current at the time of PSUR preparation.
  - Clinical trial data should be supplied only if they suggest a signal or are relevant to a possible change in the benefit-risk relationship.
  - If >200 individual case reports, submit only summary tabulations and not line listings (which may be supplied on request by the regulator).
  - For 5-year reports, follow-up information on cases described in the previous report should be provided only for cases associated with new or ongoing safety issues.
  - Inclusion of literature reports should be selective and cover publications relevant to safety findings, independent of listedness.
  - For PSURs with large numbers of case, discussion and analysis for the overall safety evaluation should be by system organ class rather than by listedness or seriousness.
  - An abbreviated PSUR saves time and resources if little or no new safety information is generated during the time period covered. Criteria for an abbreviated report:
    - No serious unlisted cases
    - Few (e.g., ≤10) serious listed cases
    - No significant regulatory actions for safety
    - No major changes to the CSI
    - No findings that lead to a new action
- PSURs: a bridging report
  - A summary bridging report is a concise document that provides no new information and integrates two or more previously prepared PSURs to cover a specified period.
  - Its format follows that of a regular PSUR, but the content should consist of summary highlights of the reports being summarized.
- PSURs: an addendum report
  - This report is prepared on special request of the regulators to satisfy regulators who require

reports covering a period outside the routine PSUR reporting cycle (e.g., if the reports are based on the local approval date in that country rather than on the IBD).

- It updates the most recently completed PSUR.
- It follows the usual PSUR format.

- PSURs: miscellaneous proposals
  - A brief (e.g., one-page) stand-alone overview (executive summary) should be provided.
  - Manufacturers should be allowed to select the IBDs for their old products to facilitate synchronization of PSURs.
  - If there is no CSI for an old product, the most suitable local labeling should be considered for use.
  - The evaluation of cases in a PSUR should focus on unlisted ADRs with analyses organized primarily by system organ class (body system).
  - Discussion of serious unlisted cases should include cumulative data.
  - Complicated PSURs and those with extensive new data may require more than 60 days to prepare adequately and the regulators should be flexible.
  - The possibility of "resetting" the PSUR clock (from annual to semiannual reports as the result of a new indication or dosage form) should be allowed by the regulators.

- PSURs: population data
  - Detailed calculations on exposure (the denominator) are ordinarily unnecessary, especially given the unreliability of the numerator; rough estimates usually suffice, but the method and units used should be explained clearly.
  - Drug exposure data are approximate and usually represent an overestimate.
  - For special situations, such as when dealing with an important safety signal, attempts should be made to obtain exposure information covering the relevant covariates (e.g., age, gender, race, indication, dosing details).

CIOMS VI (2005): Management of Safety Information from Clinical Trials

The CIOMS VI working group focused on clinical trial safety, which represents a departure from the focus of the earlier working groups that concentrated primarily on postmarketing safety issues. The report, available from the CIOMS office in Geneva, like the CIOMS V report,

runs some 300 pages. The most important points are summarized here. The reader is referred to the report itself for further detail. Keep in mind that these recommendations are quite new and have not been put into regulations in all jurisdictions.

General Principles and Ethical Considerations

- The concepts of pharmacovigilance presented here apply to trials in phases I through IV.
- Any study that is not scientifically sound should be considered unethical.
- Informed consent is the cornerstone of human subject research, but there are situations where it is either not possible or appropriate (such as in anonymous tissue sample studies, epidemiologic research, or emergency treatment protocols).

Systematic Approach to Managing Safety Data

- The concepts of pharmacovigilance, risk management, assessment, and minimization should be applied to the study phases and the postmarketing period. Sponsors must have in place a well-defined process to readily identify, evaluate, and minimize potential safety risks. The process should start before the first phase I study. A formal development risk management plan should be developed.
- A dedicated safety management team should be formed for each development program to review safety information on a regular basis so that decisions can be made in a timely manner. The review should be at least quarterly, and the team should consider changes to the investigator's brochure, informed consent, and protocol as needed.
- When licensing partners are involved, a joint safety committee should be created with clear roles and responsibilities. This should ideally be defined in the initial contract. A project management function should be set up to ensure scheduling, tracking, and timelines.
- All pertinent data must be readily available from the clinical trial and safety databases as well as preclinical toxicology, mutagenicity, pharmacokinetic, pharmacodynamic, and drug interaction data.
- Epidemiology should be incorporated into the planning process.
- Certain toxicities should be considered for all new drugs, including abnormalities of cardiac conduction, hepatotoxicity, drug interactions, immunogenicity, bone marrow toxicity, and reactive metabolite formation.

Data Collection and Management

- The investigator should report (immediately if judged critical) to the sponsor any information that is considered to be important in regard to safety even if the protocol does not call for it. The sponsor must carefully train the investigative site in this matter.

- The collection of "excessive" data can have a negative impact on data quality. Case report form fields should collect only those data that can be analyzed and presented in tabular form. All other data should be collected as text comments.

- Safety monitoring in phase IV studies may not require the same intensity as for phase I-III trials, but the same principles and practices should apply.

- If a company provides any support for an independent trial it does not sponsor (investigator-initiated studies/trials), the company should still obtain at a minimum all serious suspected adverse reactions. The company should do its own causality assessment and, if appropriate, report it to the health authorities even if the investigator has already done so.

- In the early phases of drug development, it is often necessary to collect more comprehensive safety data than in postmarketing studies. Some studies may require longer follow-up.

- Phase I data are especially important because these data are collected in healthy volunteers and are critical to the future development of the drug.

- There is no definitive way to determine causality of a particular AE. That is, its attribution to the drug or to a background finding with only a temporal association cannot be definitively done. Thus the following is recommended:

  - All AEs, both serious and nonserious, are collected whether believed to be related or not. This applies to the experimental product, placebo, no treatment, and active comparators.

  - Similarly, studies initiated during the immediate postapproval period should continue this practice. Once the safety profile is judged to be well understood, it may be possible to collect less data (e.g., nonserious AEs believed not to be due to the drug).

- The use of herbal and other nontraditional treatments should be sought when data are being collected in all studies.

- Although causality assessments based on aggregate data or case series are usually more meaningful than those based on individual cases, the investigator causality assessment should be done and may play a role in the early detection of significant safety events, especially rare ones.

- The investigator should be asked to use a "simple binary decision" for drug causality of serious AEs: related or not related; reasonable possibility or no reasonable possibility, and so on. The use of the words "unknown" or "cannot be ruled out" should be avoided.

- Causality for nonserious AEs should not be requested from investigators routinely.

- Where appropriate, the investigator should supply a diagnosis rather than signs and symptoms. However, when a diagnosis is supplied for a serious AE, the accompanying signs and symptoms should be recorded.

- Before starting a study, AEs of special interest and anticipated AEs (if known) should be communicated to the investigator. This is less critical for nonserious AEs unless they are prodromes of more serious conditions (e.g., muscle pain and creatine phosphokinase elevation as a possible prodrome of rhabdomyolysis).

- Medically serious clinical events that are recorded in a trial as clinical efficacy outcomes or endpoints should be reviewed by the sponsor and data monitoring committee even though they are not considered AEs.

- It is preferable to frame questions to patients in general terms rather than suggesting that the study treatment was responsible for reported AEs. Although a "laundry list" of AEs should not be read to the patient, patients should be alerted to known issues of medically important suspected or established AEs to alert the investigator as soon as possible.

- Data collection should start from the time of the signing of the informed consent.

- Safety data event collection should continue after the last dose of the drug for at least an additional five half-lives of the experimental product.

- General rules for data quality:

  - Cases should be as fully documented as possible.

  - There should be diligent follow-up of each case.

  - The reporter's verbatim terms should be captured and retained.

  - If the reporter's terms are considered inaccurate or inconsistent with standard medical terminology, attempts should be made to clarify them. If disagreement continues, the sponsor should code the AE terms according to its judgment but identify them as distinct from the reporter's terms and reasons for differences noted.

- Primary analyses of the data should be done using the reporter's terms. Additional analyses may be done using the sponsor's terms. Any differences must be noted and explained.

- Individual case safety reports should be categorized and assessed by the sponsor using trained individuals with broad experience. Investigators should obtain specialist consultation for clinically important events that fall outside their expertise.

- AE tables may display both the reported investigator's verbatim term and the sponsor's terms.

- The sponsor (as well as health authorities) may wish to consider the use of a listing of event terms that are always regarded as serious and important. Such events then routinely trigger special attention and evaluation.

- Cases should not be "overcoded" using more terms than minimally necessary to ensure retrieval of the cases. Similarly, cases should not be "undercoded" where the terms chosen downgrade the severity or importance of events.

Risk Identification and Evaluation

Ongoing Safety Evaluation

- Sponsors should develop a system to assess, evaluate, and act on safety information on a continuous basis during drug development to ensure the earliest possible identification of safety concerns to allow risk minimization.

- The integrity of the studies should not be compromised by the safety monitoring and analysis.

Safety Data Management

- Safety data should be handled using consistent standards and criteria with care and precision.

- Safety evaluations must be individualized for each product because there are no standard approaches to evaluating or measuring "an acceptable level of risk."

Review of Safety Information

- Safety data analysis should involve both individual case reports as well as aggregate data. Individual cases should be reviewed within specified time frames and aggregate data on a periodic basis.

- The evaluation should be done in the context of the patient population, the indication studied, the natural history of the disease, and currently available therapies.

- Causality determinations should be done for all reported cases. The investigator causality assessment should be taken into account.

- AEs of special interest should be identified in the protocol and handled as if they are serious even if they do not meet the regulatory definition of serious.

- Nonserious AEs should be reviewed to see whether there are events of special interest with particular attention paid to those associated with study discontinuation.

Frequency of Review of Safety Information

- Safety review of all data should be done frequently:
  - Ad hoc for serious and special interest AEs
  - Routine periodic review of all data whose frequency varies from trial to trial or program to program
  - Reviews triggered by specific trial or program milestones
  - At the time of study completion and unblinding

Analysis and Evaluation

- Subgroup analysis, though possibly limited by small sample size, should be done for dose, duration, gender, age, concomitant medications, and concurrent diseases.

- Data pooling should include studies that are of similar design. This can include all controlled studies, placebo-controlled studies, studies with any positive control, studies with a particular positive control, and particular indications.

- If the duration of treatment varies widely among participants, data on the effect of treatment duration should be analyzed.

Statistical Approaches

- The techniques for use of statistics for analyzing safety data are less well developed than for efficacy.

- Statistical association (probability values) alone may or may not be of clinical value. Examination of both statistical and clinical significance must involve a partnership between the statistical and clinical experts.

- It may be necessary to acknowledge when the data are insufficient to draw conclusions on safety: "absence of evidence is not evidence of absence."

- There are several large sections of this report devoted to specific statistical situations and techniques, and the reader is referred to the report for further detail.

Regulatory Reporting and Communications of Safety Information from Clinical Trials

The working group notes, in bold type, that these recommendations are only proposals and do not supersede current regulations. They represent proposals for discussion.

- The group endorses ICH Guideline E2A (see Chapter 26) and recommends the harmonization of criteria for expedited reporting whereby such reporting to authorities should include only suspected ADRs that are both serious and unexpected. Only under exceptional circumstances should other cases (i.e., expected cases) be submitted as expedited reports. If reporting without regard to causality is required, it should be done on a periodic basis with clearly defined timelines and format.

- The regulators should adopt the phrase "a reasonable possibility of a causal relationship" and not use the ICH E2A phrase of "a causal relationship cannot be ruled out" in regard to suspected ADRs.

- Once a drug is marketed, the company CSI (CCSI) document should be used as the reference safety document for determining expectedness for regulatory reporting of phase IV trials. For new indication trials the DCSI document should be used. The two documents should be aligned as much as possible.

- As with spontaneous reports, reportability for case reports from trials should be determined at the event level. That is, a case would be expedited if there is a suspected adverse reaction that is serious and unexpected.

- Suspected ADRs that are serious and unexpected and thus are expedited reports should, in general, be unblinded. There may be certain circumstances where this should not occur, however (e.g., serious AEs that are also efficacy endpoints). Such exceptions should be agreed on by the regulatory authorities and be clearly described in the investigator brochure and the protocol.

- Unblinded placebo cases should not be reported to regulatory authorities as expedited cases. Unblinded (and open label) comparator drug cases should be reported to the regulatory authorities and/or the company owning the comparator on an expedited basis whether expected or not.

- Seven-day reports should be limited to cases from clinical trials and not spontaneous reports. This should apply both in countries where the drug is approved and where it is only under clinical study.

- The sponsor should develop clear standard operating procedures for the expedited or prompt reporting of other safety issues with special attention to when the clock starts for
  - Nonclinical safety issues that might have implications for human subjects
  - A higher incidence of a serious AE for the drug compared with the comparator or the background rate in the general population
  - An increased frequency of a previously recognized serious adverse reaction
  - A significant drug interaction in a pharmacokinetic study
  - AEs that are deemed not to be drug related but are considered study related

- Contrary to established regulations, the working group recommends that routine expedited cases reported to investigators and investigational review boards (IRBs)/ethics committees (as opposed to reports to regulatory authorities) be eliminated and replaced with regular updates of the evolving benefit-risk profile highlighting new safety information.
  - For unapproved products, the reports to investigators and IRBs should include a line listing of unblinded clinical trial cases that were expedited to regulatory agencies during this time period, a copy of the current DCSI with an explanation of changes, and a brief summary of the emerging safety profile. Quarterly updates are the "default" with other frequencies as appropriate.
  - For approved products, the reports to investigators and IRBs should be quarterly if the product is in phase III trials. For well-established products, a less frequent interval would be acceptable. At some point, only investigators and IRBs would need to be updated for significant new information. For phase IV investigators and IRBs, only changes to the CCSI would be needed.
  - The reports, whether for approved or unapproved products, should include in the line listings only unblinded expedited reports from trials and include only interval data (i.e., changes since the last update). A summary of the emerging safety profile should be included with cumulative data as needed. MedDRA should be used. The listings should not include spontaneous reports, which should be described in narrative form in the update.

- Should a significant safety issue be identified (i.e., an issue that has a significant impact on the course of the clinical trial or program or warrants immediate update of the informed consent), the sponsor should promptly notify the regulatory authorities, investigators, IRBs, and, if relevant, data safety monitoring committees.

- A safety management team should review all safety data on a regular basis: quarterly before approval and coordinate with the PSUR schedule postapproval. Ad-hoc meetings would occur as needed to address urgent safety issues and signals. They would review the overall evolving safety profile to make changes to the DCSI, informed consent, and protocol as needed.

- A single Development Safety Update Report (DSUR) should be submitted to regulators annually. The format and content would be defined and would cover the drug product, not just a single study.

- For marketed products with well-established safety profiles and for which most trials are in phase IV in the approved indications, the PSUR would replace the DSUR.

- Sponsors should incorporate the DCSI into every investigator brochure, either as a special section of the investigator brochure or as an attachment. The sponsor should clearly identify the events for which the company believes there is sufficient evidence to suspect a drug relationship. These events would be considered expected ("listed") for regulatory reporting criteria.

- The investigator brochure and DCSI should be reviewed and updated at least annually.

- If the developer or manufacturer of a product is not the sponsor of a particular trial but rather supports an external clinical or nonclinical investigator-sponsored study, a provision of any agreement should be the prompt reporting to the company of all serious suspected ADRs in humans or significant findings in animals.

- As with the CCSI for marketed drugs (see CIOMS III/VI), the same threshold criteria should be applied to the DCSI and informed consent in preapproval drugs.

- Informed consent should be renewed with the subjects whenever there is new information that could affect the subjects' willingness to participate in the trial. In certain circumstances, a more immediate communication may be appropriate.

CIOMS VII (Ongoing): DSUR

This working group has been at work since 1995 and hopes to establish specifics for the format and content of the DSUR and establish links to the PSURs that will be written after the marketing of the drug. See the CIOMS website for updates on this topic.

International Conference on Harmonization Reports

> **NOTE:** (Unless otherwise noted, the word "drug" or "drug product" should be taken in this book to include "biologics" and "vaccines.")

This chapter summarizes what the International Conference on Harmonization (ICH) is and the reports issued by the various working groups that are related to drug safety. These reports have been used as the basis for the creation of certain safety regulations in North America, Europe, Japan, and elsewhere. They are worth taking the time to review. Keep in mind that not all proposals from the ICH were adopted nor were those that were adopted necessarily taken directly and without change by national regulatory authorities.

The documents in question are

- E2A: Clinical Safety Data Management: Definitions and Standards for Expedited Reporting
- E2B: Maintenance of the Clinical Safety Data Management, including the Maintenance of the

Electronic Transmission of Individual Case Safety Reports Message Specification
- E2C: Clinical Safety Data Management: Periodic Safety Update Reports for Marketed Drugs
- E2CA Addendum to E2C: Periodic Safety Update Reports for Marketed Drugs
- E2D: Postapproval Safety Data Management: Definitions and Standards for Expedited Reporting
- E2E: Pharmacovigilance Planning

They can be found at Web Resource 26-1.

■ Clinical Safety Data Management: Definitions and Standards for Expedited Reporting (E2A)

This document was adopted by the ICH in October 1994 as a "step 4" document, meaning that it is recommended for adoption by the regulatory bodies of the European Union, Japan, and the United States (US Food and Drug Administration [FDA], *Federal Register* 1995;60:11284-11287).

E2A combines many concepts from the Council for International Organizations of Medical Sciences (CIOMS) I and CIOMS II documents covering the development of standard definitions and terminology for safety reporting and the appropriate mechanism for handling expedited (alert) reporting. This document was originally developed to cover primarily the investigational phase of drug development, but its concepts have been extended to cover postmarketing (approved) drugs also. See document E2E below.

The definitions and recommendations for expedited reporting developed in this document have largely been accepted throughout the world. However, some of the recommendations have been tried and withdrawn (e.g., increased frequency reporting in the United States), inconsistently applied (e.g., breaking the blind), or never applied (reporting an expedited case to all open Investigational New Drug Applications [INDs]).

Definitions

Adverse event (AE) (or adverse experience): "Any untoward medical occurrence in a patient or clinical investigation subject administered a pharmaceutical product and which does not necessarily have to have a causal relationship with this treatment."

Adverse drug reaction (ADR): "In the pre-approval clinical experience with a new medicinal product or its new usages, particularly as the therapeutic dose(s) may not be established: all noxious and unintended responses to a medicinal product related to any dose should be considered adverse drug reactions. For marketed products: A response to a drug which is noxious and unintended and which occurs at doses normally used in man for prophylaxis, diagnosis, or therapy of disease or for modification of physiological function."

Unexpected ADR: "An adverse reaction, the nature or severity of which is not consistent with the applicable product information (e.g., Investigator's Brochure for an unapproved investigational medicinal product)." Note that this applies to nonmarketed drugs. This definition was extended to marketed drugs in E2E (see below).

"Serious" and "severe": The terms serious and severe are differentiated: The term "severe" is often used to describe the intensity (severity) of a specific event (as in mild, moderate, or severe myocardial infarction); the event itself, however, may be of relatively minor medical significance (such as severe headache). This is not the same as "serious," which is based on patient/event outcome or action criteria usually associated with events that pose a threat to a patient's life or functioning. Seriousness (not severity) serves as a guide for defining regulatory reporting obligations.

Serious: "A serious adverse event (experience) or reaction is any untoward medical occurrence that at any dose results in death, is life-threatening, requires in-patient hospitalisation or prolongation of existing hospitalisation, results in persistent or significant disability/incapacity or is a congenital anomaly/birth defect.

"Medical and scientific judgment should be exercised in deciding whether expedited reporting is appropriate in other situations, such as important medical events that may not be immediately life-threatening or result in death or hospitalization but may jeopardize the patient or may require intervention to prevent one of the other outcomes listed in the definition above. These should also usually be considered serious." Note that "cancer" and "overdose" have been removed. These terms appeared in various pre-1995 definitions of "serious."

What Should Be Reported to Regulatory Authorities as Expedited Reports?

All ADRs that are both serious and unexpected are subject to expedited reporting. This applies to reports from spontaneous sources and from any type of clinical or epidemiologic investigation, independent of design or purpose.

- Note that this means all adverse reactions (i.e., causally related to the drug) that are serious and unexpected. Thus it requires all three categories (causality, seriousness, and unexpectedness) for clinical trial cases. Although not explicitly stated in this document, for postmarketing cases the causality is implied (i.e., all spontaneous reports are presumed to be causally related), and thus only two criteria need to be examined: seriousness and expectedness.

- No international standard exists for causality classification.

- An increased frequency of a known serious ADR should be reported in an expedited fashion.

- A significant hazard to the patient population such as lack of efficacy with a medicinal product used in a life-threatening disease.

- A major safety finding from a newly completed animal study.

Reporting Time Frames

- Fatal or life-threatening ADRs: 7 calendar days by phone or fax followed 8 calendar days later with an expedited 15-day report.

- Other serious unexpected ADRs: 15 calendar days after the first knowledge by the sponsor that the case meets the minimum criteria for reporting.

Minimum Criteria for Reporting

- An identifiable patient
- A suspect medicinal product
- An identifiable reporting source
- An event or outcome that is serious and unexpected and, for clinical trial cases, a reasonable suspected causal relationship

Follow-up information should be sought and reported as soon as it becomes available.

The CIOMS I form should be used to report the cases.

Managing Blinded Cases

This report recommends that although advantageous to retain the blind for all patients before study analysis, when a serious adverse reaction is reportable on an expedited basis, the blind should be broken only for that specific patient by the sponsor even if the investigator has not broken the blind. The blind should be maintained where possible for the personnel in the company responsible for the analysis and interpretation of the results. There may be circumstances where not breaking the blind is desirable, and in these circumstances, an agreement with the regulatory authorities should be pursued.

Other Issues

- For reactions with comparators, the sponsor is responsible for deciding whether to report the case to the other manufacturer and/or to the appropriate regulatory agencies. Placebo events do not normally need to be reported.

  ➡ NOTE: (Note that some regulatory agencies do require placebo reporting and the reporting of any "study-related" cases.)

- When a drug has more than one presentation (e.g., different dosage forms, formulations, delivery systems) or uses (different indications or different populations), the expedited report should be reported to or referenced to all other product presentations and uses.

  ➡ NOTE: (Note that this is generally not the case currently. Reporting is usually to only one IND or premarketing dossier in most countries should multiple INDs or dossiers exist.)

- Poststudy AEs are usually not collected or sought by sponsors but may nonetheless be reported to the sponsor by the investigator. These events should be treated as if they were study events and reported as expedited reports should they qualify to be such.

■ Data Elements for Transmission of Individual Case Safety Reports (E2B) and Message Specification Technical Details (M2)

Two working groups were set up in the ICH to develop the means for the electronic transmission of individual case safety reports between or among companies and regulators, regulators and regulators, and companies and companies. This system would allow the (theoretical) replacement of paper-based submissions using MedWatch or CIOMS I forms. To do this the data elements, fields, and contents of the electronic report needed to be rigidly standardized. There are two series of documents in question.

The first are the E2B documents, which were prepared by the medical representatives and specified data elements for the transmission. The second are the M2 documents, prepared by the informatics representatives and that provide technical specifications for structured messaging; electronic data interchange; data definitions to incorporate structured data formats (e.g., SGML); security to ensure confidentiality, data integrity, authentication, and nonrepudiation; documents to handle heterogeneous data formats; and physical media for storage and transferability of data. These are available at Web Resource 26-2.

Several documents were issued and the nomenclature is a bit confusing.

The E2B ("Medical") Documents

- E2B (M): Maintenance of the Clinical Safety Data Management including Data Elements for Transmission of Individual Case Safety Reports
  - This document was finalized (a "step 4" document) in July 1997 and amended for Maintenance on November 10, 2000.
  - Posted on the FDA website (Web Resource 26-3) on April 4, 2002.
- E2B(R): Revision of the E2B(M) ICH Guideline on Clinical Safety Data Management: Data Elements for Transmission of Individual Case Safety Reports

- This guideline provides additional information and clarification as well as some modifications to the above ICH E2B guideline signed off in July 1997 and modified in November 2000. It incorporates adjustments based on the experience gained after the implementation of the guideline in the three regions.
  - Published by the FDA in the *Federal Register* (2005;70:57610-57611). Deadline for comments by October 28, 2005.
- E2B(M): Maintenance of the Clinical Safety Data Management including Questions and Answers
  - Since reaching step 4 and publication within the ICH regions as E2B(M) in November 2000, experiences by all parties with the implementation of the First Revision of the E2B(M) Guideline resulted in the need for some further technical clarification. This supplementary Questions and Answers document intends to clarify key issues.
  - Posted on the FDA website at Web Resource 26-4 on March 16, 2005.

The M2 (Informatics) Documents

- SGML DTD (Document Type Definition), Version 1.0 and related files for structured electronic data interchange data
- DTD Version 2.0, ICSR Acknowledgment Message and related files
- DTD Version 2.1, ICSR Acknowledgment Message and related files, which includes M2 Version 2.3 Specification Document

Personnel involved in drug safety should be familiar with the E2B documents, and the informatics personnel supporting them should be familiar with M2, in addition. The contents of the E2B transmissions determine to a certain degree how data are handled and stored in a company's database. For example, decisions must be made on whether to code laboratory data as free text or as structured fields.

We briefly review here the data elements of the E2B documents. The goal of the E2B document is to provide all the data elements needed to comprehensively cover complex reports from most sources, different data sets, and transmission requirements. Not all cases have all data elements available. Thus simple cases have very few elements transmitted, and complex cases have many or most of the elements transmitted.

Structured data are strongly recommended and are available for AE terms and other elements using the *Medical*

Dictionary for Regulatory Activities (MedDRA). However, structured vocabularies for other elements (e.g., drug names) are not yet available, finalized, or agreed on. The E2B document also allows for unstructured text to be transmitted (e.g., narratives) and in some cases allows data to be transmitted as structured or unstructured data (e.g., laboratory values).

There are two sections to a transmission. The first is the header, which contains technical information, and the second is the data elements in two parts: first the administrative and identification information and second the case information. The data elements are described briefly here.

A1. Identification of the case safety report
  - Case unique identifier number and MedDRA version
  - Source country; country where the AE occurred
  - Date of transmission
  - Type of report (spontaneous, study other)
  - Seriousness
  - Date of latest information
  - List of other documents held by sender
  - Expedited report?
  - Other identifying numbers for the case (e.g., local health authority numbers)

A2. Sources
  - Reporter name, address, profession
  - Literature reference
  - Clinical study information (name, type, study number)

A3. Sender Information
  - Type: company, regulatory authority, health care professional, World Health Organization, and so on
  - Sender identifier, address, e-mail, and so on

B1. Patient characteristics
  - Identifier, age, date of birth, age at reaction onset, weight, height, sex
  - Medical and drug history and concurrent conditions (either structured or as free text)
  - Death information
  - Parent-child report information

B2. Reaction(s)/event(s): This is a repeating section so that a new section can be created for each reaction/event.
  - Verbatim term, MedDRA lower level term, term highlighted by reporter

- Seriousness criterion
- Start and stop dates and outcome

B3. Tests and procedures (and their results) done to investigate

B4. Drug information
- Drug type (suspect, concomitant, interacting, blinded, etc.)
- Drug name, active ingredient
- Authorization (New Drug Application) holder and (New Drug Application) number
- Dose, start date, route of administration, indication for use, action taken
- Drug-reaction matrix for causality (to capture causality at the event level and a reporter and company causality)

B5. Narrative (clinical course, therapeutic measures, outcome, and additional relevant information)
- Reporter comments
- Sender's diagnosis/syndrome and comments

■ Periodic Safety Update Reports (PSURs) for Marketed Drugs (E2C)

This was adopted by ICH as a step 4 document in November 1996 and published in the *Federal Register* (1997;62:27469-27476). Note that an addendum was published and is summarized below.

This document gives guidance on the format and content of safety updates, which need to be provided at intervals to regulatory authorities after products have been marketed. The guideline is intended to ensure that the worldwide safety experience is provided to authorities at defined times after marketing with maximum efficiency and avoiding duplication of effort.

PSURs have been adopted by many countries, including those in the European Union, Japan, Canada, and others. In the United States it is not obligatory, but the FDA does accept PSURs. Companies wishing to submit PSURs in place of New Drug Application periodic reports must contact the FDA to obtain US requirements and FDA consent for their submissions.

The general principles are as follows:

- One report for one active substance. The PSUR should cover all dosage forms, formulations, and indications. There may be separate presentations of data for different dosage forms or populations if appropriate. The PSUR should be a "standalone" document.
- For combination products also marketed individually, safety information may be done as a separate PSUR or included in the PSURs prepared for one of the components with cross-referencing.
- The report should present data for the interval of the PSUR only except for regulatory status information, renewals, and serious unlisted ADRs, which should be cumulative.
- The report should focus on ADRs. All spontaneous reports should be assumed to be reactions (i.e., possibly related). Reports should be from health care professionals. For clinical trial and literature reports, only those cases believed by the reporter and sponsor to be unrelated to the drug should be excluded.
- Lack of efficacy reports (which are considered to be AEs) should not be included in the tables but should be discussed in the "other information" section.
- Increased frequency reports for known reactions should be reported if appropriate.
- If more than one company markets a drug in the same market, each marketing authorization holder (MAH) is responsible for submitting PSURs. If contractual arrangements are made to share safety information and responsibilities, this should be specified.
- Each product should have an international birth date (IBD), usually the date of the first marketing authorization anywhere in the world. This date should be synchronized around the world for PSUR reporting such that all authorities receive reports every 6 months or multiples of 6 months based on the IBD.
- The report should be submitted within 60 days of the data lock-point.
- The reference document for expectedness ("listedness" as opposed to "labeled-ness," which refers to national data sheets such as the US package insert) should be the company core data sheet (CCDS), the safety section of which is known as the company core safety information (CSI).
- The verbatim reporter term as well as standardized coding term (i.e., MedDRA, which was approved after E2C was finished) should be used.
- ADR cases should be presented as line listings and summary tabulations. That is, individual CIOMS I or MedWatch forms are *not* included.

The sections of a PSUR are as follows:

- Introduction
- Worldwide market authorization status
    - A table with dates of market authorization and renewals, indications, lack of approvals, withdrawals, dates of launch, and trade names
- Update of regulatory authority or MAH actions taken for safety reasons
- Changes to the Reference Product Information
    - The version of the CCDS in place at the beginning of the PSUR interval as the reference document. If there is a time lag between changes to the CCDS and local labeling, this should be commented on when submitting to that local health authority.
- Patient exposure
    - The most appropriate method should be used and an explanation for its choice provided. This includes patients exposed, patient-days, number of prescriptions, and tonnage sold.
- Presentation of individual case histories from all sources (except nonmedically confirmed consumer reports)
    - Follow-up data on previously reported cases should be presented if significant.
    - Literature should be monitored and cases included. Duplicates should be avoided. If a case is mentioned in the literature, even if obtained also as a spontaneous or trial case, the citation should be noted.
    - If medically unconfirmed cases received from consumers are required to be submitted in the PSUR, they should be submitted as addenda line listings and summary reports.
    - Line listings should include each patient only once. If a patient has more than one adverse drug experience/ADR, the case should be listed under the most serious adverse drug experience/ADR with the others also mentioned there. If appropriate, it may be useful to have more than one line listing for different dosage forms and indications. The headings for the listings are
        - MAH reference number
        - Country where the case occurred
        - Source (trial, literature, spontaneous, regulatory authority)
        - Age and sex

- Daily dose, dosage form and route of suspected drug
- Reaction onset date
- Treatment dates
- Description of the reaction (MedDRA code)
- Patient outcome at the case level (resolved, fatal, improved, sequelae, unknown)
- Comments (e.g., causality if manufacturer disagrees with reporter, concomitant medications, etc.)
    - Line listings should include the following cases:
        - Spontaneous reports: all serious reactions, nonserious unlisted reactions
        - Studies or compassionate use: all serious reactions (believed to be serious by either the sponsor or investigator)
        - Literature: All serious reactions and nonserious unlisted reactions
        - Regulatory authority cases: All serious reactions
        - If nonserious, listed ADRs are required by some authorities, they should be reported as an addendum
    - Summary tabulations
        - Each line listing should have an aggregate summary that will normally contain more terms than patients. It may be broken down by serious and nonserious and listed and unlisted as well as other breakdowns as appropriate. There should also be a summary for nonserious listed spontaneous reactions.
        - Data in summary tabulations should be noncumulative except for ADRs, which are both serious and unlisted for which a cumulated figure should be provided in the table.
    - MAH analysis of individual case histories
        - This section may contain brief comments on individual cases. The focus here is on individual cases (e.g., unanticipated findings, mechanism, reporting frequency, etc.) and should not be confused with the global assessment as described below.
- Studies
    - All completed studies (nonclinical, clinical, epidemiologic), planned or in-progress studies, and published studies yielding or with potential to yield safety information should be discussed.

- Other information
  - Lack of efficacy information should be presented here.
  - Late-breaking information after database lock should be presented here.
- Overall safety evaluation
  - The data should be presented by system organ class and should discuss
    - A change in characteristics of listed reactions
    - Serious unlisted reactions, placing into perspective the cumulative reports
    - Nonserious unlisted reactions
    - Increased frequency of listed reactions
    - New safety issues
    - Drug interactions
    - Overdose and its treatment
    - Drug misuse or abuse
    - Pregnancy and lactation information
    - Experience in special patient groups
    - Effects of long-term treatment
- Conclusion
  - This section should indicate which safety data do not remain in accord with the previous cumulative experience and with the company CSI
  - Any action recommended or initiated
- Appendix: Company Core Data Sheet (CCDS)

■ PSURs for Marketed Drugs (Addendum to E2C)

The Addendum provides clarification and guidance on PSURs and addresses some new concepts not in E2C but reflecting current pharmacovigilance practice needs, including Proprietary Information (Confidentiality), Executive Summary, Summary Bridging Report, Addendum Reports, Risk Management Program, and Benefit-Risk Analysis.

It was adopted by the ICH in February 2003 and published in the *Federal Register* (2004;69:5551-5552). The major points are summarized below. Refer to the document for full details.

International Birth Dates (IBDs)

- PSURs should be based on IBDs. To transition to a harmonized IBD, the MAH may submit its already prepared IBD-based PSUR plus (1) line listings and/or tabular summaries for the additional period (≤3 months if submitting a 6-month PSUR or ≤6 months if submitting a longer PSUR) with comments or (2) an Addendum Report (see below) with the same duration limits as in (1).
- In attempting to harmonize IBDs, it is possible that a drug will be on a 5-year cycle in one country and a 6-month cycle in another. If harmonization is not possible, the MAH and regulators should try to find a common birth month and day so that reports can be submitted on the same month and day whether every 6 months, yearly, or every 5 years. (Note that the European Union has changed the frequency from 5 years to 3 years.)

Summary Bridging Reports

- A summary bridging report integrates two or more PSURs to cover a specific time period for which a single report is requested. Thus two 6-month PSURs could be used to create a summary bridging report to cover the full year or 10 6-month reports to cover a 5-year PSUR. The bridging report does not contain new data but briefly summarizes the data in the shorter reports. The report should not contain line listings but may have summary tables.

Addendum Reports

- An addendum report is used when it is not possible to synchronize PSURs for all authorities requiring submissions. The addendum report is an update to the most recently completed PSUR. It should be used when more than 3 months for a 6-month PSUR and more than 6 months for a longer PSUR. It is not intended as an in-depth report (which will be done in the next regularly scheduled PSUR). It should contain an introduction, any changes to the CSI, significant regulatory actions on safety, line listings, and/or summary tabulations and a conclusion.

Restarting the Clock

- For products in a long-term PSUR cycle (e.g., 5 years), the return to a 6-month reporting schedule may occur if a new clinically dissimilar indication is approved, a previously unapproved use in a special population is approved, or a new formulation or route of administration is approved. The restarting of the reporting clock should be discussed with the regulatory authorities.

Time Interval between Data Lock-Point and the Submission

- The MAH has 60 days to prepare a submission after the data lock-point. An issue that arose was review and comment by the regulatory authority(ies) that took a long time to do and was sent back to the sponsor at a date very close to the submission of the following PSUR. If this review contains new requirements or other obligations for the MAH, the MAH may not be able to adequately complete the additional analyses requested in time for the next PSUR. Hence the Addendum notes that the regulatory authority will attempt to send comments to the MAH

  - As rapidly as possible if any issues of noncompliance with format and content are noted.

  - As rapidly as possible and before the next data lock-point if additional safety issues are identified that may require further analysis in the next PSUR. It is noted that such analyses could also be submitted as a separate stand-alone report instead of in the next PSUR.

Additional Time for Submissions

- In rare circumstances, the MAH may request an additional 30 days to submit a PSUR. This might occur if there is a large number of case reports and there is no new safety issue, if issues are raised by the authorities in the previous PSUR for which additional time is needed for further analysis for the next PSUR, or if issues are identified by the MAH needing further analysis.

Reference Safety Information

- The MAH should highlight differences between the CSI and the local product labeling in the cover letter accompanying the PSUR.

- For 6-month and 1-year PSURs, the CSI in effect at the beginning of the period should be used as the reference document.

- For PSURs longer than 1 year, the CSI in effect at the end of the period should be used as the reference document for PSURs and Summary Bridging Reports.

Other Issues

- The title page of the PSUR should have a confidentiality statement because proprietary information is contained in the report.

- An executive summary should be included right after the title page in each PSUR.

- Patient exposure data
  - It is acknowledged that these data are often difficult to obtain and not always reliable. If the exposure data do not cover the full period of the PSUR, extrapolations may be made. A consistent method of exposure calculations should be used over time for a product.

- Individual case histories
  - Because it is impractical to summarize all cases as narratives, the MAH should describe the criteria used to describe the cases summarized.
  - The section should contain selected cases, including fatalities, presenting new and relevant safety information and grouped by medically relevant headings or system organ class.

- Consumer listings
  - If required by regulators, consumer listings should be done in the same way that other listings and summary tabulations are prepared.

- The "comments" field
  - This field should only be used for information that helps to clarify individual cases.

- Studies
  - This section should contain only those company-sponsored studies and published safety studies (including epidemiology studies) that produce findings with potential impact on safety. The MAH should not routinely catalogue or describe all studies.

- The "other information" section
  - Risk management programs may be discussed in this section.
  - When a more comprehensive safety or risk-benefit analysis has been done separately, a summary of the analysis should be included here.
  - Discussion and analysis for the "Overall Safety Evaluation" section should be organized by system organ class and not by listedness or seriousness.

Postapproval Safety Data Management: Definitions and Standards for Expedited Reporting (E2D)

The guideline was finalized in November 2003 and provides a standardized procedure for postapproval safety data management, including expedited reporting to the relevant authority. It parallels and adds to the E2A document, which covered preapproval (clinical trial) safety data management by covering postmarketing safety data management. This document standardizes data management of cases from consumer, literature, Internet, and other types of postmarketing cases. The FDA published the guidance in the *Federal Register* on September 15, 2003.

Definitions

AE: The definition is nearly identical to the E2A version, leaving out the reference to clinical trials. "An AE is any untoward medical occurrence in a patient administered a medicinal product and which does not necessarily have to have a causal relationship with this treatment. An adverse event can therefore be any unfavorable and unintended sign (for example, an abnormal laboratory finding), symptom, or disease temporally associated with the use of a medicinal product, whether or not considered related to this medicinal product."

ADR: This definition is similar to the preapproval definition (E2A) but defines the causality component in the postmarketing setting ("at least a possibility" of a causal relationship). "All noxious and unintended responses to a medicinal product related to any dose should be considered adverse drug reactions. The phrase 'responses to a medicinal product' means that a causal relationship between a medicinal product and an adverse event is at least a possibility (refer to ICH E2A). A reaction, in contrast to an event, is characterized by the fact that a causal relationship between the drug and the occurrence is suspected. If an event is spontaneously reported, even if the relationship is unknown or unstated, it meets the definition of an adverse drug reaction."

Serious AE/ADR: This definition is the same as the one in E2A for preapproval issues. "Any untoward medical occurrence that at any dose that results in death, is life-threatening, requires inpatient hospitalization or results in prolongation of existing hospitalization, results in persistent or significant disability/incapacity, is a congenital anomaly/birth defect, is a medically important event or reaction. Medical and scientific judgment should be exercised in deciding whether other situations should be considered as serious such as important medical events that may not be immediately life-threatening or result in death or hospitalization but may jeopardize the patient or may require intervention to prevent one of the other outcomes listed in the definition above. These should also be considered serious."

Unexpected ADR: The definition of expedited-ness is somewhat different from that in E2A for preapproval cases because the reference documents are different (investigator's brochure for preapproval and the local labeling for marketed drugs). In addition, class labeling is discussed. This is summarized briefly:

> "An ADR whose nature, severity, specificity, or outcome is not consistent with the term or description used in the official product information should be considered unexpected.
>
> An ADR with a fatal outcome should be considered unexpected, unless the official product information specifies a fatal outcome for the ADR. In the absence of special circumstances, once the fatal outcome is itself expected, reports involving fatal outcomes should be handled as for any other serious expected ADR in accord with appropriate regulatory requirements."

Note that the term "listedness" is not applicable for expedited reporting (refer to ICH E2C for definition in which listedness refers to whether the reaction is noted in CSI for PSURs). "Class ADRs" should not automatically be considered to be expected for the subject drug. "Class ADRs" should be considered to be expected only if described as specifically occurring with the product in the official product information.

Health care professional: "Any medically-qualified person such as a physician, dentist, pharmacist, nurse, coroner, or as otherwise specified by local regulations."

Consumer: "A person who is not a healthcare professional such as a patient, lawyer, friend or relative of the patient."

Sources of Individual Case Safety Reports

- Unsolicited sources: spontaneous reports
  - These are unsolicited communications by health care professionals or consumers to a company, regulatory authority, or other organization (e.g., World Health Organization, Regional Centers, Poison Control Center) that

describe one or more ADR in a patient who was given one or more medicinal products and that does not derive from a study or any organized data collection scheme.

- "Stimulated reporting may occur in certain situations, such as a notification by a 'Dear Healthcare Professional' letter, a publication in the press, or questioning of healthcare professionals by company representatives. These reports should be considered spontaneous." (Note this contradicts to a certain degree the FDA's guidance of August 1997 [Web Resource 26-5] that requests that such cases be considered as if they were obtained from a postmarketing study and thus the triple requirements of seriousness, causality, and expectedness must be applied.)

- Consumer reports should be handled as spontaneous reports irrespective of any subsequent "medical confirmation," a process required by some authorities for reportability. Emphasis should be placed on the quality of the report and not on its source. Even if reports received from consumers do not qualify for regulatory reporting, the cases should be retained in the database.

- Unsolicited sources: literature
  - The MAH is expected to regularly screen the worldwide scientific literature by accessing widely used systematic literature reviews or reference databases according to local requirements or at least every 2 weeks. Cases of ADRs from the scientific and medical literature, including relevant published abstracts from meetings and draft manuscripts, might qualify for expedited reporting.

  - The regulatory reporting time clock starts once it is determined that the case meets minimum criteria for reportability.

  - If the product source, brand, or trade name is not specified, the MAH should assume that it was its product, although reports should indicate that the specific brand was not identified.

- Unsolicited sources: the Internet
  - MAHs are not expected to screen external websites for ADR information. However, if an MAH becomes aware of an adverse reaction on a website that it does not manage, the MAH should review the case and determine whether it should be reported.

- Unsolicited cases from the Internet should be handled as spontaneous reports.

- Regarding e-mail, identity of the reporter needs to be evaluated to see whether it refers to the existence of a real person. That is, it is possible to verify that the patient and reporter exist.

- Unsolicited sources: other sources
  - Cases from nonmedical sources, such as the lay press, should be handled as spontaneous reports.

- Solicited sources
  - This refers to cases from organized data collection systems, which include clinical trials, postapproval named patient use programs, other patient support and disease management programs, surveys of patients or health care providers, or information gathering on efficacy or patient compliance. AE reports obtained from any of these should not be considered spontaneous. For the purposes of safety reporting, solicited reports should be handled as if they were study reports and therefore should have an appropriate causality assessment.

- Contractual agreements
  - If companies make contractual arrangements to market a product in the same or different countries or regions, explicit agreements must be made to specify the processes for exchange of safety information, including timelines and regulatory reporting responsibilities, though the MAH is ultimately responsible. Duplicate reporting should be avoided.

- Regulatory authority sources
  - Individual serious unexpected ADR reports originating from foreign regulatory authorities are always subject to expedited reporting. Resubmission of serious ADR cases without new information to the originating regulatory authority is not usually required, unless otherwise specified by local regulation.

Standards for Expedited Reporting

- Serious ADRs
  - Cases of ADRs that are serious and unexpected are subject to expedited reporting.

  - For reports from studies and other solicited sources, all cases judged by either the reporting health care professional or the MAH as having a possible causal relationship to the medicinal product qualify as ADRs. Note that this now parallels the FDA's 1997 guidance on expedited reporting of solicited reports.

- For the purposes of reporting, spontaneous reports associated with approved drugs imply a possible causality.

- Other observations
  - Any significant unanticipated safety findings, including in vitro, animal, epidemiologic, or clinical studies, that suggest a significant human risk and could change the benefit-risk evaluation should be communicated to the regulatory authorities as soon as possible.

  - Lack of efficacy observations should not be expedited but should be discussed in PSURs unless local requirements oblige their being expedited.

  - Overdoses with no associated adverse outcome should not be reported as adverse reactions. The MAH should collect any available information on overdose related to its products.

  - Minimum criteria for reporting include an identifiable reporter, an identifiable patient, an adverse reaction, and a suspect product. The MAH is expected to exercise due diligence to collect missing data elements.

  - Reporting time frames for expedited reports are normally 15 calendar days from initial receipt of the minimal information by any personnel of the MAH. This is day 0. Additional medically relevant information for a previously submitted report restarts the clock.

  - Nonserious ADRs are not normally expeditable whether expected or not.

Good Case Management Practices

- Assessing patient and reporter identifiability
  - One or more of the following automatically qualifies a patient as identifiable: age (or age category, e.g., adolescent, adult, elderly), gender, initials, date of birth, name, or patient identification number. In the event of second-hand reports, every reasonable effort should be made to verify the existence of an identifiable patient and reporter.

  - All parties supplying case information or approached for case information should be identifiable.

  - In the absence of qualifying descriptors, a report referring to a definite number of patients should

not be regarded as a case until the minimum four criteria for case reporting are met.

- The role of narratives
  - The objective of the narrative is to summarize all relevant clinical and related information, including patient characteristics, therapy details, medical history, clinical course of the event(s), diagnosis, and ADR(s), including the outcome, laboratory evidence, and any other information that supports or refutes an ADR. The narrative should serve as a comprehensive stand-alone "medical story." The information should be presented in a logical time sequence; ideally, this should be presented in the chronology of the patient's experience rather than in the chronology in which the information was received. In follow-up reports, new information should be clearly identified.

  - Abbreviations and acronyms should be avoided, with the possible exception of laboratory parameters and units.

- Clinical case evaluation
  - An ADR report should be reviewed by the recipient for the quality and completeness of the medical information. This should include, but is not limited to, the following: Is a diagnosis possible? Have the relevant diagnostic procedures been performed? Were alternative causes of the reaction(s) considered? What additional information is needed?

  - The report should include the reporter's verbatim term (and, in the case of consumer reports, the consumer's description of the event). Staff receiving reports should provide an unbiased and unfiltered report of the information from the reporter. Clearly identified evaluations by the MAH are considered acceptable and, for some authorities, required.

- Follow-up information
  - The information from ADR cases when first received is generally incomplete. Efforts should be made to seek additional information on selected reports.

  - The first consideration should be prioritization of case reports by importance: cases that are (1) both serious and unexpected, (2) serious and expected, and (3) nonserious and unexpected. In addition to seriousness and expectedness as criteria, cases "of special interest" also deserve extra attention as a high priority (e.g., ADRs under active surveillance at the request of the regulators), as well as any cases that might lead to a labeling change decision.

- Follow-up should be obtained by a telephone call, site visit, and/or a written request. The MAH should provide specific questions it would like answered. The MAH should tailor the effort to optimize the chances of obtaining the new information.

- Written confirmation of details given verbally should be obtained whenever possible. Ideally, health care professionals with thorough pharmacovigilance training and therapeutic expertise should be involved in the collection and the direct follow-up of reported cases.

- Pregnancy exposure
  - MAHs are expected to follow up all reports, from health care professionals or consumers, of pregnancies where the embryo/fetus could have been exposed to one of its medicinal products.

- How to report
  - The CIOMS I form has been widely accepted. Whatever form is used should have all the appropriate elements included.
  - MedDRA should be used for coding.
  - E2B should be implemented for electronic transmission of individual cases.

- Recommended key data elements
  - The reader is referred to the Appendix of the E2D report for a list of recommended key data elements that should appear in all expedited reports.

■ Pharmacovigilance Planning (E2E)

This guideline was finalized (step 4) in November 2004 and is intended to aid in planning pharmacovigilance activities, especially in preparation for the early postmarketing period of a new drug. The main focus of this guideline is on a Safety Specification and Pharmacovigilance Plan that might be submitted at the time of the application for marketing. This report was published by the FDA in the *Federal Register* (2005;70:16827-16828).

Background and Scope

All three regions of the ICH (United States, European Union, and Japan) have been turning their attention to risk management and pharmacovigilance planning throughout the life cycle of a drug. This document reflects ICH's views.

The guidance is proposed for new chemical entities, biotechnology-derived products, and vaccines, as well as for significant changes in established products (e.g., new dosage form, new route of administration, or new manufacturing process for a biotechnology-derived product) and for established products that are to be introduced to new populations or for new indications or where a new major safety concern has arisen.

It is recommended that company pharmacovigilance experts get involved early in product development. Planning and dialogue with regulators should also start long before license application. A safety specification and pharmacovigilance plan can also be developed for products already on the market (e.g., new indication or major new safety concern). The plan could be used as the basis for discussion of pharmacovigilance activities with regulators in the different ICH regions and beyond.

For products with important identified risks, important potential risks, or important missing information, the pharmacovigilance plan should include additional actions designed to address these concerns. For products for which no special concerns have arisen, routine pharmacovigilance should be sufficient for postapproval safety monitoring, without the need for additional actions (e.g., safety studies). During the course of implementing the various components of the plan, any important emerging benefit or risk information should be discussed and used to revise the plan.

The following principles underpin this guidance:

- Planning of pharmacovigilance activities throughout the product life cycle
- Science-based approach to risk documentation
- Effective collaboration between regulators and industry
- Applicability of the pharmacovigilance plan across the three ICH regions

A Pharmacovigilance Plan for a product has three sections: Safety Specification, Pharmacovigilance Plan, and an Annex—Pharmacovigilance Methods.

Safety Specification

The safety specification is a summary of the important identified risks of a drug, important potential risks, and important missing information. It should also address the populations potentially at risk (where the product is likely to be used) and outstanding safety questions that warrant further investigation to refine understanding of the benefit-risk profile during the postapproval period.

The format and contents should focus on the identified risks, important potential risks, and important missing information. It should refer to the three safety sections in the Common Technical Document. The following elements should be considered for inclusion.

- Nonclinical
  - This section should present nonclinical safety findings that have not been adequately addressed by clinical data, for example, toxicity (including repeat-dose toxicity, reproductive/developmental toxicity, nephrotoxicity, hepatotoxicity, genotoxicity, carcinogenicity, etc.), general pharmacology (cardiovascular, including QT/QTc interval prolongation, nervous system, etc.), drug interactions, and other toxicity-related information. If the product is intended for use in special populations, consideration should be given to whether specific nonclinical data need to exist.
- Clinical
  - Limitations of the human safety database (e.g., related to the size of the study population, study inclusion/exclusion criteria) should be considered and discussed. Particular reference should be made to populations likely to be exposed during the intended or expected use of the product in medical practice.
  - The worldwide experience should be briefly discussed, including the extent of the worldwide exposure, any new or different safety issues identified, any regulatory actions related to safety, and populations not studied in the preapproval phase (children, elderly, pregnant or lactating women, patients with relevant comorbidity such as hepatic or renal disorders, patients with disease severity different from that studied in clinical trials, subpopulations carrying known and relevant genetic polymorphism, patients of different racial and/or ethnic origins).

- AEs/ADRs: This section should list the important identified and potential risks that require further characterization or evaluation. Discussion of risk factors and potential mechanisms should draw on information from the Common Technical Document and other relevant information, such as other drug labels, scientific literature, and postmarketing experience.
- Identified risks that require further evaluation:
  - More detailed information should be included on the most important identified AEs/ADRs, which would include those that are serious or frequent and that also might have an impact on the balance of benefits and risks of the product. This information should include evidence bearing on a causal relationship, severity, seriousness, frequency, reversibility, and at-risk groups, if available. Risk factors and potential mechanisms should be discussed. These AEs/ADRs should usually call for further evaluation as part of the pharmacovigilance plan (e.g., frequency in normal conditions of use, severity, outcome, at-risk groups).
- Potential risks that require further evaluation:
  - Important potential risks should be described and the evidence that led to the conclusion that there was a potential risk should be presented. It is anticipated that for any important potential risk, there should be further evaluation to characterize the association.
  - Identified and potential interactions, including food-drug and drug-drug interactions should be discussed with consideration of the evidence, and the potential health risks posed for the different indications and in the different populations should be discussed.
- Epidemiology
  - The epidemiology of the indication should be discussed, including incidence, prevalence, mortality, and relevant comorbidity and should take into account whenever possible stratification by age, sex, and racial and/or ethnic origin. Differences in the epidemiology in the different regions should be discussed (because the epidemiology of the

indication(s) may vary across regions), if this information is available.

- For important AEs that may require further investigation, it is useful to review the incidence rates of these events among patients in whom the drug is indicated (i.e., the background incidence rates).

■ Pharmacologic class effects

- The safety specification should identify risks believed to be common to the pharmacologic class.

- Summary: This should include the important identified risks, potential risks, and missing information on an issue-by-issue basis.

Pharmacovigilance Plan

The pharmacovigilance plan should be based on the safety specification and developed by the sponsor. It can be discussed with regulators during product development, before approval (i.e., when the marketing application is submitted) of a new product, or when a safety concern arises postmarketing. It can be a standalone document.

For products for which no special concerns have arisen, routine pharmacovigilance should be sufficient for postapproval safety monitoring, without the need for additional actions (e.g., safety studies). However, for products with important identified risks, important potential risks, or important missing information, additional actions designed to address these concerns should be considered. It should be updated as important information on safety becomes available and milestones are reached.

The format and content should include the following:

■ Summary of ongoing safety issues, including the important identified risks, potential risks, and missing information.

■ Routine pharmacovigilance practice should be conducted for all medicinal products, regardless of whether or not additional actions are appropriate as part of a pharmacovigilance plan. This routine pharmacovigilance should include the following:

  ■ Systems and processes that ensure that information about all suspected adverse reactions that are reported to the personnel of the company are collected and collated in an accessible manner.

■ The preparation of reports for regulatory authorities including expedited ADR reports and PSURs.

■ Continuous monitoring of the safety profile, including signal detection, issue evaluation, updating of labeling, and liaison with regulatory authorities.

■ Other requirements, as defined by local regulations.

■ Action plan for safety issues:

- The plan for each important safety issue should be presented and justified according to the safety issue, objective of proposed action, action proposed, rationale for proposed action, monitoring by the sponsor for safety issue and proposed action, and milestones for evaluation and reporting. Any protocols for specific studies may also be provided.

■ Summary of actions to be completed, including milestones:

- An overall pharmacovigilance plan for the product bringing together the actions for all individual safety issues should be presented and organized in terms of the actions to be undertaken and their milestones.

- It is recommended that milestones for completion of studies and for submission of safety results be included in the pharmacovigilance plan. The milestones should reflect when exposure to the product will have reached a level sufficient to allow potential identification/characterization of the AEs/ADRs of concern or resolution of a particular concern and when the results of ongoing or proposed safety studies are expected to be available.

- These milestones might be aligned with regulatory milestones (e.g., PSURs, annual reassessment and license renewals) and used to revise the pharmacovigilance plan.

■ Pharmacovigilance methods

- The best method to address a specific situation can vary, depending on the product, the indication, the population being treated, and the issue to be addressed. When choosing a method to address a safety concern, sponsors should use the most appropriate design.

■ Design and conduct of observational studies

- Carefully designed and conducted pharmacoepidemiologic studies, specifically observational (noninterventional, nonexperimental) studies, are important tools in pharmacovigilance.

- A protocol should be finalized and experts from relevant disciplines (e.g., pharmacovigilance experts, pharmacoepidemiologists, and biostatisticians) should be consulted. It is recommended that the protocol be discussed with the regulatory authorities before the study starts. A study report after completion, and interim reports if appropriate, should be submitted to the authorities according to the milestones within the pharmacovigilance plan.

- The sponsor should follow good epidemiologic practice for observational studies and also internationally accepted guidelines, such as the guidelines endorsed by the International Society for Pharmacoepidemiology.

Annex

■ A detailed discussion of pharmacovigilance methods is appended to the document to which the reader is referred for further details.

Pharmaceutical Companies

There are many types of companies and institutions in the pharmaceutical world with responsibilities regarding drug safety. A summary of various types of institutions follows.

■ Big and Somewhat Big Pharma

There are many large drug companies in the world that sell billions of dollars of product each year. Although the number has decreased through mergers and acquisitions, there still remain some 43 publicly traded companies with annual sales of over $1 billion per year and roughly another 400 with sales under $1 billion per year. The largest has sales over $50 billion per year (Source: Morningstar.com stock screener performed 1-Nov-2005). In addition, there are many other small and mid-sized privately held companies involved in pharmaceuticals. As noted throughout this book, companies have obligations to report animal and human safety data (among other information) to health authorities, ethics committees, investigational review boards, and so on.

Big Pharma generally refers to the dozen or so large "full-service" companies with revenues in the billions of dollars. These companies are multinational, with headquarters in the United States or Europe primarily but with some located in Japan and elsewhere. They usually have scientists doing drug discovery in an attempt to come up with new patentable drugs that will hopefully become "blockbusters" (drugs with sales of over a billion dollars a year by some definitions). The companies have the capacity to do their own preclinical studies (pharmacology and toxicity) and clinical trials (phases I-IV). They have large marketing and sales divisions with thousands of "representatives" or "sales reps" or "detailers." The Big Pharma company does much of its own manufacturing in factories throughout the world. There are large departments to handle regulatory issues, legal issues, and patents. Many have subsidiaries in the major markets (50 or more) throughout the world. Some are only sales organizations, whereas others are staffed to do clinical research as well. Some functions may be located outside the mother country (e.g., home office in the United States but a phase I clinical research unit(s) in the United Kingdom or Asia or vice versa).

And, of course, there is a large drug safety department. The safety department is often, but not always, located in the corporate headquarters in the mother country. This is the major center for drug safety with receipt of some or all of the individual case safety reports for data entry as well as preparation of MedWatch and CIOMS I forms, New Drug Application (NDA) periodic reports, Investigational New Drug Application (IND) annual reports, Periodic Safety Update Reports (PSURs), annual clinical trial reports, and other aggregate reports.

The servers for the safety database are located at a central location as a rule. There are usually drug safety departments in most or all subsidiaries to receive local safety reports (in the local language) and make submissions (sometimes in English, sometimes in the local language).

These subsidiaries, depending on size and function, may have a separate physician serving as safety officer or have the medical director (often the only medical doctor in the local company) also serve as the safety physician. The subsidiaries often serve as "pass through" points for adverse events (AEs) to be sent to central or regional data centers for data entry into the safety database. Sometimes a subsidiary (or regional center) will have expanded functions covering multiple countries. For example, some companies (e.g., whose headquarters are located in the United States or Japan) will set up a major center in the European Union to do data entry and to prepare PSURs and other documents for submission to the European Medicines Agency and national health authorities. In other situations where the corporate headquarters are located in a smaller country (e.g., Switzerland), one of the "subsidiaries" will become the dominant center for drug safety (e.g., in the European Union or United States). There is a tendency for safety departments to now be located in major English-speaking countries, such as the United States or the United Kingdom, which, coincidentally or not, are the regulatory sites for the two major world pharmaceutical markets (the United States and the European Union).

There is also a trend to out-source some nonsafety business functions even by large pharmaceutical companies. This includes the manufacturing of certain specialty products (e.g., delayed-release formulations), some animal toxicology and pharmacology studies, and phase I studies requiring inpatient settings. As a rule, drug safety functions are out-sourced with much hesitancy, though this may be changing. Some companies have totally separate safety departments for prescription and over-the-counter products.

Generic Companies

Some national and multinational companies are devoted only to generic products and thus have little or no drug discovery or clinical research capacity. They may do small studies to show bioequivalence. Occasionally, they do formal phase II, III, or IV clinical trials but usually out-source them.

These companies create safety departments according to the functions needed, but they tend to be less involved with critical issues than the companies that deal with new chemical entities. By the time a drug is generic, most of the safety issues have been addressed and AE reporting and pharmacovigilance tends to be a "maintenance function" with few new data or signals appearing. In addition, because it is often hard to identify the manufacturer of a generic product, the AEs tend to get reported to the originating company that first created and sold the product whether the actual AE occurred with that product or not.

Some Big Pharma companies have generic divisions in addition to the innovator divisions. This is done to both make money selling generics but also to be in the position to manufacture generics to the branded products they sell after these products go off patent. That is, a company may sell a branded and a generic version of the same product.

Mid and Small Size Pharma

Some pharmaceutical companies are mid-size (sales in the hundreds of millions of dollars) and located in a single country. They thus do not have to establish the worldwide expertise in the safety department and can concentrate on the safety analysis and reporting in their market alone. These companies range from those that have significant sales figures (e.g., hundreds of millions of dollars) down to small biotech start-up companies with only one product in clinical research and no sales. These companies usually establish a safety function either as a stand-alone unit with a handful of people if the volume warrants it or combine the function with the medical/clinical research group or the regulatory affairs group. Some companies out-source some or all of the function (e.g., data entry, aggregate report writing) to clinical or contract research organizations (CROs) or other out-sourcing firms.

Sometimes these companies have contractual agreements for research or sales with other companies both inside and outside their home country. These contracts oblige the company to conform to safety and regulatory requirements if the partner is outside the home country. That is, they must send AEs to the contracting business partner in a timely manner and in the proper format so that the business partner can remain in compliance with its local laws and regulations.

Clinical or Contract Research Organizations

CROs are companies that handle some or all clinical and regulatory functions that pharmaceutical companies do, including phase I-IV studies, regulatory submissions, safety data, and IND and NDA preparations. There are large "full-service" CROs, such as PPD (Web Resource 27-1) and Quintiles (Web Resource 27-2), that are almost mini-pharmaceutical companies, and there are "niche" or "boutique" CROs that specialize in one or two functions in the pharma world, such as Sentrx (Web Resource 27-3) handling primarily safety data and Orbis Drug Safety (Web Resource 27-4). These CROs usually set up whatever safety system(s) are needed for their functions. If they are doing primarily clinical research, they often set up a database for entry of the individual case safety reports that are either sent to the sponsoring company or to the US Food and Drug Administration directly. They may prepare IND annual reports, handle investigator notification, and so on. Others that handle safety as their primary function may set up multiple safety databases so that they are able to use the same one that the sponsoring company(ies) use. As technological change spreads (e.g., E2B) it is likely that worldwide standards will be developed to make data exchange easier and less complex.

There are multiple other types of service organizations that serve the pharmaceutical industry. A listing in the Drug Information Association's 2003 publication, "Contract Service Organization Directory," includes companies providing the following services: abstract preparation, advertising, specific types of trials (e.g., AIDS), analytic laboratories; bibliography preparation; contract management; validation of assays and laboratories; specimen storage; preparation of NDAs, Biologic License Applications, CANDAs, PSURs, clinical study reports, investigator brochures, expert reports, publications, drug master files; cardiovascular monitoring; case report form preparation; central laboratories; chemistry-manufacturing-control is-

sues; studies: phases I, II, III, IV, investigator initiated trials, compassionate use trials, epidemiology trials, pharmacoepidemiology trials, claims support studies, safety studies; information technology services (server management, programming and software development, data migration, data management, validation); clinical pharmacology, clinical packaging; clinical supply management; study management; focus groups and consumer testing; auditing; ethics committees and investigational review boards; data safety monitoring boards; digitized QTc analysis; dissolution testing; DNA diagnostics; document imaging, paper and electronic data management; translations; environmental assessments; formulation development; compliance Good Clinical Practices, Good Manufacturing Practice, Good Laboratory Practice, Good Pharmacovigilance Practices; home infusions; intranet, Internet, and website development; investigational site finding; setting up investigator meetings; licensing and acquisitions; market research; medical communications; call centers; medical science liaisons; microbiology testing; nursing; patient compliance, education, recruitment; preparation of labeling and patient information leaflets; process validation; project management; quality assurance and quality control; quality of life assessment; randomization; regulatory affairs, registries; remote data entry; prescription to over-the-counter switch; stability testing; standard operating procedure development; statistical services; toxicology; training; transportation; and reengineering and process redesign. Not all these organizations deal with safety or pharmacovigilance issues, although occasionally issues do come up and the drug safety department may need to work with these companies on safety-related projects.

The business models in the pharmaceutical world are changing. Innovation is tending to come now from small start-ups and biotechs as well as from large pharmaceutical companies. Whether the multi-billion dollar companies transform into development and marketing companies, leaving innovation to the smaller companies, remains to be seen. How this will touch the world of drug safety also remains to be seen.

Universities and Academic and Nonacademic Medical Centers

Universities and academic medical centers have multiple areas in which they interact with the drug safety world:

- Discovery and licensing
- Specialized clinical research units (CRUs) that run studies
- Other clinical divisions that run studies
- Training medical students, pharmacists, nurses, epidemiologists, and other health care professionals
- Ethics committees/investigational review boards (IRBs)
- Data safety monitoring committees
- Consultation to the industry
- Reporting adverse events (AEs) that occur in the hospital

Discovery and Licensing

The Bayh-Dole Act, or Patent and Trademark Law Amendments Act, was passed in 1980 (35USC200-212 and 37CFR401). See Web Resource 28-1. Among other provisions, it gave universities the right to hold patents for discoveries from research that they performed that also had federal funding. Government agencies had been hesitant about letting universities and small businesses obtain or license government-held or -sponsored patents. This act encouraged universities and small businesses to move discoveries into the marketplace. Examples now abound:

- New York University: Prof. Jan Vilcek and colleagues at the New York University School of Medicine developed the drug infliximab (Remicade©) from which many millions of dollars in royalties were made. Prof. Vilcek donated $105 million to the medical school (*New York Times*, August 12, 2005).
- Emory: Emory University receives significant sums of money from the sales of emtricitabine (Emtriva©). (Source: Emory University; Web Resource 28-2)

The development of university-held patents has, of course, in the American setting produced lawsuits over royalties. In 1999, Glaxo Wellcome Inc. agreed to pay the University of Minnesota royalties on the company's worldwide sales of Ziagen©, an antiviral AIDS drug, to settle a lawsuit brought by the university over royalties for patents held by a College of Pharmacy professor and subsequently licensed to Glaxo (Source: University of Minnesota; Web Resource 28-3).

Depending on the type of work and studies done, the universities and medical centers also have obligations to report certain safety information to health authorities, ethics committees, and IRBs as well as to contractual partners in the course of due diligence investigations.

Clinical Research Units and Centers

Many universities have established CRUs, including the University of Chicago, University of Buffalo, University of Medicine and Dentistry of New Jersey-New Brunswick, Duke University, University of Miami, University of Pennsylvania, University of Arizona, and University of Kentucky. In addition, there are units in the United Kingdom, Belgium, Canada, Germany, and other countries.

These units may perform both inpatient and outpatient studies in phases I, II, III, and IV. When functioning as sponsors, the CRU takes on all sponsor responsibilities as outlined in the regulations (and local institutional policies) for the study as if it were a pharmaceutical company or a large consortium running trials (e.g., cancer trials, National Institutes of Health etc.). When functioning as a study site for a pharmaceutical company, its safety functions revolve primarily on sending AEs (particularly serious ones) to the sponsor and notifying the IRB of serious cases.

Other Divisions Running Studies

Frequently, individual investigators within universities or medical centers contract with companies, consortia, the National Institutes of Health, and others to run studies or participate in multicenter clinical trials. These trials are run separately from the CRU (if such a unit exists in the institution). In such a case the investigator is responsible for complying with all safety obligations under the regulations and local university policies. Many universities now set up offices within the administration that handle such "extramural" research activities. They offer assistance to the investigators and ensure that the university collects the appropriate fees for use of their facilities.

Training Medical Students, Pharmacists, Nurses, Epidemiologists, and Other Health Care Professionals

In general, there is little training in US and Canadian medical schools in pharmacovigilance and drug safety. The training that does occur usually involves classical pharmacology and treatment with minimal (if any) discussion of the pharmaceutical industry, US Food and Drug Administration (FDA), and the subjects addressed in this book. Similarly, nursing and other allied medical programs also have little emphasis on drug safety. Some pharmacy schools and public health training programs are now beginning to touch on drug safety and epidemiology in their curricula and may establish rotations through industry or health agencies during the training of the students.

In several western European countries, drug safety teaching seems to be well integrated in those university hospitals where a pharmacovigilance reporting center, a drug information center, a poison control center, or a pharmacoepidemiology or epidemiology department exists. Obviously, it is in everyone's interest for drug safety and pharmacovigilance to become topics in which all health care professionals are trained and skilled.

Ethics Committees and IRBs

There are extensive FDA regulations and guidances for IRBs (ethics committees) to follow regarding their requirements and obligations in clinical studies. See the FDA website at Web Resource 28-4 and 45 CFR Part 46 at the Department of Health and Human Services website (Web Resource 28-5) for requirements and frequently asked questions. See also the FDA website (Web Resource 28-6) for a 2005 draft guidance on centralized IRBs. Such committees are also addressed in the International Conference on Harmonization E6E Good Clinical Practice guidance (Web Resource 28-7). Similar requirements exist in most other countries where clinical research is done.

The IRBs and ethics committees must review and approve clinical trial protocols to ensure the maximum patient protection that is possible. This includes a review of the safety procedures in these trials and ongoing monitoring of the conduct and results of the trial. They review the informed consent and the investigator's brochure as well as the protocol. These requirements oblige investigators (primarily in the United States) or sponsors (primarily in the European Union) to submit certain serious AEs to the IRBs/ethics committees either as they occur or in aggregate summary reports. In the United States, such committees may be attached to medical institutions (e.g., hospitals, medical schools) or may be unattached and free standing, which in itself has led to some controversy.

IRBs are subject to inspections by the FDA. When violations are found, the FDA may act to force the IRB to alter its procedures or may even shut it down. See, for example, a Warning Letter issued by the FDA to an IRB at Web Resource 28-8.

Data (Safety) Monitoring Committees

Over the years, in addition to IRBs, the concept of a separate independent data monitoring committee (DMC) has developed. This was codified as a draft guidance by the FDA in 2001 (Web Resource 28-9) and by the European Medicines Evaluation Agency in 2003 at Web Resource 28-10.

As stated in the FDA document: "A DMC is a group of individuals with pertinent expertise that reviews on a regular basis accumulating data from an ongoing clinical trial. The DMC advises the sponsor regarding the continuing safety of current participants and those yet to be recruited, as well as the continuing validity and scientific merit of the trial." They are not required in all studies but only those in which there is believed to be the need for additional patient safety, efficacy, and scientific validity monitoring such as "a trial that is large, of long duration, and multi-center." The committees should contain at least three members and include clinicians experienced in clinical trials as well as, in some cases, ethicists, toxicologists, epidemiologists, laboratory scientists, and even nonscientists. The DMC is usually set up to receive both aggregate blinded data and unblinded data. The DMC should have the capacity to do interim analyses and to indicate to the sponsor that the study should continue or be stopped. See the FDA guidance referenced above for full details.

In practical terms this forces the sponsor to set up a system to send both aggregate safety reports and some or all individual case safety reports for serious AEs (and sometimes nonserious AEs as well) to the DMC on an ongoing basis. This may pose logistical problems for the sponsor because the drug safety department has the unblinding information that it sends to the DMC but must keep all code breaks from the clinical research group and anyone else involved in the study.

Consultation to the Industry

When academic researchers (physicians primarily) and health care workers consult to the pharmaceutical industry, it results in much controversy. This can include giving (for a fee) opinions on clinical trial programs, protocols, clinical development, and drug safety issues. In particular, a sponsor may ask one or more academic clinicians or pharmacologists to review one or more case reports of AEs reported with the use of a drug. The review would help determine whether the AE in question is related to the drug or not.

Recent reports have indicated that some physicians involved in clinical trials have been consulting with Wall Street financial analysts (for a fee). It appears that the analysts want some indication of how the particular drug is faring in the clinical trials.

Consultation also includes giving scientific marketing talks to other physicians and health care workers on marketed drugs that the sponsor also makes. The controversy here revolves around the independence and impartiality of consultants who are also receiving sums of money for scientific marketing activities. Some believe that full disclosure of all financial ties, even remote, does permit objectivity. Others believe that objectivity in such a circumstance is never truly possible and that comments on clinical trials or drug safety are not unbiased. Because this practice is fairly widespread, it has produced, in some cases, difficulties in finding consultants with no industry ties to serve on FDA advisory committees.

Much has been written on this topic. See articles by Marcia Angell, MD, and Jerome Kassirer, MD, both formerly editors of the *New England Journal of Medicine*, and, in particular, the article, "Health industry practices that create conflicts of interest: a policy proposal for academic medical centers," by T. Brennan et al. (*JAMA* 2006;295:429-433).

Reporting AEs That Occur in the Hospital

The Joint Commission on Accreditation of Healthcare Organizations standard COP.11.6 requires organizations to monitor the effects of medications on patients. See Web Resource 28-11. However, the requirement is not explicit on reporting adverse drug reactions (or medication errors) to the FDA, although this is encouraged by the FDA via the MedWatch Program. Thus hospitals must develop some level of drug safety expertise, usually via the pharmacy department or the formulary committee (the group that decides which drugs will be kept on formulary and which will not).

Organization and Structure of a Typical Safety Department

This description covers a "standard" safety department found in a large multinational pharmaceutical company. Some functions and divisions do not exist in smaller companies or in companies that do not have international or research functions. Some functions are combined with others. Some functions may work with other divisions in the corporation in addition to the safety department.

■ The Standard Units and Functions

Management

Generally, companies have a physician who is designated "chief safety officer," "chief medical officer," or "qualified person" at a senior-level physician (e.g., executive or senior vice president) who is responsible for the final decision on medical issues for the corporation. This job includes decisions on product withdrawals, stopping clinical trials, amending protocols, changing product labeling,

and so forth for safety reasons. This person either is in the senior management of the company or in regulatory affairs or clinical research.

There is also a functional head of drug safety who ensures that the department runs in a timely, orderly, and professional manner. In smaller companies the chief safety officer and the functional head may be the same person. In larger companies they tend to be separated, especially if the company has several major safety units around the world.

Triage Unit

The triage unit is responsible for receiving, often at a single central point, all incoming adverse events (AEs) plus, in many cases, product complaints, requests for information from consumers and health care professionals, requests for reimbursement, and other medical information functions. Each incoming contact is routed to the appropriate department for handling. Decisions have to be made if a single incoming contact has several components: "I took your pill which was red instead of its normal blue color; I had chest pain after I took it—is that normal? And I want my money back." This is a product quality complaint, an AE, a question, and a request for reimbursement. In general, the priority should go to the published AE. Routes of entry of AEs include e-mail, "snail" mail, case reports of clinical trial AEs, reports from the US Food and Drug Administration (FDA) and other health authorities, and phone calls. Triage must be rapid and in real time because expedited (15-day) reports need to be acted on immediately.

This group is usually made up of both professional and clerical personnel whose job is to do the first-level screening of incoming written AEs. Telephone calls are usually screened initially by medically trained personnel (pharmacists, nurses). Mail and e-mail may first be seen by clerical staff but must be routed rapidly to medical professionals to perform the medical triage. In multinational companies, there is usually a triage group locally to handle phone calls and written communications arriving in the local language. US phone centers should be able to handle calls in English and Spanish and sometimes other languages. In Canada, English and French are required. Many companies are now moving call centers "off-shore," especially to India and Latin America, where English and Spanish language medical professionals (respectively) are available at costs that are much lower than that in the United States. Obviously, these centers must function at the same level and under the same regulatory requirements as if they were in the United States. The FDA holds them to US standards if they receive calls from American patients and physicians.

Case Assessment and Prioritization

A medical professional should rapidly review the cases for seriousness, labeledness, and causality (for clinical trial cases). Priority then goes to AEs that are 7- and 15-day expedited reports.

Data Entry Unit

After triage, cases must be medically evaluated (if not already done) and entered into the safety database. Cases that are expedited reports are usually prioritized for immediate data entry. Cases that are not expedited reports are put into a queue for handling and data entry. Serious cases are usually entered within 7-15 days and nonserious cases within 30 days. Companies' procedures vary widely.

The initially received information is entered into the drug safety database after screening for duplicates is done. Data entry is usually performed by clerical personnel who have been trained on how to enter cases into the company's safety database and sometimes after training in medical terminology.

Case Processing Unit

This unit is made up of health professionals, usually nurses and pharmacists, but occasionally also podiatrists, dentists, and other health care professionals. This group does the initial evaluation for expedited cases (as noted above, usually before data entry) and then reviews and/or prepares the case medical information. In particular, this involves the creation of the "narrative," which is a stand-alone text summary of the case that appears on the MedWatch and CIOMS I forms, and the verification of drug names, dosages, past medical history, and so on. The case-processing group also prepares medical queries (with the assistance of the physicians) to be sent to the reporter or investigator to obtain further information if the initial data are incomplete, including the final outcome for ongoing cases.

Medical Case Review

This group is almost always composed of physicians with expertise in drug safety and case review. They generally review the assessment, the AE coding, and the medical content of the narrative to ensure that the medical story is cogent and that it is a true reflection of the source data supplied. These physicians may also handle other work, including the preparation and review of signals, aggregate reports, and ad hoc queries (see Medical Affairs, below).

Transmission Unit

This group ensures that the appropriate cases are sent to the appropriate recipients. Expedited reports either go directly to the FDA or to the regulatory department for transmission to the FDA and other health authorities. Other cases may be sent within the company to other interested parties (e.g., clinical research, legal, etc.) and to associated business partners who also market and/or study the drug either in the United States or abroad. This function may be assumed by a unit that handles all "traffic" matters, including triage, routing, and transmission.

Regulatory Unit

Usually, this unit is not a part of drug safety but is a separate division. In some companies, expedited cases are reviewed by the regulatory group before transmission to the FDA as a final quality check. Many companies prefer to have all communications in and out to the FDA and other health authorities handled by the regulatory division rather than by drug safety and other groups to ensure tight tracking of all governmental contacts.

Legal Unit

Like the regulatory unit, this unit is never a part of drug safety. The legal unit interacts with drug safety in two primary areas. First, in some companies the legal department reviews all cases (MedWatch forms) that are sent to the FDA. The second area involves litigation or potential litigation based on AEs. In these cases, the drug safety and legal areas work very tightly together in defense of the litigation and in obtaining any follow-up from the suing party. Such follow-up is often done via the attorneys rather than directly from drug safety. The legal unit may also be a source of AEs that arise in lawsuits against the company that first arrive in the legal department.

Signaling, Pharmacovigilance, Pharmaco-epidemiology, or Medical Affairs Unit

This function may be called many things, as noted in the heading. This unit is made up of physicians and other health care workers. Their primary function is to review the safety data (AEs, medical errors, and product quality complaints) collected by the company and to evaluate whether new signals are popping up or old ones resolving or worsening. They may use tools available commercially or developed in-house for "data mining." (Data mining is the examination of data using statistical or database tools to look for patterns, relationships, and trends.) When an issue is found, they begin an initial safety investigation that includes a review of the published literature, the company's clinical research database (if different from the safety database), toxicology, and pharmacology and any other relevant information to prepare a summary report for presentation to the decision makers (e.g., the senior corporate safety committee) for resolution.

They may handle other functions, including, as noted above, review of individual cases, preparation of Investigational New Drug Application (IND) annual and New Drug Application (NDA) periodic reports, Periodic Safety Update Reports (PSURs), integrated safety summaries, responses to ad hoc queries from the FDA and other health authorities, pharmacoepidemiology studies and analyses, advertising review for medical content, review of communications to the public ("Dear Doctor or Dear Health Care Professional" letters), review of labeling and package inserts, medical testimony in litigation, and consultation on drug withdrawals.

Aggregate Report Preparation

This unit, comprised of physicians and other health care professionals, sometimes separate from the pharmacovigilance unit, prepares aggregate or summary reports of data derived from individual case safety reports. These reports include NDA periodic reports, IND annual reports, PSURs, ad hoc queries from health authorities, and other corporate departments.

Labeling Review and Update for Safety

This function is sometimes done within drug safety and sometimes separately by the labeling group and/or regulatory affairs. It involves the continuous monitoring of the labeling of the company's products to ensure that all the safety information is fully up to date. This includes examination of the core safety information document as well as local labeling sheets (e.g., Summary of Product Characteristics, US package insert) and patient information leaflets. Areas of interest include AE, warnings, precautions, contraindications, pregnancy and lactation, overdose, and drug interactions. This may be a very substantial task if the company sells multiple drugs with multiple formulations in many countries around the world.

It may also require the monitoring of the safety labeling of products of other companies of drugs in the same class as well as drugs that may have interactions with the company's drugs. For example, if company B adds a statement to its drug's labeling stating that there is a drug interaction between the company B drug and a company A drug, company A should determine whether it should add a similar statement to its labeling. The function of labeling creation, maintenance, and review is a critical one for a company (and regulatory authority) and is beyond the scope of this book.

Archive/File Room

Although there is a trend toward the so-called paperless office, the amount of paper used and the number of photocopy machines do not yet appear to be decreasing. The safety department must make sure they have an adequate archive/file room system such that all safety information is saved in the appropriate place and is readily available for review whether by the company or during a health authority audit. Several logistical decisions need to be made concerning such things as follows:

- The storage of documents in a multinational company where serious AE reports may come in multiple languages: Should they be kept in the country where they are received (and able to be read) or centrally or both?

- Are the storerooms adequately protected from fire, flood, and other hazards? Should sprinkler systems specifically not be installed but rather an alternative system used for fire protection?

- Storing paper charts for tens of thousands of cases per year (in a large company) can require very large physical storage areas. Should these cases be kept on site or archived in a document storage facility off-site?

- What tracking system will be used? Should bar codes or chips be used for paper files and, if so, for the folder jacket or for every document inside also?

- How long should documents be retained? Note that retention rules may differ for the United States, European Union, and other jurisdictions. In general, documents should be retained for the longest time required by any country whose documents are stored in that archive. Some companies keep all safety data forever.

- Who has access to and control of the file room?

- What backup methods are used (e.g., in case of fire or water damage)?

- If contract facilities (outside vendors) are used, who supervises them and ensures the safe keeping of the files and the ability to retrieve needed files (e.g., for a health authority audit) within 24 hours?

Information Technology/Informatics Liaison

Almost all drug safety departments use a commercial or home-grown database to store safety data and produce MedWatch, CIOMS I forms, and PSURs. There is usually a dedicated informatics/information technology (IT) support and development group that works with drug safety ("the business owners") to support the database and handle changes, bugs, new hires and access levels, upgrades, *Medical Dictionary for Regulatory Activities* (MedDRA) and other dictionaries, testing, and validation. Sometimes the IT group reports to the drug safety group and sometimes not. Usually, the IT group is fully versed in the IT aspects of the database but needs business input from a "superuser" or drug safety expert who understands the safety business and issues and who can speak the "IT language" to facilitate communication. This "IT liaison" function has various titles from company to company but is found in nearly all companies because the need to bridge the gap between the computer experts and the safety experts is real and ongoing.

Standard Operating Procedure (SOP) Creation and Maintenance

Written formal SOPs, working documents, and guidances are obligatory in drug safety departments under Good Clinical Practices (GCP) requirements from the International Conference on Harmonization (ICH), the FDA, the European Medicines Agency (EMEA), and elsewhere. In addition, there may be manuals, guidances, and job aids that accompany the SOPs (e.g., a data entry manual). The first thing an FDA, EMEA, or internal company inspector will ask for at the start of an audit is a copy of the organizational chart of the safety department and list of the SOPs in place. The SOPs govern the handling of safety data, report preparation, training, database and computer issues, and crisis management. It is not uncommon for a company to have 50 to 100 such SOPs and guidances. The creation, review (yearly at least), maintenance, and updating of SOPs is a function that must be ensured in a safety department. The issue of version control of SOPs must also be addressed so that everyone has access to and is working from the latest versions of the SOPs and guidances. This may mean controlled distribution of paper copies or availability of SOPs on-line only (and not as paper copies).

Training

Another requirement of GCP and quality systems is that training be done and documented. The training, based on the SOPs, guidances, and working documents, covers:

- The concepts of drug safety, pharmacovigilance, and risk management
- The laws, guidances, and regulations in place
- The specific procedures in that organization or division and others if appropriate (e.g., clinical research)
- The computers and software

In addition, there is the more general training offered by the organization on corporate values and workplace behavior, equality issues, physical safety in the workplace, and so on.

There is usually a formal training function or department within drug safety with a dedicated trainer (sometimes "certified" by some training body or organization either internal to the company or outside) who develops formal curricula and courses for the various people (based on job function) who need to be trained. This applies both to new hires and update training for current employees. The training involves both the drug safety department workers as well as others in the organization who might receive AEs in the course of their own jobs (e.g., in clinical research, regulatory, legal, telephone operators, customer relations, etc.). Each person in the safety department should have an up-to-date and accurate training folder documenting all training that person has had. This will often need to be produced during a health authority audit.

Quality Assurance/Control

The concepts of "quality assurance/control and quality systems" are relatively new to drug safety and GCP compared with their use in the manufacturing and laboratory areas. Quality is broadly broken up into two phases.

The first is quality assurance (QA), which, as we refer to it in drug safety, refers to actions taken *during* the process of handling safety data to ensure that the work is correct and complete. During the preparation of a MedWatch or CIOMS I form for submission to a health authority by a pharmacist, the QA might be done by his or her supervisor.

The second phase is quality control (QC), which usually refers to a review of the (final) deliverable. This is done to ensure that the deliverables (e.g., the completed MedWatch or CIOMS I form) were correctly and completely prepared and that no data are lost or changed along the way. QC may include formal audits by third parties from outside or inside the company or organization. Such audits are routinely done at the end of the process. The difference from QA is that the review is usually done after the case is completed.

Organizations should have both quality functions in place. During the processing and analysis of safety data, QA should be performed at the appropriate stages in the process. After the work is done, a review or an audit may be done on selective cases routinely or periodically (e.g., monthly) to see that the entire process is done correctly. Many safety departments in companies have a yearly audit done by the quality group (separate from the drug safety group). And, of course, the FDA does periodic pharmacovigilance audits (as do the EMEA and other health authorities) to check the quality of the safety department's work (see Chapter 45).

AE Exchange Agreement Function: Creation and Maintenance

Many pharmaceutical companies, both large and small, now enter into agreements with other companies to outsource or share certain responsibilities, such as comarketing in the same country, marketing in other countries, clinical trials (including development, monitoring, and data analysis), manufacturing, and safety data handling. As with other business arrangements, it is obligatory that all parties involved have written contracts specifying the safety functions and requirements of all partners. The contract should set specific terms for the exchange of all needed safety data, both individual case safety reports and aggregate reports such as PSURs and NDA periodic reports as well as labeling, investigator brochures, advertising, and regulatory communications. This must be done so that all partners are able to stay in full compliance with all regulations and laws (see Chapter 44).

Literature Review

US and European Union regulations, as well as those elsewhere, require periodic review of the worldwide literature to ensure that published reports of safety information on a company's products are found and reported to health authorities. This usually involves the computer (weekly to monthly) review of large databases that scan hundreds to thousands of medical journals and then report on "hits" (i.e., citations containing the drug in question or any other key words designated in the search). Once a safety case is found that meets reporting criteria (drug, AE, patient, reporter), the usual reporting requirements (e.g., 15 calendar days for an expedited report) apply. The safety department must ensure that this function, usually done in conjunction with the corporate library or an outside vendor, is performed in a correct and timely manner.

Data Dictionary Maintenance

In this sense of the word, a "dictionary" is a listing of standardized and fixed terms that companies and regulators agree to use. This is particularly important when data are exchanged electronically. If an unknown term is used in the sending of a case from one company or health authority to another, the receiving computer system often rejects (or at least notes or "flags") the case for attention.

MedDRA is an example of a dictionary used for the coding of AE terms (see Chapter 38). Other (now largely outmoded) AE dictionaries include COSTART, WHO-ART, and HARTS. Other dictionaries exist for the standardization of drug names (e.g., WHO-Drug Dictionary), abbreviations, laboratory measurements and units, and so forth.

A more global dictionary now being used primarily in the United States and the United Kingdom is SNOMED (see Web Resource 29-1 and Web Resource 29-2). The latter site is an attempt by the US Department of Health and Human

Services to expand SNOMED's use to build "a national electronic health care system that will allow patients and their doctors to access their complete medical records anytime and anywhere they are needed, leading to reduced medical errors, improved patient care, and reduced health care costs."

Coding Unit

Again related to dictionaries, this in particular to MedDRA, the use of a standardized coding dictionary also implies the use of this dictionary in a standardized manner. That is, every member of the drug safety staff (and any other unit that does coding such as clinical research) should be taught to code in the same manner using the same methodology and conventions to achieve internal consistency. This is done through a central coding unit (within or outside of drug safety) that either does the actual coding or verifies the coding done by the drug safety personnel.

Planning and Project Management/Operations

Many pharmaceutical companies are now integrating project planning directly into the drug safety unit to oversee and facilitate the multiple and ongoing changes that now seem to be a part of the daily life in drug safety. This includes the ensuring of a smooth integration of ongoing safety work with the introduction of new procedures, software and hardware, and dictionaries. For example, regulations change frequently around the world and all of them must be adhered to—even though they may sometimes be contradictory. Other usual occurrences include MedDRA upgrades twice a year, safety database upgrades or transfer to a new platform, and new contracts signed with business partners. To coordinate the successful implementation of these ever-changing requirements, a solid operations and project planning/management function must be in place to manage contingencies, timing, personnel, and communications.

Liaison to External Organizations

Many companies and health authorities are regular attendees at meetings held by international organizations that examine and develop new guidances and procedures. These include the ICH, CIOMS, Pharmaceutical Research Manufacturers of America, and the International Society of Pharmacoepidemiology. Pharmaceutical companies send personnel from their drug safety units to these meetings. Attendees are either employees whose sole or primary function is to represent the company at external organizations or ad hoc representatives chosen because of the duties they perform in their company.

Participation in these meetings is critical for the future of pharmacovigilance because these are the organizations that continue to spearhead the changes and advances in drug safety. ICH has produced many guidances that now form the basis for pharmaceutics in the United States, the European Union, and Japan. CIOMS developed the "CIOMS I form" and "CIOMS II line listings," among others.

This group may also serve as a "safety intelligence unit," gathering information on new laws, regulations, and guidance that touch drug safety. They then disseminate this information to relevant departments in the company.

CHAPTER 30

Business Partners and Adverse Event Exchange Agreements

In today's globalized pharmaceutical world, the nature of relationships between and among companies is changing. In the past, a single company would develop, study, and market a drug. If the company was multinational, it would sell the drug in its foreign markets and in the home country. Occasionally, it would license it out to one or more companies in countries where the originating company did not have sales offices.

This has changed. We are now seeing large, small, and mid-sized companies creating contractual arrangements with one or multiple other pharmaceutical companies and contract research organizations to handle development, sales, marketing, safety handling, regulatory matters, and manufacturing. These contracts may be short term or long term and involve companies all over the world.

Examples of contracts that concern safety departments include agreements covering licensing, development, clinical trial research, consultants, contract sales forces, distributors, health and disease management programs, manufacturing, patient support programs, promotion and copromotion, research, speakers bureaus, services and vendors, and any other agreements where there is a possibility that the parties may receive adverse event (AE) reports for the drug covered by the contract. These contracts may cover all possible permutations: prescription drugs, over-the-counter drugs, drugs that are prescription in one country and over-the-counter in the other, biologics, blood products, devices, and combination products (a device with a drug in it, such as a pre-filled syringe, or a drug-impregnated gauze pad).

It is critical that a written contract is set up between all parties to cover the exchange of all appropriate safety information. A good example of this is an article by Fieldstad et al. (*Drug Information J* 1996;30:965). Although a little out of date, it still covers the basics, which are summarized below.

The negotiation and maintenance of safety agreements is a complex endeavor that should be done by a person or team that is fully versed in US and international drug safety rules, practices, and guidelines. The persons must also fully understand their company's functions and needs during negotiations so that realistic and doable agreements are reached. They must know when and how to compromise and where they cannot compromise. They must also be good communicators and teachers within their own institution to train and update in-house personnel. They must search out contracts that may not always be sent to drug safety from the business people and marketers in far-away parts of the company. Knowing additional languages is useful.

In large companies with multiple agreements, it may be wise and necessary to create a database either as a spreadsheet or a more complex relational database to track the multiple commitments that the company must adhere to and that may vary from drug to drug, country to country, and company to company. The issue of storage and maintenance of the contracts should be clarified within the company. Although the safety department may not collect and store all contracts, staff should collect and store all safety agreements or, at the very least, have them available (in English) for a regulatory inspection within 24-48 hours. In companies with multiple subsidiaries, each of which has the authority to make deals, the tracking, collection, and maintenance of safety exchange agreements may be a very difficult task. The legal department is usually an excellent ally in this battle because almost all contracts go through the law department(s) at one time or another.

A "safety exchange agreement" or "AE exchange agreement" should ideally go into effect the moment the full contract (covering manufacture, drug supplies, sales and marketing, money, etc.) goes into effect. In practice, the full contract is often done in secret (for proprietary and economic reasons) and the drug safety department, unfortunately, is often brought into the picture at the moment of signing ("Could you please review the safety section of this contract because the CEO wants to sign it tomorrow?"). In cases like this, if there is not an adequate safety section, the best the drug safety reviewer can hope for is to remove an incorrect or inadequate safety section and add wording to the effect that both parties will sign a full safety exchange agreement within a specified time period (usually this should be no more than 60-90 days) if there is no risk of being out of compliance during this interval period (i.e., no drug sales or studies). If there is an immediate impact, the drug safety department should have minimal "boilerplate" wording that can be incorporated directly into the contract to cover the minimal safety exchange requirements (e.g., exchange of all expedited reports, all serious AEs, and all aggregate regulatory submissions such as New Drug Application [NDA] periodic reports, Periodic Safety Update Reports, etc.). This should be drawn up by the safety and the legal departments and kept on file. Ideally, the legal department contract reviewers should be sensitized to include the safety boilerplate automatically in all contracts that cross their desks.

Hubs versus Direct Party-to-Party Exchange

The safety agreement itself may be made between two or more companies. The more companies involved, the harder it is to get an agreement and gain consensus. In general, contracts with three or more parties should be handled differently from bilateral (two-party) agreements. If three or more parties are involved in the exchange of AEs, particularly serious AEs, the decision must be made whether the exchange will be direct from party to party or via an intermediate "hub," akin to the way airlines arrange flights. One may fly directly city to city or one may fly to a hub where many flights arrive and passengers switch flights to the city they need to reach. In terms of AE exchange, all AEs (or serious AEs as the case may be) are sent within a set time period to the hub company that receives all of them, enters them into its database, performs some level of quality control and analysis, and then retransmits the cases to all other parties. This implies "ownership" of the process by the hub company. In practice, this mechanism is often easier than direct company-to-company transmissions, especially when there are more than three companies involved.

Using a hub requires active work by the hub owner to ensure format and content consistency as well as a quality check. The hub company enters the data into its database, corrects errors or lack of clarity (one hopes), and then retransmits the case in the same format (e.g., CIOMS I form, MedWatch form, E2B file) to everyone. Being a hub is more than just a pass-through. If the timing is well worked out and all partners hold to the timelines, the system can work very efficiently, especially if the hub database is capable of E2B or batch transmissions of many cases automatically.

Timing and Documents Exchanged

Note that in the discussion that follows, all timing refers to days after the first receipt by the first partner of safety information anywhere in the world. That is, the clock starts when any person (not just the safety department) in the first company first receives safety data. Although some countries start their regulatory reporting clock when the case arrives in that country (i.e., at the company in that country), many countries do not. The safety agreement, in order to keep all parties in full compliance, must then adhere to the toughest rules in place in any of the territories involved.

The most time-sensitive issue in safety exchange is the need to be on time for expedited reports. The timing in almost all areas of the world follows that of CIOMS/

International Conference on Harmonization. The worst case scenarios are 7 calendar days for a death or life-threatening, unlabeled, possibly related, clinical trial, serious AE and 15 calendar days for a serious, unlabeled, spontaneous AE.

The decision must then be made whether source documents (raw data including the "AE transmittal form," see below) will be exchanged or whether a completed CIOMS I or MedWatch form will be transmitted. If source documents are exchanged, then each partner will create its own MedWatch or CIOMS I form for submission to its health authority based on the source documents. The contents of these two forms will most likely differ, in particular, regarding the narrative and coding. There is usually not enough time to harmonize or reconcile the two (or more) partners' documents. This may or may not present problems. If this method is chosen, then source documents should be exchanged (by fax, or scanned and e-mailed preferably over secure networks or encrypted over the Internet) rapidly because little or no preparation of the documents is needed by the sender. Usually, if this method is used, all documents must be in English or translated into English. Translations are often labor intensive, time consuming, and costly, especially if out-sourced. Exchange is usually 1 to 2 working days for potential 7-day reports and 2 to 5 working days for all other serious AEs. Nonserious AEs are usually less time sensitive and can be exchanged once or twice a month unless one is nervous about missing a serious AE misclassified as nonserious in the nonserious transmission. In this case, weekly transmission should be done.

If the exchange between or among the partners is done with completed CIOMS I or MedWatch forms, then exchange should be by calendar day 8 to 10 to allow the receiving partner time to enter it into its database, make corrections (if any), or add local information (e.g., the Investigational New Drug Application (IND) or NDA number for US submissions) and transmit the case by calendar day 15.

As noted above, all documents and all transmissions should be in English. This is sometimes difficult with certain source documents that may be very long and difficult to translate. Some countries still require all domestic reporting to be in the language of that country.

All cases transmitted should have receipt verified and should be reconciled. That is, if 12 cases totaling 100 pages are transmitted (by whatever means), then 12 cases totaling 100 pages should be received. This verification should be done either at the time of each transmission or weekly (at most) to ensure that no cases are missed or lost. Reconciliation is done to ensure that all AEs sent are, in fact, received. Reconciliation can be done after each case is sent with the receiver sending a fax or e-mail indicating receipt of the AE. Alternatively, reconciliation can be done

in batches at weekly, biweekly, or monthly intervals. The longer one waits to reconcile, the greater the risk of having a late expedited report should that case be picked up only on reconciliation after a faulty initial transmission.

E2B transmissions between and among companies (not just from companies to regulators) are becoming more widespread now that transmission to regulatory agencies is obligatory in the European Union. This promises to standardize and facilitate transmissions, although the start-up period has the potential to be time consuming, costly, and painful.

■ Other Issues That Must Be Addressed in Safety Agreements

- ■ Database
  - ▪ Is there an "official database" from which signaling will be done and regulatory reports prepared? This database should be complete and include all the data for this drug. Are there multiple databases or one database available to all parties? If there are multiple databases, should they be reconciled?
  - ▪ Timing of *Medical Dictionary for Regulatory Activites* (MedDRA) updates. If one party updates its database 45 days after the new MedDRA release and the other party at 60 days, for 15 days the parties will be using different versions of MedDRA. How will this be handled and does it matter? Will there be reconciliation or will the parties "agree to disagree"?
  - ▪ Drug dictionary and other standard dictionaries used. Will the same or different ones be used? If different, will there be reconciliation?
- ■ Regulatory Status
  - ▪ The countries where the drug is under study (e.g., IND, CTC, CTX) or sold (marketing authorizations, NDAs, NDSs) must be noted and listed by country and company. In addition, any special conditions should be noted (e.g., compassionate use, multiple marketing authorizations).
  - ▪ The regulatory representative for each company, including subsidiaries, if appropriate should be spelled out in an appendix.
  - ▪ Reporting responsibilities by each party should also be very clearly defined and assigned to each party.
- ■ Regulatory Documents
  - ▪ Who owns, updates, and controls which documents (CCSI, DCSI, Investigator Brochure, SmPC, US PI, other labeling for marketed products)?

- Exchange and coordination of responses to documents received from health authorities. Who prepares the responses and who must agree to them from one or both parties? Is there mutual review of documents before submission to health authorities or are documents exchanged only after being sent to the authorities (i.e., no presubmission approval by the other party)?

- Exchange of AEs
  - Preagreement legacy databases. Should legacy data be exchanged and stored by each drug safety unit? If so, how will exchange be done? How will cases be changed if they are in older versions of MedDRA or if different drug dictionaries are used?
  - Case identification numbers. Does each company track all other companies' numbers for each case?
  - Mode of transfer: E2B, e-mail, PDF, secure network, Internet, encryption, etc.
  - Format: E2B, MedWatch, CIOMS I, serious AE transmission sheet (contents agreed on by all parties).
  - Source documents. Are they exchanged? What if they are not in English? Must they be translated?
  - Language(s) permitted. Must all documents be translated or can they be stored and translated at a later date if needed?
  - Clinical trials: Exchange serious AEs only? Nonserious also? Only related cases (and as determined by whom)? Only unexpected cases (and by whose label)? Timing and clock start date for 7- and 15-day and nonexpedited reports. Blind breaking rules. Investigator and Investigational Review Board/ethics committee notification.
  - Postmarketing, compassionate use, stimulated reports, etc. Timing and clock start date. Serious and nonserious. These should be mentioned and procedures and responsibilities defined.
  - Follow-up and new information procedures, handling, and transmission. Do the parties define follow-up procedures and information differently? Do they treat all follow-up data as reportable to health authorities or is only certain "medically significant" follow-up information reported to the authorities? Must both parties use the same approach or is it acceptable that one party then submits more information to their health authority than the other partner?
  - Health authorities' requests for additional information on specific cases and more general issues. Who answers, approves, timing?

- Aggregate Reporting
  - Who prepares and approves Periodic Safety Update Reports, IND annual reports, NDA periodic reports, etc.?
  - Exchange of documents. How and when is it done? Is e-mail acceptable with PDF attachments or E2B files? What level of encryption is required if the Internet is used?

- Literature Review
  - Who does it? Centrally versus having each country review local language journals? Avoidance of duplication. Who does follow-up, especially if in a far-away non-English-speaking country? Language and translation issues. Is it done weekly, twice monthly, monthly?

- Third Parties and Subcontractors
  - How are they handled? Responsibilities.

- Signaling and Pharmacovigilance
  - Who is responsible? How can duplicate signaling by each party be avoided? Should it be avoided? Are there periodic meetings of the two signaling groups to discuss signals? How are differences resolved if one party identifies a signal and the other disagrees?
  - Product quality complaints and their handling. How are these tracked, investigated, and resolved? Where should returned product be sent and by what shipping method? How are all parties kept up to date on analytic investigations done on returned or retained samples?
  - Medication errors and their handling.

- Dispute Resolution
  - Case level disagreements on seriousness, expectedness, relatedness, especially in regard to tight reporting time frames.
  - Responses to health authorities.
  - Labeling changes and worldwide consistency.

- Crisis Management
  - Recalls, withdrawals, stopping trials, changing protocols, and investigator brochures.

As noted at the beginning of this chapter, as companies globalize, complex business arrangements are becoming more and more common. The US Food and Drug Administration and other health authorities (the European Medicines Agency in particular) are putting great store in the timely reporting of AEs from all over the world. They fully expect that modern communication and technology can bring safety information from the "ends of the earth" to them within 7 or 15 days as required.

Computers, Informatics, Validation, and Data Entry

Any company that receives more than a handful of adverse events (AEs), whether for marketed products or for products only in clinical trials, needs a database to collect, assemble, and report on these AEs. As the rest of the chapters in this book indicate, the regulations and reporting requirements are voluminous and follow tight standards in terms of content, format, and timing for reports to health authorities (HAs). It is thus necessary to have an AE database that allows, at the minimum, easy data entry, preparation, and printing of MedWatch and CIOMS I forms and various other aggregate data reports for Periodic Safety Update Reports (PSURs), Investigational New Drug Application (IND) annual reports, and New Drug Application (NDA) periodic reports. This, however, is just the tip of the iceberg. Many more functions are needed for a modern drug safety department, especially if the department has worldwide data in-

put and reporting obligations. This chapter reviews the issues and specialized needs around safety databases.

■ Database Needs and Functions

The following list represents a high-level view of the functions that a safety database must have to meet the needs of a multinational drug safety department. For smaller single-country departments, the needs are somewhat less. There will surely be other requirements needed now or in the future that are not listed here. The ability to change and customize the database as requirements change is critical.

- Data Entry
  - Case data entry to include all needed fields to produce a completed MedWatch form, CIOMS I form, PSUR, CIOMS line listing, E2B transmission, etc.
  - Tabular entry of laboratory data.
  - Multiple narratives for the same case (e.g., short narrative, long narrative, non-English narrative, case comments, blinded narrative, etc.). Mechanism to handle follow-up information in

the narrative (overwrite vs. append). Size limitations on the field.

- Seriousness, expectedness (labeledness), causality at the case, and AE level.
  - Ability to handle multiple labels (e.g., Summary of Product Characteristics, US package insert, etc.) producing different expectedness classification depending on label.
  - Ability to handle reporter and multiple partners giving different classifications.
- Versioning with multiple versions possible for each case.
- Tracking of information in and out (case log).
- Support of the *Medical Dictionary for Regulatory Activities* (MedDRA) (multiple versions and languages), WHO-ART (and other) drug dictionaries, as well as dictionaries for other functions (such as abbreviations, laboratory units, SNOMED, etc.).
- Handling of devices, drugs, biologics, medication errors, product quality complaints, blood products as needed.
- Duplicate check.
- Ability to add fields as needed (e.g., new business partner case reference numbers).
- Ability to close/complete a case and reopen it as needed.
- Ability to have scanned source document attached or linked to a case.
- Required fields customizable by users.
- Edit checks (e.g., system will not allow entry of data to show that a 50-year-old patient has a birth date of 12-Jan-2005).
- Ability to handle clinical trial, spontaneous, solicited, named patient, literature, and other types of cases.
- Spell check in multiple languages.

- Work Flow
  - Ability to track and move a case through its processing using customized business rules set up by the users.
  - Communication ability at the user and case level (e.g., a reviewer can electronically ask a question of the person who entered the case data).
  - Version tracking of each case.
  - Metrics to measure status of groups of cases with groups customized by the user (e.g., each work team has its own metrics and management has aggregate metrics).

- Duplicate checking and ability to duplicate a case or archive a case.
- Ability to handle customized case identification numbering with each case having multiple numbers.
- Multiple clock start dates (e.g., varies by country).
- Follow-up letter generation.

- Administration
  - Customized access limits at user, country, group, case, drug level (e.g., France cannot read Germany's cases, team handling drug X cannot see drug Y cases, etc.).
  - Security and passwords.
  - Scalability (able to add more users, countries, drugs, etc. easily).
  - International (if needed) use.
  - Multiple language support.
  - Tickler (reminder) system.
  - Audit trails. Validation.
  - Tracking of submissions for expedited and aggregate reports to multiple HAs.

- Vendor Support and Information Technology (IT) Issues
  - User groups.
  - Support from vendor and internal IT colleagues at home-base and worldwide user sites.
  - Ability to customize if new regulations put in place (e.g., US Food and Drug Administration's [FDA's] "tome").
  - IT support capability in-house.
  - Upgrade policy and support for older versions.
  - Hardware needs and compatibility with other hardware and software.

- Validation
  - A fully validated system and validation strategy in place going forward. 21CFR11 compliance.
  - Change control in place.
  - Acceptable to US, European Union, and other inspectors.
  - Complete audit trails.

- Labeling Functions
  - The database should be able to store the AEs that are labeled/listed for each drug and formulation and be able to identify which cases, based on the labeling, seriousness, and causality (for clinical trial cases) are 7- and 15-day reports to HAs in various countries.

- Labels for multiple countries should be storable and useable in this manner.
- Reporting Functions
  - Draft and final versions of all usual reports: MedWatch, CIOMS I, PSUR tables, listings etc., NDA periodic and IND annual tables, Investigator Letters.
  - Less common reports: UK yellow card, French inputability in English and other languages.
  - Ability to identify, based on algorithms that are entered into the database, which cases are 7-day and 15-day reports and which cases go into PSURs, NDA periodic reports, etc.
  - Ability to pull in data from the database and other sources and place into templates (e.g., MS Word documents).
  - Ability to query easily (e.g., Query By Example) on all fields to produce queries that can be made into reports. Batch printing, transmission of MedWatch forms, or line listings of query or report results.
  - Ability to save queries and reports at the user level.
  - Ability to do Structured Query Language queries.
  - Ability to anonymize reports and queries (e.g., no initials, no reporter names or addresses, etc.).
- Data Export and Import
  - E2B import with strategy on how to triage or "accept" a case before adding it to the database, especially if an earlier MedDRA version or different drug dictionary used.
  - E2B export to multiple sources with automated receipt acknowledgment and multiple headers and/or content changes (e.g., different file for Japan, United States, and European Union for each case).
  - Automated transmission of cases based on business rules to internal and external recipients (e.g., a particular drug's cases go to licensing company externally and recipients internally 10 calendar days after first receipt date).
  - Ability to generate other formats for data export (Excel, pdf, etc.).
- Pharmacovigilance Functions
  - Ability to produce pharmacovigilance reports, data mining both defined in the software and customized by the user.
  - Drug usage data stored and used in queries and reports.

- Ability to export data to be used in a third party's data mining software.

IT/Informatics Support

With a complex safety database in place, the drug safety group will need dedicated support from the technical services handling computers and information within an organization (be it a health agency or a pharmaceutical company). This will usually require one or more people working full time with the drug safety group. This is critical as the IT personnel, in order to better serve, must learn a significant amount about how the safety business runs.

The IT group will serve in multiple functions, including administration of the hardware and software, upgrades, user access and security, ad hoc queries (by the programmers), ongoing maintenance, bug fixes, new reports and projects, and validation and change control. In addition, there will be many behind-the-scenes personnel (e.g., database administrators, server maintenance, network personnel etc.) involved in support of the drug safety database.

It is usually good for both the drug safety medical staff and the IT personnel to have "one-stop shopping." That is, requests for IT support for new projects should go through one person within the drug safety department to manage the flow or work and requests, track projects, and clarify needs. The IT person will then coordinate the behind-the-scenes needs he or she has (e.g., network personnel, database administrators, etc.). Similarly, the drug safety personnel should be able to go to one IT person for any computer issues and not have to figure who to go to in IT: the database coordinator, the software support team, or the hardware support team.

Privacy

The database must support all privacy and security requirements from around the world. In particular, the European Union has in place very strict privacy regulations (Directive 95/46). The United States has Health Insurance Portability and Accountability Act requirements in place as well (see Chapter 12). Whatever database is used must be able to handle multiple and sometimes conflicting privacy and data protection requirements. This may involve storing personal identifier information (names, addresses, reports, etc.) in separate files in separate servers, sometimes within the European Union.

These rules are complex and changing. Most companies now have dedicated privacy officers who can assist in these issues.

Data Entry Strategy

Companies must make strategic, organizational, and operational decisions on where data entry should occur, especially if they are multinational companies. Single-country companies are able to have their safety data entered centrally in one or at most two facilities. This streamlines operations and allows for standardization across all data entry personnel and for backup data entry if one site should go out of service (e.g., fire, loss of electrical power, etc.).

Multinational companies must deal with issues of multiple languages, the need for follow-up on AE cases by local personnel in the local language, local reporting requirements (again, often in the local language), and the need for consistency and a single message (say the same thing to all HAs in each AE case). Companies respond to these needs in multiple ways:

- Headquarters data entry: For small companies or AEs from only one or two countries, it is sometimes feasible to ship all AEs to the main drug safety department for data entry.

- Geographic data entry by region: One data entry center each for North America, Europe, South America, and Asia/Africa. Follow-up of cases is done locally in the local language and the data transmitted to the regional data center for entry into the corporate safety database. This requires careful timing and coordination to remain in full compliance.

- Country data entry: Some companies have more dispersed data entry than by region. They may designate major affiliates or subsidiaries, particularly those with high volumes of AEs, to do data entry for their country (and possibly other countries nearby), thus having data entry done, for example, in the United States, Canada, Mexico, France, the United Kingdom, Germany (also handling Austria), Spain, Benelux (all done out of one site), Australia, South Africa, Japan, Singapore (covering the rest of Asia outside of Australia and Japan), and so forth.

- Out-sourcing for some or all data entry: Companies may hire Contract Research Organizations to do data entry for them, shipping completed cases for review back to the company. This could occur for all cases or only for those cases in a country where the company chooses not to set up a data entry function.

The critical issues in whichever mechanism is chosen are as follows:

- Maintaining standards and consistency across multiple and diverse sites, often speaking different languages and working under different conditions, is always challenging.

- Organizational reporting may also present issues if the safety personnel abroad report only locally and not "dotted line" to the head safety office.

- Training is harder over greater distances even with on-line and other high technology tools.

- Quality is harder to measure and maintain.

- IT issues occur in terms of storage, networks, security, data transmission speed, and support.

- Time zones interfere with workflow. It is almost impossible to arrange a simultaneous teleconference between Japan, the United States, and Europe due to time differences. The international dateline also presents some dating problems ("this report came into the United States today from Japan where it was received tomorrow").

E2B

See Chapter 26 regarding the E2B documents issued from the International Conference on Harmonization. In this section, the practicalities of setting up E2B for data import and export are discussed.

E2B export of individual case safety reports is now obligatory for manufacturers to HAs in Japan and the European Union. The United States is still in a test phase, but the FDA has encouraged the use of E2B by manufacturers for post-marketing expedited reports. The FDA has indicated that at some point in the future it will make E2B transmission of postmarketing expedited reports obligatory.

There are several issues in E2B export:

- There is no longer a true international consensus on the E2B file. A separate file for each case must be prepared for Japanese reporting, because the so-called J-File is required by the Japanese HA in addition to the standardized E2B file. The European Union and the United States also have some differences in requirements that are forcing some companies to prepare three separate files, one each for the United States, Japan, and the European Union.

- The database structure of some old databases is not fully compatible with E2B transmissions. For example, the European Union prefers laboratory data to be entered into structured fields rather than as free text. Some companies have dozens of years of laboratory data stored as free text. The question of whether companies will have to convert these data (sometimes from hundreds of thousands of cases) is not fully answered at this time. The European Medicines Agency has requested that companies send them legacy data (i.e., data on older cases), back to 1995, and for companies with format issues, this is a complex question.

- Technical issues exist on gateways, drug dictionaries, and MedDRA versions.

- A process must be set up within a company to verify that all appropriate reports have been sent to the appropriate HAs (and/or business partners) on a timely basis and that they were received and successfully uploaded into the receivers' database(s).

Clearly, all these issues can be overcome as many companies, both large and small, are doing E2B transmissions to the FDA and the European Medicines Agency and the Japanese HA. Out-sourcing companies are able to do E2B transmissions for companies that have not set up the system and processes needed for direct E2B transmission themselves.

There are corresponding issues in regard to E2B import. In addition, there are other issues:

- How to screen and triage a report coming in. Should it be uploaded automatically into the receiver's database or should it be kept in a "holding area" until drug safety personnel are able to review the file for content and format to ensure that it meets the appropriate criteria for entry into the database?

- How is the file actually reviewed by the staff? The data can be loaded into a MedWatch form, but this only covers a part of the data transmitted. It is not practical to review the XML/STML transmission itself, so some sort of reader must be created to view the file.

- Screening for duplicates may be done in the triage area or after uploading. Duplicates are defined as receipt of the same case containing no new information whatsoever.

- A strategy must be found for identification, handling, and versioning of follow-up reports for cases already in the database.

- Dictionary incompatibility. If the sender has not yet upgraded to the latest version of MedDRA and the receiver has, how is the case handled? If different, and possibly incompatible, drug dictionaries are used, how are the data handled?

- How is security handled regarding encryption, viruses, and so on?

As with export, many companies are receiving E2B transmissions from other companies, showing that it is possible to use E2B for company-to-company exchange of serious AEs. Usually, this has involved the expenditure of very large amounts of time by the drug safety and IT groups to customize the exchange business rules and IT functionality.

It is anticipated that as more and more companies and HAs use E2B, the procedures, processes, hardware, and software will be standardized and allow the use of E2B for both import and export with less up-front expenditure and customization.

There are four major database products on the market currently:

ArisG by ArisGlobal®. See Web Resource 31-1.
Argus by Relsys Inc. See Web Resource 31-2.
Clintrace by Phase Forward, Inc. See Web Resource 31-3.
AERS by Oracle Inc. See Web Resource 31-4.

Each has its strong and weak points but all seem very acceptable for AE database use.

Standard Operating Procedures and Guidelines That a Drug Safety Group Must Have

U S regulations require that companies have written standard operating procedures (SOPs). These are documents that describe the general or specific steps to be done in a process, job, or function to ensure that the result is obtained in a fashion that is complete, reproducible, and delivers what is sought. The procedure should be descriptive and may be used for training and as a reference document.

The following is from the US Food and Drug Administration's (FDA's) document for inspectors doing adverse event (AE) audits (Chapter 53: Post-Marketing Surveillance and Epidemiology: Human Drugs, Enforcement of the Post-Marketing Adverse Drug Experience Reporting Regulations, September 30, 1999, Field Reporting Requirements. See Web Resource 32-1):

"The regulations (21 CFR 211.198) require that...manufacturers... have written procedures for complaint files including provisions for determining whether a complaint represents a serious and unexpected ADE. The regulations (21 CFR 211.25) also require that qualified person-

nel investigate and evaluate ADEs. If serious deficiencies are found during the inspection, obtain copies of the procedures and determine personnel qualifications and staffing, especially if the firm utilizes computerized reporting. Effective April 6, 1998, any person subject to the ADE Reporting regulations, including those that do not have approved applications, shall develop written procedures for the surveillance, receipt, evaluation, and reporting of postmarketing adverse drug experiences to FDA" (21 CFR 314.80(b) and 21 CFR 310.305(a)).

Similar requirements apply in the European Union (EU) and elsewhere.

One of the first requests that an inspector from the FDA or the EU will make at the beginning of a drug safety audit is for written copies of the SOPs and related documents (such as guidelines, working documents, manuals, etc.) covering drug safety. Usually, the company has an index or listing of these documents that is given to the inspector, who then chooses which ones to examine. Companies then must expect that the FDA, corporate auditors, and others will read the SOPs in great detail and expect those governed by the SOPs to follow them scrupulously. Auditors may also look at manuals and guidelines and other documents (see below) that groups prepare to aid in their work. The auditors also expect the staff to adhere to these guidelines too, especially if they are approved by some formal or semiformal company mechanism.

Companies or health agencies may create multiple levels of procedures. For a large company, there may be a very high level (or "global" or "corporate") SOP that states the scope and mission and broad outlines of the policy. Then, each division within the scope may develop its own localized policy, and subdivisions may then develop theirs. Usually, two to three layers are the practical limit of this hierarchy. For example, for a large multinational company, one way to approach this is to create three levels of SOPs:

1. High-level corporate policy that applies to all divisions of the company: This is the corporate policy to collect, analyze, and report to the appropriate health authorities and internal and external clients all AEs, product quality complaints, and medication errors that the company learns of with its products that occur in humans and animals.

2. Division level: Each division of the company then prepares a more detailed version of the high-level policy that applies only to that division:

   - Human products division: Creates a broad policy to put the high-level policy into effect. This would cover all research and marketing in the United States and abroad (directly or via subsidiaries or affiliates) and direct them to prepare their own local SOPs (in their local language with a translation into English for review by the quality group).

3. Subdivision level: Each section (e.g., the French affiliate) within a division then creates its own SOPs to put the policies noted above into place. There may be multiple policies needed to accomplish this, and they should specifically cover such things as responsibility by job title (e.g., the medical monitor is responsible for...), timing (e.g., all serious AEs from investigational sites sent to the company within 1 working day of occurrence by fax, e-mail...), and so on. For example, the following units could create one or more SOPs to cover the following:

   - The US drug safety unit SOPs would cover the specific details of the handling of spontaneous serious AEs, spontaneous nonserious AEs, literature AEs, clinical trial AEs from phase I-IV studies, clinical trial AEs from in-

vestigator-initiated trials, AEs from business partners, or AEs from consumers in the United States. If this is the corporate headquarters, this policy might also apply then to all other company units.

   - The clinical research unit SOPs would cover instructions to investigators and monitors on what and when to send AEs using what form or electronic process.

   - The animal toxicology/pharmacology unit(s) should have SOPs covering how and when animal findings regarding safety and toxicity should be reported and to whom, because in many jurisdictions animal findings that may result in safety issues in humans must be reported within 15 calendar days as expedited reports.

Other documents at any level can also be created. At any point, a unit may create documents to assist staff in doing their daily jobs. These documents might be manuals (e.g., a data entry manual explaining screen by screen how to enter AE cases into the safety database), guidelines, guidances, "cheat sheets" (e.g., a table of all AEs listed in a drug's package insert to aid in the rapid determination of whether an AE is labeled/listed or not), process guides, and various other work aids. Ideally, these should be done in a somewhat formal manner and verified to be correct and consistent from person to person within a group.

■ Version Control, Numbering, Updating, and Training

SOPs must be kept in tight control because they represent the "bible" and instructions to the employees that must be followed. Only the latest version of the SOP should be used and available to all employees. In theory, keeping only the latest versions of SOPs on-line ensures that employees do not use older outdated versions. However, in practice, especially if there are many SOPs, employees print out copies rather than looking on-line every time they have a question (e.g., they might have to log out of a case they are entering into the database to look up an SOP question). This tends to defeat the purpose of SOPs but is probably unavoidable. In that case the printed version should contain a statement to the effect: "This printed copy does not necessarily represent the latest in-force version of this SOP. The current in-force copy may be found on-line at [give link or URL]." Alternatively, the SOP group may issue to every employee covered loose-leaf binders containing numbered and dated versions of all SOPs. When a new version of an SOP is published, a member of the SOP group goes to each binder and replaces the old version with the new version.

Clearly, very tight version control must be maintained. This should be spelled out in the SOP governing SOP creation and maintenance. It should cover how and by whom it is determined that an SOP is needed and its creation, review, approval, and updating. A system of version control and numbering should be described. It should also mandate the training of the appropriate employees on the new procedures.

Training on SOPs is obligatory. Training should not be simply distribution of the SOPs and having someone read to him or herself, line by line, the contents. Efforts should be made using dedicated trainers (e.g., employees who have some skills in teaching and training) to develop methodology to ensure that training is effective. This includes setting up training and retraining schedules and curricula, using effective technology (interesting presentations, video, web-based training, etc.), and testing after the training to ensure that the content was absorbed. Many companies now have formal training departments that "certify" trainers ("train the trainers") within divisions of the company. The trainers themselves may not train on all SOPs but may enlist subject-matter experts to do the actual training. The trainers may review and approve the training materials. In addition, detailed records of training must be kept. They should be at the employee level and at the SOP level so that it can be easily demonstrated (with written records) to an auditor that every employee was successfully trained. Copies of the training materials must also be kept.

Quality

It is not sufficient to write and publish SOPs. They must be followed. The quality department should review (audit) SOPs on several levels:

- Do the SOPs meet the mission and standards they set? For example, if a safety SOP requires adherence to US and EU expedited reporting requirements, the SOP should be audited against the US and EU regulations, laws, and guidelines. This is often a difficult job for an auditor, because it requires that he or she must be quite familiar with these laws and regulations. Historically, the groups doing pharmacovigilance audits also did clinical research audits as well as, in some cases, financial, Good Laboratory Practice, and Good Manufacturing Practice audits. This would often mean that the auditors had only a superficial knowledge of safety requirements. Companies are now beginning to develop auditing units that have employees with specific specialties, including pharmacovigilance. Thus the auditor is able to make a learned judgment on whether the SOP meets FDA and EU requirements.

- The second level of review is the more common and, in general, easier level to audit: Are the employees adhering to the requirements of the SOP? If the SOP is clear and prescriptive, the auditor is easily able to verify whether the procedures are done appropriately. For example, if the SOP requires that each AE report coming into the safety department is date stamped immediately on receipt and then entered into the database within 2 working days, it is relatively straightforward for the auditor to check the date stamp and compare it with the date of data entry.

- Another level of review is internal consistency. If each subsidiary in the countries where a multinational company sells the drug has a safety SOP, these SOPs should be reviewed for consistency with the higher level SOP and, if desired and appropriate, with each other.

Working with Business Partners

In our age of globalization, it is now very common for companies to work with many other companies in codevelopment, comarketing, and other joint arrangements. Some of these can involve multiple companies throughout the world. Although the Council for International Organizations of Medical Sciences (CIOMS) and the International Conference on Harmonization (see Chapters 25 and 26, respectively) have done much work to harmonize requirements and regulations, there are still significant differences between and among each company's SOPs. These differences, on the working level, can be substantial and very difficult for companies to work out in a manner satisfactory to all parties.

Sometimes companies may not permit their (highly proprietary) SOPs to leave their building. The other company may see them but only by physically visiting the site where the first company keeps the SOPs.

The specific requirements of SOPs may also present problems. If one company uses only MedWatch forms and the other only CIOMS I forms, there will be issues to resolve. Or, if two companies agree to exchange completed CIOMS I forms for all serious AEs with each other and one company bases its procedure on completing the forms by calendar day 7 and the other by calendar day 11, there may be significant timing and process issues forcing one of the companies to alter its procedure to accommodate a shortened preparation schedule. One company may require a legal review of each case and the other may not. At some point most companies harmonize as much as they can and "agree to disagree" on the remainder of the issues. Generally, the larger the company, the less flexible it is.

■ SOPs for Drug Safety

Below is a list of some of the basic SOPs that should exist for a drug safety department. This list is not complete and will be tailored by each organization. Some organizations will be "lumpers" and others will be "splitters," creating fewer or more SOPs, respectively:

- Handling of AEs in clinical research, including investigator-initiated trials as well as phase I-IV studies
- Handling of AEs from marketing and sales, legal, telephone operators, and the mail room
- Reporting requirements for employees not normally involved in safety to specify that all AEs must be sent to drug safety within certain time frames (i.e., if an accounting department employee hears from a neighbor over the weekend that one of the company's products made him sick, that AE should be reported to drug safety)

- Handling of AEs in animals
- The mechanics of the drug safety department:
  - Receipt of AEs from trials, from spontaneous reports, from consumers, electronic data capture, logging, database entry, quality review, narrative preparation, the *Medical Dictionary for Regulatory Activities* coding conventions, drug naming conventions, breaking the blind in clinical trials, literature review, medical review, querying, and follow-up
  - Handling of 7-day expedited reports
  - Handling of 15-day expedited reports (clinical trial and postmarketing)
  - How to develop safety agreements with partners; handling of reports sent to business partners and internal clients
  - Preparation of Investigational New Drug Application annual reports, New Drug Application periodic reports, Periodic Safety Update Reports, and other aggregate reports
  - Contacts with the FDA and other government agencies
  - Crisis management and disaster recovery
  - Database management and access
  - How to handle an audit
  - Archiving and filing; record retention
  - Signaling
  - Medication error handling
  - Product quality handling
  - Quality assurance and quality compliance
  - SOP preparation and maintenance
  - Litigation
  - Training

Training

Two broad and related areas are addressed here: training of the drug safety staff and training of the other employees in the organization.

■ Drug Safety

In any organization there are two broad areas of training required. The first includes the corporate/organizational requirements and includes such things as using the computer systems, corporate ethics, behavior and mission, equality in the workplace, getting along with coworkers, safety in the workplace, filling out needed forms for payroll and benefits, and how to use the library. These programs are usually taught to all workers in the organization by the corporate-level training group. These are not addressed further here.

The other area of training, discussed in detail in this chapter, involves job-specific drug safety training. Nearly all drug safety groups now have a training function, and many groups now have full-time dedicated trainers whose job it is to handle all the aspects of training. This group sets up a training system with tailored curricula depending on the job being trained and customized for it.

The training group sets up schedules for training and make-up sessions for those who missed the first session. Although they may do much of the training themselves, especially on high level or more general subjects, they create a roster of subject matter experts who will be called on to train in highly specialized or technical areas that the trainers cannot teach. The training group works with the quality and compliance groups as well as with the drug safety group to determine which employees should be trained in which areas. They determine which training can be "one shot" and which requires updating or refresher training. Some groups with high turnover require frequent training sessions of new employees (e.g., the sales force), whereas others are often more stable and do not require training sessions as frequently.

The training job may require significant travel if training is done at various sites around the United States or the world. This is particularly true for multinational organizations and those that have employees working at home or off-site. The levels of training for full-time employees versus consultants should also be taken into account.

Issues of training of non-English-speaking employees outside (and even inside) the United States need to be addressed, especially now that English is required for international communications in drug safety and international business in general.

The group should have a good understanding of the newer technologies for training, including web-based training and distance learning. The use of out-sourcing in the appropriate circumstances should also be considered.

The training group sets up a recordkeeping system, both for the training department to document globally who was trained and for employee-specific training files, which usually remain within each employee's employment (or dedicated) training dossier. Copies of the training materials should also be retained in the master file. Thus during an audit the training group can demonstrate that training of a particular function (e.g., handling 7-day expedited reports) was done to the appropriate groups (e.g., drug safety, clinical research, regulatory affairs) with the training documentation (slides, handouts) on file. In addition, the training group can go to each employee's file and show the record indicating that that employee was trained on this function on this particular date.

The training group should work with the departments to be trained as well as drug safety to prepare a matrix of which employees (by title or function) need which training modules and at what frequency. They should determine which employees need refresher training even if the standard operating procedures (SOPs) and processes have not changed.

Other Groups

Many companies now have a general corporate policy that requires all employees and agents of the company (including consultants and temporary employees) to report adverse events (AEs) to the drug safety group if they hear about them during and outside of work. This usually refers to marketed drugs and covers such items as when a neighbor or relative casually notes that he or she took your company's drug XX and had a bad reaction. The policy requires the employee to report this to the drug safety group by the next business day with sufficient contact information to allow drug safety to follow up on the report and get the details of the case.

On drug safety issues, it is necessary to train several groups ("feeder groups") within the company on their duties in regard to sending AEs to drug safety and then the handling and distribution of the cases. Groups that require training include the marketing and sales groups, the legal department, the mailroom staff, the telephone operators, senior corporate management and their administrative staff (who often receive complaint letters addressed to the chief executive officer or President), all clinical research and support groups, medical affairs, the product complaint department, the quality and compliance groups, regulatory affairs, medical information/services, the new business development group, the library, and any other groups identified as being involved with AE or safety reports.

Outside groups include clinical or contract research organizations doing work with or for the company as well as all other contractors and out-sourcers (e.g., hired sales forces, such as "rent a rep"), investigators doing clinical research who need to report AEs to the company, outside legal counsel, and other business partners who, by contract, need to adhere to the company's SOPs. This may sometimes be difficult to determine.

As the training needs of the organization increase due to both new hires, expansion, and changes in regulations and requirements, it is unlikely that the personnel and travel budget in the training department will increase proportionately. This forces the group to increase productivity and to "work smarter." There are many ways to do this, including video recording of procedures that rarely change so that a training course or module remains valid and useful for an extended period of time. Other techniques include web-based training, distance learning, delegation of training ("train the trainer"), and self-training modules.

The issue of testing arises frequently. It is generally accepted that it is not sufficient to simply train people by having them read materials or attending live classroom sessions or one-on-one training. Some determination of whether the material has been absorbed is usually required. This can be done by formal testing at the end of training or at some point after training is completed (e.g., yearly at the same time each year). The testing may be anonymous or the testee known. The results may be given only to the testee or may be seen by the testers or drug safety trainers. Retraining and retesting for people who fail may be required. Training may be self-training on-line or paper-based. In all cases, good pedagogic techniques must be followed such as "praise publicly, reproach privately."

Typical Curriculum for a New Hire in Drug Safety

The training group typically prepares modules covering each section or subsection listed below and can thus pick out which modules should be used to train which employees as a function of the employee's job and experience. For example, internal hires may need less training than hires new to the company.

Organizational Structure and Site Information

- New employee orientation (usually done by Human Resources)
- Introduction to staff and organization
- Review of training curriculum
- Site information
- Telephone, password, voice mail, web portal functions
- Safety department overview—structure and functions, teams, support staff
- Subsidiary and country operations
- Duties and responsibilities of the position
- Performance objectives and measures; goal setting
- Support groups
- Training from other divisions (e.g., as provided by clinical research, legal, regulatory affairs, informatics, etc.)
- Emergency procedures if the site is not accessible or the computers are down

Computer, Forms, Electronic, and Print Resources

- Computer and Internet accounts and password
- Applications
- Help desk
- E-mail policies
- Storage drives
- Corporate website and portal
- Services accessible on-line: library, benefits, forms.
- Wireless use (if available)
- Logging on from off-site

What Is Pharmacovigilance?

- Governing US and ex-US regulations, laws, guidelines, directives
- SOPs, manuals, job aids, guidelines
- Terminology
- US Food and Drug Administration (FDA) and European Medicines Agency functions and duties

- Mission of drug safety
- Labeling (summary of product characteristics, package insert, investigator brochure, company core safety information, development of core safety information)

Corporate and Drug Safety SOPs

- High-level corporate SOPs
- Divisional SOPs
- Drug safety SOPs
- Other departments' SOPs that touch on drug safety
- International Organization for Standards requirements if applicable (This group produces SOPs and standards that are accepted and followed in many fields, including device manufacture in the United States. See Web Resource 33-1.)

Medical Dictionary for Regulatory Activities (MedDRA) and Other Dictionaries

- Introduction to MedDRA
- The MedDRA browser
- Coding AEs: Maintenance and Support Service Organization and FDA conventions
- Requesting new codes and periodic updates
- Drug dictionary
- Other dictionaries (e.g., abbreviations) and conventions

Safety Database

- Access to the database: IDs and passwords
- Screen by screen training on data entry
- Pregnancy cases, mother-child cases, and other special situations
- Data privacy
- Laboratory data
- Source documents and scanning
- Archiving and deleting cases
- Clock start date and other date issues
- Duplicates
- Transmission of expedited reports to the FDA or other regulatory agencies
- Transmission of cases to business partners
- Workflow
- Quality checks

- Requesting follow-up information from the reporter/investigator
- Preparing reports, cover letters, investigator letters
- Ad hoc queries, structured query language, query by example
- Device, combination product, vaccine, biologics, blood product issues
- E2B import and export

Workflow

- Handling 7-day clinical trial expedited reports
- Handling 15-day Investigational New Drug Application (IND) expedited reports
- Handling 15-day New Drug Application (NDA) expedited reports
- Ex-US expedited reports
- Nonexpedited serious reports
- Nonserious reports
- Pregnancy cases
- Literature reports

- Stimulated reports and investigator-initiated study reports
- Medication errors
- Product quality reports
- Medical (physician) review
- Quality checks
- Aggregate reports, including IND annual reports, NDA periodic reports, and Periodic Safety Update Reports
- Interactions with other departments (e.g., clinical research, regulatory)
- Breaking the blind in clinical trials: individual cases and at the end of the trial for all cases

Signaling and Pharmacovigilance

- Signal generation, handling, and workup
- Crisis management
- Drug withdrawal, protocol changes, stopping studies, tampering, and other urgent issues
- Label changes
- Media training

The Safety Department's Role in Clinical Research, Marketing and Sales, Labeling, Regulatory, Due Diligence, and Legal Issues

The drug safety department plays a vital and major role in the daily activities of other sections of a pharmaceutical company. The roles and interfaces are discussed here.

Clinical Research

The clinical research (or medical research) department is the section of a company that does clinical trials and studies. There are many ways to structure such departments. Some companies have their research department only do phase II and III (developmental) trials with a separate group handling phase I (clinical pharmacology) studies and another group handling phase IV (postmarketing) studies. Alternatively, there may be separate groups handling different types of products: biologics, drugs, devices, or over-the-counter products. Other structures are by country or geographic region: US studies, European Union (EU) studies, and "rest of the world" studies.

Whatever the structure of the clinical research division may be, the drug safety department must play a continuous role in these groups' day-to-day activities because clinical studies almost always produce adverse events

(AEs). The drug safety group must ensure that it receives all appropriate AEs from all trials. "Appropriate" usually means all serious AEs (SAEs), some or all non-SAEs, and all pregnancy cases (not AEs, of course, but in practice handled like AEs from a logistic point of view; see Chapter 36). In most countries of the world, there is a requirement to report certain SAEs to the health authorities in either 7 or 15 days (expedited reports) or periodically (e.g., yearly). Unless the clinical research divisions are able to receive and process such AEs themselves, these cases must be sent to the drug safety department.

The clinical research and drug safety groups must establish a process to ensure that all SAEs are reported to the company within 24 to 48 hours after occurrence at a clinical site. This allows the company to process them and report the cases to the US Food and Drug Administration (FDA) and other agencies, particularly for the 7- or 15-calendar-day SAEs.

The investigators must be trained and sensitized (on a continual basis) to report SAEs. Usually, this means reporting all SAEs, although some companies only collect unexpected SAEs on an expedited basis, receiving the others weekly or monthly. The process involves the electronic transmission (fax, e-mail, electronic data capture) of a report form with all the necessary information regarding the

SAE and the patient for the company to enter the data into the safety database and prepare a MedWatch or CIOMS I form (or E2B file) for submission to the FDA, clinical investigators, and other health authorities, respectively. This process often involves queries to the investigator (done either by drug safety directly or via the clinical research department). This process can become exceedingly complex if SAE volume is very high, if multiple worldwide sites are involved, if a clinical research organization or other intermediaries are involved, if a cooperative group is involved (e.g., in oncology studies), or if a governmental agency (e.g., National Institutes of Health) is involved.

Some studies generate very large numbers of SAEs, such as oncology studies in very ill patients receiving toxic study drugs. For such studies, various protocol customizations may be done to ensure that the important SAEs (those that are unexpected and/or related to the study drug) reach the company within 1-2 days and the health agencies within 7 to 15 days. SAEs that are expected or clearly not related to the study drug may be reported to the company in a less urgent fashion (e.g., monthly or even at the end of the study). Most health agencies (including the FDA) are willing to negotiate such arrangements. For large multinational trials, this may require negotiations with multiple national health authorities to reach a workable consensus that meets all needs. For example, a protocol might state that because drug X in previous trials has been shown to produce gastrointestinal, urinary, and pulmonary hemorrhage in this patient group, these cases will not be reported until the end of the trial unless the patient dies. Hemorrhage from other body sites would be reported to the company in 1-2 days.

Many companies, especially the larger ones, maintain two safety databases. One very common model has a safety database maintained by the drug safety department and a clinical trial database maintained by the clinical research/statistics groups. The drug safety database holds only the SAEs from clinical trials plus all spontaneous serious and nonserious reports. This database is used for the regulatory reporting of expedited reports and Investigational New Drug Application (IND) annual reports. The clinical research department maintains the other database that holds all safety and efficacy data from clinical trials (but no spontaneous reports) and is used in preparing the final clinical study report for each study as well as integrated safety summaries for New Drug Application (NDA) submissions and the equivalent for submissions in the EU and elsewhere.

The data in the two databases for any given patient may vary. One reason is due to different mechanisms of data collection. The drug safety database usually receives data from the investigator using a dedicated one- or two-page SAE reporting form rather than multiple pages from the case report form (CRF). Thus the same SAE information is collected in two different places for each patient. In addition, the drug safety group receives a clinical trial SAE within 24-48 hours after the investigator first notes it. The clinical trial database may not receive the CRF data for several weeks if the CRFs are "harvested" only every 6 weeks or so by the medical monitor. The use of electronic data capture promises to decrease this issue (see below).

Other differences between the databases may occur if different people code each case differently (one person in the drug safety department and one in the clinical research department). Follow-up information or corrected data may reach one database and not the other. More subtle differences may arise in the data that are collected. For example, for the clinical research department, the drug compliance (what percentage of the study drug was actually taken by the patient and which doses were missed) is critical. To the safety department it is less important that the patient took 75% of the study drug versus 85% or 95%. To drug safety, it is a much more binary (yes/no) question of whether the drug was ingested at all or not. Thus drug safety usually spends less time clarifying the dosing schedule followed by the patients than the clinical research department.

It is thus necessary to reconcile the cases within the two databases to ensure that the data, or at least the key data, are identical. This can be done at the end of the trial or during the trial as each patient or groups of patients complete the study. This can be a very time-consuming procedure requiring attendance at meetings by both drug safety and clinical research. Differences must be ironed out, and sometimes new queries to the investigative sites are generated from the reconciliation. Another vexing problem that occurs periodically, for 15-day alert cases, concerns important follow-up information that arrives in clinical research and is not sent to the drug safety group for submission to the FDA as a follow-up alert report. This produces a late alert report because the data were in-house for weeks or months before the 15-day alert is sent to the FDA and other health agencies.

The drug safety group may be involved in the creation by clinical research of the final study report for each individual study. This includes data reconciliation as well as supplying the "narrative" (and/or "capsule summary") or other data sets prepared for each case to clinical research to aid them in the preparation of their final study reports.

The clinical research and drug safety groups usually collaborate when a signal is being worked up or an ad hoc health authority question arises. For example, if a health agency asks about a particular AE or groups of AEs (e.g., acute pancreatitis or all pancreatic AEs), it is usually necessary to pull the non-SAEs from the clinical research database and the SAEs from the drug safety database to capture all the AEs in question. Because of the way data are entered into the clinical research database (either at the end of the study or when batches of data arrive at the data entry site), the drug safety database is usually more up to date at any one time because drug safety usually enters data immediately upon receipt and clinical research may enter data periodically or when a group of CRFs arrive or even at the end of the study.

The use of electronic data capture, where each investigator enters data into a database in real time, making it available immediately to clinical research, statistics, drug safety, and others involved in the study, promises to change the way data are handled and analyzed in companies and health authorities. The concept of a single (or distributed) central database (or data warehouse) holding all data that can be viewed by any party that needs to see it is being developed by software companies and some drug companies. Thus an investigator could enter a patient's study data into a local computer on-line to the company website/database. The efficacy and safety data would go ("be pushed") to the clinical research department's database, the safety data to drug safety's database, the administrative and enrollment information to the corporate accounting department to pay the investigator, and so on. Alternatively, all the data go into one central site and each department can "pull" the data it needs when it needs them.

Although the concept is welcomed by all, the devil is in the details and the central warehouse successes to date have been primarily in small companies with few studies and marketed products. Nonetheless, it is highly likely that data storage, handling, centralization, and viewing over the Internet will develop over time, making data available to all who need to see it.

The clinical research department and the safety department also interact at development and project planning meetings, signaling meetings, training sessions, preparation of annual reports, investigator brochure updates, and so on. The drug safety group is also charged with sending blinded or unblinded safety information to drug safety monitoring committees or data monitoring committees. These are outside groups that evaluate the safety profile and status of a study on an ongoing basis during the study to ensure patient safety and data integrity. This may become very tricky if the drug safety group breaks individual patients' blinding codes to report the case unblinded to the FDA and data committees but,

at the same time, endeavors to maintain the blind for the clinical research and biostatistics departments (see Chapter 26 on E2A). Drug safety may also assist the clinical research department in the preparation of data for meetings with health authorities, FDA advisory committee meetings, and responses to ad hoc queries.

Marketing and Sales

Drug safety and marketing interact in various ways. At some level in each company, a medical group (sometimes drug safety, sometimes medical affairs, sometimes another group) must review advertising and promotional copy for drugs to be sure that the medical and safety claims being made are correct. That is, the claims made by the company correctly reflect the information contained in the official labeling (the approved package insert in the United States).

Marketing will often ask drug safety for information on AEs for their own uses (to help sell more product). Although it is hard to refuse to supply such data, drug safety should remind the marketers that spontaneous drug safety data cannot, in general, be used for promotional activities or safety claims.

Drug safety may also be asked to supply data that the customer relations department (often within marketing where technical and scientific questions are asked) uses to prepare responses to patients' or health care professionals' medical queries ("Have you ever seen pulmonary emboli with this drug in young women? If yes, how did they do and how were they treated?").

In the evaluation of signals and in the production of certain reports, including Periodic Safety Update Reports (PSURs) and some FDA required reports, it is necessary for drug safety to obtain drug use data, such as sales data, patients using the drug, tonnage shipped, or prescriptions written, to estimate a reporting frequency of AEs. These data are kept by the marketing and sales departments. Sometimes they are generated internally and sometimes they are purchased from outside vendors who track prescriptions and sales. This is another area of interaction between drug safety and marketing/sales.

Drug safety often does training of sales representatives, advertising copywriters, and others in the marketing and sales departments in regard to the reporting of AEs. Although the sales force generally believes that its job is to sell drugs and not collect AEs, it is now generally understood by all parties that sales representatives, when they hear of AEs on their products, have an obligation to report them to the safety department for follow-up and regulatory reporting.

In a more subtle way, drug safety must also influence and reinforce its ethical and legal role with marketing and sales. Many sales people, particularly those handling over-the-counter products, do not fully comprehend that the pharmaceutical industry, along with the financial and nuclear industries, are among the most regulated industries in the world. The limitations, reporting obligations, and safety issues are often not in the mindset of marketers and sales people whose job (and pay) is dependent on product sales. It is drug safety that often must set the limits on what marketing and sales can and may do. For this reason, the marketers often call the drug safety department the "sales prevention department" and the head physician "Dr. No."

The drug safety department is a cost center that never produces revenue and profit for a company. This tends to produce, in some drug safety people, a siege mentality because they carry little weight in the corporate hierarchy and are continually "fighting" to get their message out. The primary goal of the safety department, of course, is to prevent patient harm and to protect the public health. This viewpoint is sometimes not shared by others in the company who believe that the safety department's primary job is to protect the company's products at all costs. In fact, by doing correct and complete safety work, the safety department is protecting the company's products so that at some point down the road, when the safety issues do arise, they will not produce drug withdrawals, lawsuits, and patient harm. However, this is often a hard concept to "sell to the sales department." Potential dollars not lost in the future do not appear on balance sheets or get people raises and bonuses.

Labeling

The drug safety department will have some role in label creation and maintenance. At the simplest level, drug safety supplies AE information, particularly on treatment emergent AEs for marketed products, to the department (e.g., regulatory affairs, medical writing, dedicated label departments) that creates and maintains the label. The safety department may also be charged with periodic or continuous label review to ensure that the label contains the latest scientific and medical information. This may mean that the safety department must notify the appropriate departments of new AEs worthy of being put into the label (usually with prior approval by a labeling or safety committee), changes in the pregnancy status of a drug, new warnings, contraindications, and precautions both for the product itself and for the whole class of drugs ("class labeling"). It is also worthwhile for the drug safety

or labeling department to scan the drugs labels of other companies' products for the appearance of a new drug interaction with other marketed drugs in these other drugs' labeling. The actual division of these duties is not clearly standardized and varies from company to company.

Legal

The drug safety department may be involved with the legal department when AEs are reported in cases under litigation or when there is threat of litigation. In such instances, the lawyers usually forbid the drug safety department to have direct contact with the patient or health care providers. All contact, to obtain further safety information, is usually done through the company's legal department. In addition, one or more people from the drug safety department (usually physicians) may be subpoenaed to testify in cases involving the company and safety issues related to its products. This involves "witness training" for those at risk to be called on to testify at depositions or in court.

It is also very common, when a company is being sued, for the plaintiff's attorneys to request copies of safety information. This process is called "discovery." The safety department may be forced to stop work to prepare or assist in the preparation of photocopies or diskettes of hundreds to thousands of pages of material needed in a very tight time frame. In the worst case, the drug safety department may have its paper and/or electronic files sealed to prevent any changes or the adding of new information. Drug safety is also heavily involved in the preparation of the company's defense in such cases and in the evaluation of claims that have not yet reached litigation.

Regulatory Affairs

Although usually reporting to the clinical research department in a company, the drug safety department's function is primarily a regulatory one. Drug safety is responsible for the preparation and submission of MedWatch forms, NDA periodic reports and such to the FDA, and similar reports to business partners and health agencies abroad. Usually, expedited IND reports and sometimes expedited NDA reports are transmitted to the regulatory department for transmission to the FDA and elsewhere. This requires careful and detailed procedures to ensure that reports are not lost or sent in late. Regulatory affairs is usually the intermediary in any direct contacts between the FDA and the safety department as well as other departments in the company because most companies prefer to carefully control and monitor all communications with health authorities. Most company employees are not permitted to contact the FDA directly but must go through regulatory affairs.

The FDA may approach the company and request that a labeling change be made. This usually results in the company setting up a task force, including drug safety, clinical research, regulatory, and animal toxicology, to respond to the request.

■ Quality and Compliance

The drug safety group interacts with the quality group and the compliance group both in regard to the safety department's duties but also in regard to assisting in technical matters when these groups are dealing with safety issues in other departments. This might involve assistance in audits of investigator sites, vendors and contract research organizations, review of business partner standard operating procedures and safety data, and manufacturing safety issues. This is highly variable from company to company.

■ New Business Due Diligence Reviews

When a company wishes to purchase or license in a drug product to sell, it usually examines the entire data set for the drug to be purchased. This includes the review of manufacturing data, standard operating procedures, animal toxicology and pharmacology data, clinical data, and regulatory correspondence with the FDA, European Medicines Evaluation Agency, and others. The drug safety department may be called in during this "due diligence" review to examine the clinical safety data, including MedWatch and CIOMS forms, NDA periodic reports, IND annual reports, PSURs, rapporteur responses to PSURs, and all sorts of other safety data. Sometimes the data are available electronically, sometimes on paper, or both. Sometimes it is aggregate data primarily, and other times it is less well-organized individual patient safety information. For a drug that has not been tested in humans or only minimally so, the data may be sparse; for a marketed drug it may be extensive.

In general, the safety evaluation of a drug should include all clinical trial and postmarketing safety data, regulatory correspondence, and animal toxicology data. Attention should be paid, in clinical trial data, to dropouts, deaths, lack of efficacy, and lost-to-follow up cases and any other areas where safety data might be lurking. The safety department should take the view that the information supplied to them are data intended to "make the sale" and as such it will highlight the favorable information and put the less favorable data in the background. Although the outright hiding of safety data is rare, it is not unheard of, and the safety reviewer should approach the due diligence duty with a healthy skepticism. The safety reviewer cannot say yes or no to the company's in-licensing a product but must spell out the safety and risk part of the "benefit-risk" analysis that the company performs.

■ Manufacturing (Complaints)

In the signal analysis of a product, it is not sufficient to simply examine AE data. The signal reviewer must also review product quality complaints. It is entirely possible that the AE is due to a problem in the manufacturing process that produced an impurity, an unstable product, an excipient issue, a manufacturing process, or vendor change producing unforeseen bad effects. This is surprisingly common as companies change vendors frequently for raw materials and product containers and make process changes when efficiencies or new machines are available. These are all done under appropriate change control (or should be), but unintended consequences can occur. For this reason the signal review must include product quality complaints and communicate frequently with colleagues in the manufacturing area when issues arise.

The physicians in the safety group may also be called on to give a medical opinion in cases where a product may need to be withdrawn from the market. Rarely, this is a major issue (e.g., Phen-Fen, Vioxx). Usually, it involves a single batch or lot of product that does meet manufacturing and release specifications. The company and the FDA will need to do an analysis to determine whether the issue is sufficiently severe to withdraw the lot in question from the market, issues warnings, or do nothing. The physicians may be asked to give an opinion on whether the problem could cause patient harm either through lack of efficacy or safety problems. For example, companies will test retained samples of individual lots that have been released to the market over the shelf lifespan. If a capsule that is sold is claimed to have a shelf-life of 2 years but is found to have a dissolution level or an assay level lower than that of the FDA-approved specifications at the 1-year after lot release testing, the company must evaluate whether to recall this lot or not. The physician must judge whether the lower available level of product may be harmful to the patient or not. Or if a particular contaminant (e.g., an organic compound leached out of a rubber stopper) is noted, an evaluation of the potential toxicity of the compound must be made. This is a most interesting but difficult aspect of the drug safety function.

Adverse Event Volume, Quality, and Medical Records

In spite of all the difficulties inherent in the system for collecting and analyzing adverse events (AEs), the number of AEs received by companies and health authorities is rising dramatically. This may be due to several reasons:

- An increased awareness by health care practitioners that reporting AEs is of critical importance to public health, and better communications to the US Food and Drug Administration (FDA), European Medicines Agency (EMEA), and other health authorities is needed.

- An increased awareness among patients and consumers of the importance of reporting AEs, at least in the United States and Canada where these reports are encouraged. This is generally not the case elsewhere, although this may be changing as the United Kingdom and other agencies are extending their AE reporting system to the general public.

- More clinical trials producing more AEs.

- Increasing prescribing of drugs by physicians and the increasing use of drugs by the general population (both prescription and over the counter), producing more AEs.

- More toxic (and more efficacious) drugs being produced treating diseases that, 20 years ago, were untreatable by drugs (e.g., AIDS, certain malignancies).

- More drug use by the elderly as assistance programs are being increased both by governments (e.g., Medicare in the United States and pharmaceutical company assistance programs for the poor).

- Better communications and easier methods of AE reporting (Internet, fax, e-mail, etc.).

- Better training in pharmacy, nursing, and medical schools as well as increased awareness in hospitals and other health care facilities of the need to report AEs.

- People are living longer.

The quantity of AEs received by the FDA on marketed products has increased from 170,000 in 1996 (Goldman and Kennedy, *Postgrad Med* 1998;103:3) to 426,000 in fiscal year 2004 (of which 69,000 were submitted electronically). The AEs submitted are increasing by about 50,000 reports per year (see the FDA's 2004 Office of Drug Safety Annual report for further details and a review of the office's 2004 activities (Web Resource 35-1)).

It should be kept in mind that non-US non-serious AEs and non-US serious labeled AEs do not have to be reported to the FDA by companies, so the numbers cited above are less than the total AEs captured. These requirements may change in the future.

Because of the press of AEs reported, the FDA and the industry are embarking on multiple initiatives to streamline the reporting and collection process. Some of the impetus for this has come from the International Conference on Harmonization, the Council for International Organizations of Medical Sciences, and the *Medical Dictionary for Regulatory Activities* (MedDRA). In particular, the electronic transmission (E2B) of MedDRA-coded serious AEs is now voluntary in the United States and will likely become obligatory at some point in the near future. Previously, the FDA would receive paper reports, recode them, and manually enter them into the FDA database. E2B reporting is now obligatory in the European Union and Japan.

■ Quality and Completeness

The FDA expects that manufacturer-submitted MedWatch forms will be complete and of high quality. In its document, "Enforcement of the Postmarketing Adverse Drug Experience Reporting Regulations," dated September 30, 1999 (Web Resource 35-2), the FDA instructs its inspectors to

"Verify the completeness and accuracy of the selected reports against other information in the firm's files as follows:

1. Was information on the form available at the time of submission?
2. Was all relevant information included on the form?
3. Was the initial receiving date supplied to the agency (FDA Form 3500A Section G Item 4) the same date as the initial receipt of information by the manufacturer?
4. Was new information obtained by the firm during the follow-up investigation and was this information submitted to the agency?
5. Where feasible, particularly when hospitalization, permanent disability or death occurred, did the firm obtain important follow-up information to enable complete evaluation of the report?"

In addition, the document further instructs the auditor:

"Document deviations from the ADE regulations. Clear deviations such as, failure to submit ADE reports, failure to promptly investigate an ADE event, inaccurate information, incomplete disclosure of available information, lack of written procedures or failing to adhere to reporting requirements, should be cited..."

These violations are cited in a "483" (see Chapter 45) addressed to the company. More severe violations may produce a "Warning Letter" (again, see Chapter 45):

"The following violations are considered significant to warrant issuance of a Warning Letter:

1. Failure to submit ADE reports for serious and unexpected adverse drug experience events (21 CFR 314.80©(1) and 310.305©).
2. 15-day alert reports that are submitted as part of a periodic report and which were not otherwise submitted under separate cover as 15-day alert reports. This applies to foreign and domestic ADE information from scientific literature and postmarketing studies as well as spontaneous reports (21 CFR 314.80©(1) and 310.305©).
3. 15-day alert reports that are inaccurate and/or not complete.
4. 15-day alert reports that are not submitted on time.
5. The repeated or deliberate failure to maintain or submit periodic reports in accordance with the reporting requirements (21 CFR 314.80©(2)).
6. Failure to conduct a prompt and adequate follow-up investigation of the outcome of ADEs that are serious and unexpected (21 CFR 314.80©(1) and 310.305©(3).
7. Failure to maintain ADE records for marketed prescription drugs or to have written procedures for investigating ADEs for marketed prescription drugs without approved applications (21 CFR 314.80(i) and 211.198).
8. Failure to submit 15-day reports derived from a postmarketing study where there is a reasonable possibility that the drug caused the adverse drug experience."

In other words, the auditors will cite lack of standard operating procedures as well as late, incomplete, inadequately followed-up, or unsent 15-day reports. It thus behooves the company to be sure that quality and compliance procedures are in place to ensure the following:

■ All cases are received where the receipt is within the company's control. For example, sales representatives and other company personnel, if told about an AE, must report these cases to the drug safety department for the appropriate handling. This must be documented in standard operating procedures, with training provided and documented and violations noted and corrected.
■ Cases must be rapidly triaged in the drug safety unit (or elsewhere if appropriate) to ensure that they are handled in the appropriate time frame. This applies

most markedly to cases that may be 15-day postmarketing expedited reports (and, of course, those clinical trial cases that may be 7- or 15-day expedited reports). In practice, this means that all serious AEs should reach drug safety within 1 to 2 (working) days after receipt anywhere in the company.

- Serious AEs should be promptly entered into the database, medically reviewed, and, those cases which are 15-day expedited reports, promptly sent to the FDA. Follow-up should be requested in those cases where there is incomplete information. It is highly unusual for a case to be complete with the initial report, and, in practice, all serious AEs will have follow-up performed.

- Data should be reviewed against the source documents for completeness and accuracy.

- Data should also be reviewed by a physician for medical content.

Audits and inspections performed by the EMEA or other European Union (EU) health authorities are similar in their fundamental nature but have certain EU twists that are different from the United States. In any case, all the points noted above would apply to an EU audit as well.

Medical Records and Archiving

The drug safety department must maintain an archive of all paper records for each case whether serious or not, whether submitted to the FDA or not, and whether important or not. These records should be kept in a secure and protected (intrusion, fire, water, etc.) file room. Access to the file room should be limited, and files that leave the file room to be worked on by the staff or examined by someone else should be formally signed out and tracked. The files should be treated the way a library treats rare and expensive books.

Old cases may be archived off-site, if need be, in a similarly protected environment but must be available for an audit within 1 working day. Hence the filing, indexing, and retrieval system must be very clearly worked out and efficient.

Source documents and cases from outside the United States, especially those not in English, may be kept at the source (i.e., the company's subsidiaries or affiliates or business partners, etc.) but must be available by fax or courier within 1-3 days at most for an audit or other safety review.

Electronic records must also be kept and available for examination by an auditor. The issues of electronic databases, electronic signatures, and validation are beyond the scope of this book. Suffice it to say, however, that as more and more recordkeeping is moving to computeri-

zation and away from paper, the computer system must be rock solid. A close coordination and working relationship with the computer department (information technology group, informatics group, etc.) is obligatory.

All paperwork, including scrap paper, jotted notes, and telephone logs, must be kept in the permanent files of the company. These documents, where appropriate, should be kept in the paper folders for each individual case safety report and easily retrievable during an inspection or audit by internal auditors, the FDA, or the EMEA. Pencils, erasers, and whiteout should also be banned from the drug safety department. All notes should be in pen. Yellow sticky notes should also be avoided because they may fall off or disappear and may contain important data. Data corrections or changes should be done by putting a single line through the incorrect value (leaving it still readable) with the new value written nearby and dated and initialed or signed.

There are various time limits that have been established, usually by the legal department or by the records retention department of a company, for all documents. Various companies have various time frames for keeping records, allowing their destruction after certain dates, such as 25 years, 3 years after the Investigational New Drug Application and New Drug Application are closed, 2 or 3 years (depending on product lifespan) after the last product is sold or used in a clinical trial, and so on. In practice, many safety departments keep all safety records forever. One never knows when one might need the records either for health authority issues or litigation. Keep in mind that diethylstilbestrol produced AEs in the offspring (and even granddaughters) decades after the original patients took diethylstilbestrol (see Chapter 6).

The best form and format of archiving should be left to professional archivists. Paper retention produces enormous volumes of files, especially if a company or health authority is receiving tens or hundreds of thousands of cases and hence hundreds of thousands to millions of pieces of paper per year. Thus nonpaper archiving appears to be a practical solution. The problem here is the obsolescence of the electronic storage systems. Data stored on 3½- or 5¼-inch floppy disks are now probably useless because the diskettes themselves may no longer be readable if stored badly and because there are very few computers that still have disk drives that can read such disks. Other storage methods (e.g., zip drives) have also come and gone. Any decision made in regard to archiving should be discussed with the appropriate experts (archivists, regulatory, legal) in the institution and reviewed periodically to see if the methods and procedures in use are still appropriate.

How an Adverse Event Is Handled in the Company from Start to Finish

This chapter (and those that follow) traces an adverse event (AE) through its course in a company from start to finish. The focus of this chapter is on process. Below a typical case handling process is outlined. It varies from company to company, but all such processes must have written procedures for data receipt, case assessment for expedited reporting, data entry, coding and data review by medical professionals (initially often by a nurse or pharmacist), and a final data review by a physician. The processes illustrated here are not necessarily better than other processes used in the industry. Nor is there a mandated process from the US Food and Drug Administration (FDA) or any other health authority. Rather, whichever process is implemented, it should ensure a smooth workflow and full compliance to all laws, regulations, and directives.

■ Mission and Goals

The mission of the AE processing unit is to ensure that all cases are processed in a timely and accurate manner such that all cases are sent to the appropriate departments within the company, to other companies, and to health authorities on time. The goals are to ensure prompt expedited reports and prompt Investigational New Drug Application (IND) annual, New Drug Application (NDA) periodic, Periodic Safety Update Reports (PSURs), and any other obligatory report. Because late reports to the FDA and business partners are usually easily and immediately noted, this statistic tends to be the one that drug safety groups, management, and even health authorities look at to "grade" companies. The goal is 100% compliance all the time, but reality tends to suggest that, in an imperfect world, anything over 95% is more or less acceptable. Nobody will actually write or say this. More importantly, cases that are late should not be late for the same reason twice. Errors, lack of following the standard operating procedures, and so on should be tracked down and corrected.

Many companies put maximal effort into keeping the expedited report score around 100%, often at the expense of case quality or delays in the processing of nonexpedited cases. Companies often build up backlogs of unprocessed or partially processed cases when resources are insufficient to be fully compliant with both expedited and non-expedited cases. Sooner or later, this situation produces a disastrous result unless corrective actions are applied.

There are many ways to handle cases. In some companies there is ownership by an individual drug safety specialist (e.g., a nurse or pharmacist) who is responsible for the completion of the case from start to finish, making sure that any other personnel involved in the case (e.g., medical reviewers) handle the case and return it to the specialist who "owns" it. Other companies have less individual ownership of a case and rather move a case from task to task in the workflow with a separate "pool" of workers responsible for a particular step, such as one group that just performs data entry, another that just does coding, and another that just writes narratives.

■ Arrival of AEs from Various Sources

Serious adverse events (SAEs) and non-SAEs may arrive in a company from multiple sources (feeder groups). Standard operating procedures must be in place to ensure that these AEs arrive in a timely manner (usually 1-2 days) in the drug safety department if they first arrive elsewhere in the company.

Spontaneous SAEs and non-SAEs arrive by telephone (usually the most common route of arrival), mail, fax, e-mail, company websites, reports to sales representatives, reports to other company representatives, the legal department, the FDA, other companies who receive AEs on their own drugs in which one of your drugs is involved, and other miscellaneous sources such as newspaper or TV stories. They are received primarily from consumers, health care professionals, and lawyers. It should be kept in mind that such AEs may arrive at any location in the company such as the manufacturing facilities (especially if the product package says something to the effect: "Manufactured by XXX Pharma in YYY City, Ohio" or if an address or phone number is on the package or patient information), subsidiaries and affiliates, contractors, outsourcers, and business partners with whom safety exchange agreements are in place.

■ Call Centers

These departments are staffed to receive phone calls from a particular region. Usually, they cover a whole country but not more than one country because labeling, indications, precautions, and warnings may differ from country to country and the appropriate information must be given to residents of the appropriate country. There may also be language issues. For example, any phone center covering Canada must be able to respond in English or French. In the United States, though not required by law, many phone centers have Spanish-speaking personnel available in addition to English speakers. Phone centers may be available Monday through Friday during business hours or sometimes 24 hours a day, 7 day a week. Multiple time zones must also be taken into account (for the United States, Alaska, and Hawaii). Call centers may be kept in-house or out-sourced to companies that specialize in handling medical phone calls.

Call centers are usually set up to receive calls from consumers, patients, physicians, and other health care providers. They usually cover questions about the products, requests for reimbursement, reporting of AEs, and product quality defects and problems. The call center must be set up in such a way as to ensure that all AEs and quality complaints are captured and sent to the appropriate departments for handling (e.g., the AEs to drug safety and the quality complaints to manufacturing quality). In addition, any questions or requests for reimbursement must be handled rapidly and correctly. Callers who are complaining or agitated must also be handled carefully and diplomatically. Thus a clear protocol must be set up to ensure that customers are served quickly and well, that their requests are met, and that all AEs and complaints are captured. The call should be picked up on the first or second ring, the caller should not be kept on hold for any significant length of time, and the caller should not have to give his or her name and address and the product issue more than once and should not be bounced to multiple departments.

All this requires a well-thought-out system to handle all issues (especially when a caller has multiple issues: "I took your pill which was supposed to be red but was blue; it smelled bad; I developed a headache; I want my money back and I have a question."). The decision about when to have medically trained personnel take the call must be clarified: Should all calls come directly to a nurse or pharmacist or should there be some level of nonmedical screening before sending the call to the health care professional? If nonmedical professionals are used, an algorithm and/or script is often used to ensure that no incorrect information is given to the caller. In addition, the priorities must be considered: Should the AE be handled first (most drug safety people would say yes to this but marketers would not)? Because there are multiple company stakeholders involved (drug safety, information technology, product quality, marketing, reimbursement, medical information, and others), the development of the call center is complex and expensive.

Other sources of AEs include:

- **Clinical studies**: Clinical study events may come in from the company's clinical research and clinical pharmacology departments as well as any other group that might (often unbeknownst to the drug safety department) run studies. Such groups might be in marketing, subsidiaries, affiliates, market research, pharmacoepidemiology, pharmacoeconomics, or other companies that are studying the drug with your company or are studying the drug without your company's consent and knowledge. AEs may also arrive from contract research organizations. Often, much to the chagrin of the safety group, the first awareness that a study is being run in some far-off outpost of the company is the arrival of an SAE. In the most egregious of such cases, an event may arrive for a drug that the safety department does not even know to be owned or sold by the company. It might, for example, be studied (or marketed) only in one subsidiary far away.

- **Legal**: Lawsuits are sometimes the unfortunate first notification to a company that there is an SAE. These cases usually come in through the legal department, which should be sensitized to the fact that they must not only defend a lawsuit but also report the AEs to the drug safety department. These AEs are usually on marketed products but may sometimes involve clinical trial patients. Rarely, a company may be notified of an issue by the arrival of a subpoena to provide evidence in a lawsuit to which the company is not a party such as a malpractice case in which there is also a drug issue. Normally, the receipt of AEs via lawsuits is limited, but in certain circumstances such cases may be very voluminous. At this writing (November 2005) there are approximately 6,400 pending lawsuits regarding Vioxx® in the United States (Source: CNN/Money website, see Web Resource 36-1, accessed November 29, 2005).

- **FDA**: The FDA has a program (MedWatch to Manufacturer) in which it sends copies of spontaneously received MedWatch reports of SAEs on newly approved NDAs to the manufacturer of the product. The drug must be a new chemical entity. This program lasts 3 years and is done at the request of the manufacturer. See Web Resource 36-2. These reports do not have to be resubmitted to the FDA by the company unless additional information is obtained.

- **Literature reports**: US and European Union regulations require that companies search the medical literature for SAEs. Such publications are usually on marketed products or occasionally clinical trials of new uses for old drugs unknown to the company or publications of trials done by the company a year or more earlier. Reports may be of SAEs or non-SAEs.

- **Stimulated reports**: Many companies have patient support programs in which company representatives or outside representatives (e.g., nurses, physicians) contact patients to encourage them to continue to take their medications. During the course of discussions, AE reports may be obtained. If the company is involved in these support programs, a mechanism must be created to ensure that the SAEs reach the company in a timely manner. Other programs such as speaker programs, named-patient programs, and compassionate use may also stimulate reports.

■ AE Triage (Case Assessment)

After the arrival, by whatever route, of the AE in the drug safety department, it must be properly classified for processing. The report should be date stamped upon entry into the drug safety department. For paper cases, this is a manual rubber stamp with the date (and possibly the time) of arrival. For electronic reports, presumably whatever system is used automatically date stamps the information. Thus clerical personnel can date stamp the cases in or print out or electronically transfer cases to a medically trained person for further triage. This should be done within 24 hours of receipt.

The initial triage should be to determine whether the report needs urgent processing in order to be transmitted to the FDA, other health authorities, or business partners. The triage should be done by someone with a medical skill set to make an accurate determination. Many companies have nurses and pharmacists in this critical role. Triage or case assessment should be standardized and trainable. Some companies use dedicated personnel for this function and others rotate clerical and/or medical staff in to do the triage. For difficult or controversial cases, the triage personnel may request assistance from the drug safety physician.

Triage should cover, at the least, the following:

- Which drug(s) involved?
- Case type: spontaneous, clinical trial, stimulated, other

- Serious or nonserious
- Causality (for serious clinical trial cases, not for spontaneous cases)
- Expectedness (labeledness) for serious and nonserious cases
- Determination of which reports are expedited reports using this algorithm:
  - 7-day IND report: serious and death/life-threatening, unlabeled, and associated (possibly caused by) with the drug in question
  - 15-day IND report: serious, unlabeled, and associated with (possibly caused by) the drug in question
  - 15-day NDA report: serious and unlabeled (no causality determination required)
  - Other reports requiring urgent processing such as those cases requested by the FDA to be transmitted to them in an expedited fashion but that do not meet the formal criteria above
- Pregnancy cases (some companies examine for pregnancy cases at triage and others do it later on in the case processing)
  - With an accompanying AE/SAE
  - No accompanying AE/SAE
- Product quality complaints (if handled in drug safety)
- Are the four elements of a valid case (reporter, patient, AE, drug) present and identifiable?

One method to handle paper cases is to create a rubber date stamp that has the eight categories listed in the box below. The drug safety specialist circles the correct category and initials and dates it. It is understood that this is a preliminary triage and the seriousness, labeledness, and causality (if needed) may be altered during the workflow. In general, the triage should be conservative so that serious cases and, in particular, 15-day expedited cases are not misclassified.

SUN	SUR	SEN	SER
	Date: _____		
NSL	NSU	SL	SU

where SUN = serious, unexpected, not related for clinical trial cases; SUR = serious, unexpected, related for clinical trial cases; SEN = serious, expected, not related for clinical trial cases; SER = serious, expected, related for clinical trial cases; NSL = nonserious, labeled; NSU = nonserious, unlabeled; SL = serious, labeled for spontaneous cases; SU = serious, unlabeled for spontaneous cases.

Alternatively, a separate tracking form, either paper based or electronic, may be used for each case where this is more convenient.

Some companies log all cases into a spreadsheet or database to track them and ensure that they are not lost in transit within the safety department. It may be most useful for "incomplete cases" or those that do not have the four required elements of a case yet but may later on. Logging them in at the outset prevents their "slipping through the cracks." A case number may be assigned at this point or at time of data entry.

After triage, each case should be assigned to the appropriate work channel. Each company develops various channels. They should roughly run along these lines:

- Rapid processing of the death/life-threatening clinical trial cases for submission to the FDA (and other health authorities) within 7 calendar days from first receipt by anyone in the company. This usually means completing the case within approximately 5 days and attempting to get whatever follow-up information is needed immediately.
- Processing of 15-day expedited reports to the IND and/or NDA. These are serious cases for which processing must be completed by calendar day 15 but preferably sooner to allow quality review, transmission to business partners, and transmission to the FDA. Many companies develop workflow such that all cases are completed by, say, calendar day 10 after initial receipt. Completion dates tend to range from 8 to 12 days in companies, though most companies pick one time frame for all cases and stick to it. This makes for simpler processing and tracking within the drug safety group.
- Processing of other serious cases that are not expedited reports. These cases do not have to be sent to the FDA within 15 calendar days. Rather they are sent in NDA periodic reports (every 3 months or yearly), IND annual reports, and PSURs. Thus there is usually the potential for a longer time frame for processing if needed. However, this is not always the case in practice.
- Serious cases that are to be sent to subsidiaries, business partners, and others may require rapid processing also if contractual arrangements require this. Many companies exchange all serious cases within 10 calendar days whether expedited or not.

- Sometimes a case is not an expedited report in one country but is an expedited case in other countries (e.g., the local labeling or reporting regulations are different there). This case must be transmitted to the subsidiary or business in time to meet 15-day reporting rules. It is often the situation, especially in large multinational companies, that the sending company (e.g., drug safety in the home office) is not able to know whether any particular serious case is an expedited report or not. Thus many companies process these cases as if they were expedited reports and use a completion date of 8-12 calendar days (as noted above).

- Nonserious cases may be processed more slowly (e.g., 30 days) because they are not reportable at all or are reportable only in aggregate reports. Nevertheless, it is wise to screen nonserious cases rapidly upon receipt, especially if they come from "less than reliable sources," to ensure that no serious cases are misclassified (presumably not intentionally) as nonserious cases. This could lead to late expedited reports.

- Similarly, the "other" cases, such as literature, legal, and MedWatch, should be processed as appropriate for the company's needs. It is a general rule of thumb that the process should be kept as simple as possible and that "exceptions to the rule" be kept limited. As few as three fundamental procedures could serve: 7-day cases, all serious cases, and all nonserious cases.

Data Entry

At this point the case should be entered into the computerized safety database. If a case number (also called a "control number" or "medical reference number") has not been assigned to the case at the triage or logging level, it is assigned now. If the data collection form used for collection of clinical trial and spontaneous data is standardized to a one- or two-page form, then data entry should be fairly easy to do. In practice, however, even if a standardized form exists in the company, all sorts of AE source documents arrive: case report forms, handwritten notes, Council for International Organizations of Medical Sciences I forms, MedWatch forms, typed notes, hospital records, and physicians' notes. Sometimes data entry is easy; sometimes it is not. Some companies have an initial review by a medical professional who highlights items for data entry; other companies have the source documents sent directly to the

data entry group (nonmedical professionals) and have medical review only after that is completed.

MedDRA coding of AEs, medical history, and other required MedDRA fields is done either by the drug safety group or by a dedicated coding group. Drug coding using a standardized dictionary is also done.

Data Review and Quality Checks

At this point, a drug safety specialist (usually a nurse or pharmacist) reviews the data entry against the source documents and prepares or reviews the case narrative. Any changes or additions to the case are made at this time. A clear methodology on the quality check should be developed so that it is done in a standardized and repeatable way. Those fields, if any, that are not reviewed (e.g., height) should be defined in the methodology up front in addition to those fields that are. The quality review should look at content, grammar, and format. In general, one does not need to be a perfectionist regarding grammar; however, sentences that are unclear or do not convey the desired meaning should be corrected. Short simple sentences should be used because many of the readers (outside the United States) may not be native English language speakers.

Follow-up information should be requested when the initial case is incomplete or unclear. Rarely does a case have complete information, especially if the AE just happened and/or is ongoing. Thus, it is almost always required that follow-up queries be sent to the reporter to complete the case data. The need for follow-up is also mentioned in 21CFR312.32(d) for IND reports and 314.80©(1)(ii) for NDA reports. Follow-up data should be entered into the database using a similar procedure to the one used for initial data. Care must be taken to ensure that the data are not mistaken for a new case but rather are clearly identified as follow-up to a case already received.

Medical Review

At this point in the case, after it has been completed and reviewed by the drug safety specialist and after it has undergone a quality review, some or all cases should be reviewed by the drug safety physician. Historically, physician review was limited to serious cases, but many companies are now having all cases undergo physician review to ensure that no serious cases are misclassified as nonserious ones.

The medical review should generally cover the medical content of the case with particular attention paid to the narrative, the suspect and concomitant drugs (including dosages), the past medical history, and coding. It is generally not the role of the physician to do a source document quality review unless he or she needs to refer to the source documents for clarification of a medical point.

Case Closure/Completion

In one sense, a case is never really closed as new information could arrive weeks, months, or even years later, requiring the case to be updated. But for practical purposes, once the above steps are concluded and follow-up requested, a case may be considered closed or completed for operational purposes. If and when follow-up arrives, the case can be reopened and processed.

Distribution and Submission

Cases are next distributed to those in the company who need to see them (e.g., clinical research, legal, etc.) and to other companies with whom safety exchange agreements are in place. Cases may also be submitted directly to the FDA or European Medicines Agency (by paper or E2B files) or distributed to others in the company such as the regulatory department for submission to the health authorities. Cases may also be sent to subsidiaries or affiliates worldwide for their submission to local agencies—often with a cover letter in the local language and, in some instances, with a translation of the case itself into the local language if English is not accepted.

Tracking and Metrics

It is critical to have markers in the database such that cases can be tracked in their trip through the processing system. Each drug safety specialist and manager should be aware of all the cases pending, their status in the trip toward completion/closure, and, in particular, the deadlines for each case. It is critical that all 7- and 15-day reports be tracked so that none is submitted late to the FDA and other health authorities, subsidiaries, or business partners. The manager can reallocate cases or other work to ensure that the time-critical cases are handled appropriately in the case of absence, vacation, or overload of his or her staff.

Similarly, nonexpedited cases that need to be completed for aggregate reports should be tracked so that they are completed by the time of data lock. This can be as frequent as every 3 months for NDA periodic reports or every 6 months for PSURs.

In general, tracking reports should be electronic and generated automatically from the drug safety database. Most modern drug safety databases have a tracking function with customizable reports. Manual tracking on spreadsheets is time consuming and usually unsatisfactory once AE volume grows and the staff becomes large.

In addition to tracking the AEs that arrive and are processed, it is wise to track the following:

- Total number of AEs
- SAEs
- Non-SAEs
- Clinical trial AEs/SAEs
- Spontaneous AEs/SAEs
- Expedited reports to the IND and to the NDA:
  - Those submitted on time
  - Those submitted late, by how much, why, and corrective actions taken
- Cases submitted to business partners and others
- Time to process cases depending on case type (expedited, serious nonexpedited, nonserious, etc.)
- Time to submission to the FDA, European Medicines Agency, and so on
- Tracking by drug or class of products or drug safety teams depending on how the drug safety group and the company are organized
- NDA periodic and IND annual reports and PSURs

It is useful to graph and publish these metrics periodically for the entire drug safety staff. Such data can also be used for resource allocation, budgeting, projection of future work (e.g., AEs for allergy drugs peak twice a year and more staff may be needed then), and justification for more resources. The metrics may aid in identifying problems or "rough spots" and help to institute changes to prevent recurrence of such problems.

Publicly posted data should not identify individuals or point out "nonproducers" to shame them into speeding up. Praise should always be done publicly, but chastisement should be done privately.

■ Timing

The timing, sequence, and duration of each step in the processing of an AE should be clearly spelled out. If the company determines that, say, all SAEs will be completed within 10 calendar days and all nonserious cases within 30 calendar days, this timing should be built into each case. This should be done automatically in the database with a tickler, e-mail, or similar reminders to the concerned individual telling him or her of the timing and due date for each case. The due dates would be updated as needed (e.g., it is determined to be or not to be a 15-day expedited report or a case is upgraded from nonserious to serious). Attention must be paid to weekends and holidays in calculating due dates. Thus the schedule for a typical SAE that arrives in the company on 1-Dec-2005 to all personnel involved in the case could be as illustrated In Table 36-1. Had this case been determined to be a 7-day case or a nonserious case, the timing would change as appropriate.

Each person in the workflow knows when his or her task is due and the manager is able to track the case through each step to ensure its completion. Other companies have "pools" of people handling each step rather than having one drug safety specialist "own" the case. In the pool situation, for each step listed above, the first available team member handling that step processes the case.

■ Special Situations

Database Lock

Presuming that a fairly rigid work schedule is put in place to ensure the timely completion of each case, it is necessary to set up rules for follow-up information or for new data that arrive while a case is being processed. As an example, if new data (which need to be added to the case) arrive on 8-Dec-2005, using the case illustrated in Table 36-1, the question then is whether the drug safety group should attempt to immediately add these data to the case or to complete the initial case and add the new data as follow-up. If the data are added immediately, much of the processing may need to be redone from the beginning with data entry, data review, and so on. On the other hand, if the case is nearly ready for transmission to the FDA, adding this new information immediately may be quite disruptive to the processing of the case.

Companies handle this situation differently. One method is to create a "database lock" for each case on a particular day after case processing starts for that case. Thus all data received by calendar day 4, say, will be incorporated into the initial case and all data received after day 4 will be added to a follow-up version of the case with the day 4 data starting the new version at day 0. Doing it this way ensures orderly flow of all data (presuming it is well tracked) at the expense of multiple follow-up versions for each case.

Others make all attempts to incorporate the newer data into the case even if it means rushing and scrounging on day 9 or 10. This method decreases the numbers of follow-up versions for each case. If working on a 10-day processing cycle is done, there is some extra time built into the system for 15-day reports, allowing an occasional case to go out on day 15 instead of day 10. Others handle each situation individually, updating at the last moment only those cases that have medically significant new information (e.g., deaths, change in outcome, worsening of the patient's condition, etc.).

Investigator Notification

Fifteen-day IND expedited reports require the notification of all "participating investigators" (21CFR32C(1)) as well

Table 36-1 Case No. USA-2005-108765			
Task	**Due Date**	**Day of the Week**	**Calendar Day**
Received in the company	1-Dec-2005	Thur	0
Received in drug safety	2-Dec-2005	Fri	1
Triage to be completed	6-Dec-2005	Tues	5
Data entry to be completed	7-Dec-2005	Wed	6
Data review and quality checks	8-Dec-2005	Thur	7
Medical review	9-Dec-2005	Fri	8
Case closure	9-Dec-2005	Fri	8
Transmission to the FDA—paper or E2B	12-Dec-2005	Mon	10

as the FDA. Most companies prepare an "investigator letter" that either contains the case information as text or is a cover sheet for the attached MedWatch form. In addition, 21CFR32(B)(ii) requires that "the sponsor shall identify all safety reports, previously filed with the IND concerning a similar adverse experience, and shall analyze the significance of the adverse experience in light of the previous, similar reports." This analysis of similar cases is usually prepared by the drug safety group from the safety database and either incorporated into the MedWatch form, the cover letter, or a separate sheet attached to the MedWatch form. Sometimes the safety department prepares the investigator letter for review and sending by the clinical research department and/or the regulatory department.

The decision as to whether to include the similar case analysis in the MedWatch narrative itself or as a separate sheet is usually made as a function of where the MedWatch form is going. If its only destination is the NDA, some companies put this information into the MedWatch narrative directly. If the form, however, is going to other health agencies or companies or if there is concern that this information will be available to the public and competitors under the Freedom of Information Act, companies often elect to put the analysis on a separate piece of paper.

15 Calendar Days and Day 0 Versus Day 1

The FDA in its draft guidance (Web Resource 36-3), "Post-Marketing Safety Reporting for Human Drug and Biological Products Including Vaccines" of March 2001 (page 10), refers to the completion of box G4 on the MedWatch 3500A form as the date the company has knowledge of the four criteria for a valid AE (reporter, patient, event, drug) and that this is day 0 of the 15-day time clock. This then gives 16 calendar days for a case. The document also notes clearly that the case must be *submitted* by day 15, which means it will be received at the FDA in a few days if sent by mail or the next day if sent by overnight courier. If the 15th calendar day is a weekend or US federal holiday, the report may be submitted on the first working day after the weekend or holiday. However, if a company has submission obligations in countries outside the United States, the federal holiday (and possibly even the weekends) should not be allowed to permit a delay in submission. Although not (yet) adopted by the FDA, this guidance does reflect the agency's latest thinking on AE submission—at least as of March 2001—and is worth reading and absorbing.

37

Seriousness, Expectedness, and Causality

The drug safety associate and the physicians involved in individual case evaluation generally have to make several decisions regarding each case. These decisions must be made rapidly on receipt of an individual case safety report because this determines how the case is handled in drug safety and whether, how, and when it is reported to the US Food and Drug Administration (FDA), other health agencies, and business partners.

◼ Seriousness

The generally accepted definition of seriousness is as follows:

"A serious adverse event (experience) or serious adverse reaction is any untoward medical occurrence that at any dose:

- *results in death,*
- *is life-threatening,*

(NOTE: The term "life-threatening" in the definition of "serious" refers to an event in which the patient was at risk of death at the time of the event; it does not refer to an event that hypothetically might have caused death if it were more severe.)

- *requires in-patient hospitalization or prolongation of existing hospitalization,*
- *results in persistent or significant disability/incapacity, or*
- *is a congenital anomaly/birth defect.*

Medical and scientific judgment should be exercised in deciding whether expedited reporting is appropriate in other situations, such as important medical events that may not be immediately life-threatening or result in death or hospitalization but may jeopardize the patient or may require intervention to prevent one of the other outcomes listed in the definition above. *These should also usually be considered serious.*

Examples of such events are intensive treatment in an emergency room or at home for allergic bronchospasm; blood dyscrasias or convulsions that do not result in hospitalization; or development of drug dependency or drug abuse" (ICH E2A).

Over the years, these definitions have been discussed, parsed, and clarified by health agencies, companies, and other interested observers. In general, the most conservative interpretation is the one-drug safety groups should use. Some comments follow:

■ Death: Although one would believe this binary concept (alive—dead) would be rather straightforward, there have been some discussions relating to the timing of the death and the circumstances around the adverse event (AE) and the death.

It is fairly clear that if a patient has a myocardial infarction (the serious AE) and then over the next several hours or days goes into shock, has severe arrhythmias, and dies, this death is related to the serious AE and this is a "fatal myocardial infarction." It gets trickier, however, if the patient has a myocardial infarction and during a cardiac catheterization goes into an intractable ventricular arrhythmia and dies. Is the myocardial infarction to be classified as a fatal one or is the death a sequelum of the catheterization? There is no clear answer, and it may vary from case to case. The most conservative call is often used by drug safety units that is, the death is a part of (or consequence of) the serious AE. However, if a medically defensible call is made that is less conservative, this should be noted somewhere in the case along with the reasoning behind this decision.

Another example would be that of a fall. If a patient trips while walking on a level surface, falls, and scrapes his or her knee, this is most probably a nonserious AE. If, however, he or she falls while standing on a ledge or walking down a staircase and dies as a result of the fall, the decision on whether this fall should be reported as a serious and fatal case needs to be made. Again, there is no clear answer; many would take the conservative approach and consider this case (if during a clinical trial) as serious, fatal, unlabeled (presuming fatal fall is not in the investigator brochure), and unrelated to the study drug (unless it is believed to be related perhaps due to accompanying dizziness, which should also be coded).

■ In a 1996 report on a survey done at the US and European Union (EU) Drug Information Association meetings in 1993, Dr. Win Castle and Dr. George Phillips reported marked transatlantic differences in the interpretation of seriousness and expectedness. For example, "total blindness for 30 minutes" was believed to be serious by 89% in the EU survey and 44% in the US survey compared with "mild anaphylaxis," which was believed to be serious by 37% of the EU responders and 98% of the US responders. Whether this is still the case remains to be seen, but the results nonetheless are most interesting and suggest the need for harmonization and training of safety reviewers (Castle and Phillips, *Drug Inform J* 1996;30:73–81).

■ Life-threatening: This concept is also interpreted as to whether the serious AE would truly kill the patient if untreated. A mild myocardial infarction with no cardiac function compromise or arrhythmias might be considered serious (medically significant, see below) but not life-threatening, whereas a myocardial infarction that progresses over the next hour or 2 to pulmonary edema would be considered life-threatening. This definition thus may overlap to a degree with "medically significant." Again, most would take a conservative approach.

■ Hospitalization: Much debate occurred over what actually constitutes "hospitalization" (at least in the United States). Some patients may be kept overnight (even up to 24–36 hours) in the emergency department for observation and treatment but not "formally" admitted to the hospital as an inpatient. Thus this patient would *not* qualify as serious based on a stay in the emergency room. (See the FDA's 2001 draft guidance on AE reporting, Section IV.A.3. Note this is still a draft and not a finalized guidance [Web Resource 37-1]).

■ Significant or persistent disability/incapacity: A relatively uncommon criterion in practice. The FDA gives an interesting example in its 2001 draft guidance:

"Persons incarcerated because of actions allegedly caused by a drug (e.g., psychotropic drugs and rage reactions) have sustained a substantial disruption in their ability to conduct normal life functions. Thus, these adverse experiences would qualify for the significant or persistent disability/incapacity outcome."

■ Congenital anomaly/birth defect: Usually rather straightforward. It would include even mild birth defects. The FDA also notes that this includes those defects "occurring in a fetus," thus covering abnormalities discovered before birth.

■ Important medical events (also called "significant medical events"): This criterion has often been difficult to handle for pharmacovigilance departments because the definition relies on medical judgment. The examples given (allergic bronchospasm, blood dyscrasias, or convulsions) do not necessarily help to clarify other less dramatic situations. The FDA also gives the examples of drug dependency or drug abuse as important events.

Often, cases elicit hours of debate in drug safety units on whether to consider it medically important or not. Is a mild focal seizure medically important? Is a platelet count 10% below the lower level of normal medically important? Other examples abound. Various rules of thumb have developed:

■ If it happened to you or a family member, would you consider it important or medically significant?

■ If you discuss or debate whether a case is medically important or not, it is.

■ Another method involves using the FDA's "always expedited" list as published in "the Tome" (see Chapter 42) or the equivalent lists from other health authorities.

■ If a member of the marketing or sales department or a nonmedical professional believes it is not important, it is important. (This "rule," though somewhat jocular and cynical, has developed to note the real observation that sometimes there are nonmedical pressures put on personnel in the safety department to interpret cases or make decisions based on sales, financial, or other nonmedical criteria. This is an unfortunate fact of life—not just in the pharmaceutical world but in the world of clinical medicine where many judgments are now made on a cost-effectiveness basis. Always keep in mind that the primary mission of the drug safety department is to protect the public health.)

■ Expectedness (Labeledness)

The US regulations governing expectedness are fairly straightforward:

"For a pre-marketed product: Any adverse drug experience, the specificity or severity of which is not consistent with the current investigator's brochure; or, if an investigator brochure is not required or available, the specificity or severity of which is not consistent with the risk information described in the general investigational plan or elsewhere in the current application, as amended. For example, under this definition, cerebral thromboembolism and cerebral vasculitis would be unexpected (by virtue of greater specificity) if the investigator brochure only listed cerebral vascular accidents" (21CFR312.32(a)).

"For marketed products: Any adverse drug experience that is not listed in the current labeling (package insert or summary of product characteristics) for the drug product. This includes events that may be symptomatically and pathophysiologically related to an event listed in the labeling, but differ from the event because of greater severity or specificity. For example, under this definition, hepatic necrosis would be unexpected (by virtue of greater severity) if the labeling only referred to elevated hepatic enzymes or hepatitis.

"AEs that are 'class-related' (i.e. allegedly seen with all products in this class of drugs) which are mentioned in the labeling (package insert or summary of product characteristics) or investigator brochure but which are not specifically described as occurring with this product are considered unexpected" (21CFR314.80(a)).

In theory this concept is rather straightforward, but in practice it becomes somewhat harder when synonyms and overlapping concepts are considered. In the report cited above by Castle and Phillips, 72% of the EU responders believed that if the labeled event is "dizziness," then "vertigo" would also be considered expected (labeled), but only 50% of the US responders believed vertigo was labeled. Similarly, 18% of the EU responders and 3% of the US responders believed that if "hypotension, wheezing, and urticaria" are labeled, then a reported term of "anaphylaxis" would also be expected. Whether these differences persist, some 12 years after the survey, is unclear. However, it does highlight the fact that well-trained experienced medical personnel doing pharmacovigilance can take the same set of facts and come up with differing and even opposing views.

In general, one should decide expectedness without thought to seriousness. That is, just because a case is nonserious and the AE in question is of mild severity and little medical import (e.g., a maculopapular rash) compared with a serious AE (e.g., severe hepatitis), the decision on expectedness should be made purely on the basis of the wording in the label and not on the seriousness. Give each AE its due.

It should be kept in mind that with clinical trial drugs, especially those not yet marketed, there may be minimal or no human experience (e.g., the first study in humans or the first phase II study after phase I studies that showed no AEs). In this case, there are no labeled events in the investigator brochure and everything is thus "new" and unexpected. Anticipated events based on the pharmacologic properties of the drug should not be considered expected until actually reported in a patient and put into the brochure.

In some cases, it is necessary to consider the route of administration, dosage, or indication being studied when assessing the expectedness. This usually depends on how the investigator brochure or marketed labeling is written. Some describe a different set of AEs for different indications, dosages, or routes of administration. Care must be taken to apply the correct label to each case when doing expectedness.

The general advice would be, as with seriousness, to decide on the side of conservatism. Then, if there are questions as to whether an AE is expected or not, consider it unexpected.

■ Causality (Relatedness)

Of the three criteria revolving around the regulatory reportability of an individual case (seriousness, expectedness, and relatedness), this one is often the most difficult to do for the multiple reasons explained below. Causality may be determined initially at the individual case level after the receipt of an individual case safety report and again after the review of aggregate data in a case series as is done for signaling, risk management, and various regulatory reports such as Periodic Safety Update Reports.

First, some basic "housekeeping" points should be cleared up to ensure that cases are always handled and collected in the same manner. In doing case assessment, one should be sure that cases are coded using the *Medical Dictionary for Regulatory Activities* (MedDRA) (usually the latest version) with trained coders who use consistent methodology and synonym lists. For aggregate reports, the search criteria for the case series should be complete and standardized (using searches from the MedDRA Maintenance and Support Services Organization or Council for International Organizations of Medical Sciences [CIOMS]). Cases should be followed up (rap-

idly upon receipt, not at a later date) as appropriate to ensure the maximum amount of high quality data.

In practice, many companies have two sets of standards and classifications for causality assessment of individual case safety reports. The first is the one used in clinical trials by the medical research group. As noted below, there is no standard system, so various categories (usually three to six) are used in case reports in clinical trials along the lines of: related, probably related, possibly related, weakly related, unrelated, and unassessable. This is very useful in later analysis of signals and in the creation of tables for investigator brochures, product labeling, and monographs to give a feel for the certainty or lack thereof in regard to the AEs and the drug in question. However, for the drug safety group, which has to make a determination of whether a clinical trial case meets the three criteria (seriousness, expectedness, causality) for expedited reporting, the decision is a yes or no decision. That is, the drug safety group must make the choice between unrelated and related. There is no middle ground or gray zone for causality here. Thus the drug safety group has to make a rapid decision on whether the case is clearly unrelated (absolutely, positively) and everything else (possibly, probably, unlikely, weakly, etc.). Some drug safety groups consider "unlikely related" to be unrelated and other groups consider it in the broad "related" category. Whichever way is decided, it should be made clear to everyone in the company what is done. Many drug safety officers believe that unless a case is clearly and absolutely unrelated, the causality should be, for reporting purposes, "related." To put it another way, the default causality for all cases is "possibly related" until there is evidence that the case is "unrelated." It is realized that this may not ultimately agree with the case analysis in the final clinical research study report where a more nuanced opinion may be recorded. So, to summarize, in drug safety there are two causality choices for reporting purposes: unrelated (thus making the case not reportable as an expedited case) and everything else.

Because there are no clear standards or classifications for causality, two broad methods have been developed for causality assessment. The first is known as "global introspection," which is a somewhat jocular description of having one or more smart experienced drug safety experts (usually physicians) read the case details, in particular the narrative, and decide on "introspective" grounds whether the case is caused by the drug or not. Obviously, all the expected difficulties exist when the decision is left to one or more human beings using subjective criteria:

different training, different experience, untested inter-rater reliability, biases, and pressure from nonmedical sources within the company or institution. Yet experience has also shown that when solid, smart, ethical individuals with thick skins and a strong desire to protect the public health do this job, it is generally well done. Algorithms, the second method and the usual alternative to global introspection, have generally not succeeded as well (see below).

Finally, there is another general rule: If there is disagreement between two or more evaluators (e.g., the clinical research team, the investigator, and the drug safety department), the most conservative judgment should be used; that is, if one believes the case is not related and the other believes it is possibly related, the case is considered to be related. This has been clarified in the guidelines cited below for situations where the investigator disagrees with the company. But this rule should apply within the company also when there is disagreement. Conservatism and over-reporting is preferable to under-reporting of serious AEs.

For a short and useful summary on how a health authority expert on pharmacovigilance approaches causality from a clinical, pharmacologic, and epidemiologic perspective, see the article by Diemont (*Netherlands J Med* 200;63:7, accessed on 6-Dec-2005 at Web Resource 37-2).

There is no international standard for causality assessment or classification. The US and EU recommendations are summarized below.

US FDA

Current US regulations require a causality assessment for Investigational New Drug Application (IND) expedited 7- and 15-day reports. These regulations require an IND safety report:

> "The sponsor shall notify FDA and all participating investigators in a written IND safety report of: (A) Any adverse experience associated with the use of the drug that is both serious and unexpected" where the definition of "*Associated with the use of the drug*" is: "There is a reasonable possibility that the experience may have been caused by the drug" (21CFR312.32).

Unfortunately, the FDA does not give a further definition of causality.

For New Drug Application (NDA) 15-day expedited reports, there is "implied" causality for spontaneous reports. What this means is that if a health care professional or consumer takes the time to report an AE to the manufacturer of the drug or to the FDA, then there is an implication that the reporter believes that to some degree the drug may have caused the AE. This is not clearly stated in the regulations that require 15-day expedited reports as follows:

> "Postmarketing 15-day 'Alert reports.' The applicant shall report each adverse drug experience that is both serious and unexpected, whether foreign or domestic, as soon as possible but in no case later than 15 calendar days of initial receipt of the information by the applicant" (21CFR80(1)(i)).

Note that the "associated with the use of the drug" phrase is missing. This has been interpreted to mean that a causality assessment is not required for these reports. The FDA has clarified this in draft guidances though not in the regulations per se.

In the draft "Guidance for Industry Postmarketing Safety Reporting for Human Drug and Biological Products Including Vaccines" of March 2001, the FDA notes the following:

> "For spontaneous reports, the applicant should assume that an adverse experience or fatal outcome was suspected to be due to the suspect drug or biological product (implied causality). For clinical studies, an adverse experience or fatal outcome need not be submitted to the FDA unless the applicant concludes that there is a reasonable possibility that the product caused the adverse experience or fatal outcome (see §§ 310.305(c)(1)(ii), 337314.80(e)(1), and 600.80(e)(1))" (Web Resource 37-3).

In the draft "Guidance for Industry: Good Pharmacovigilance Practices and Pharmacoepidemiologic Assessment" of May 2004 at Web Resource 37-4, the FDA notes the following:

> "For any individual case report, it is rarely possible to know with a high level of certainty whether the event was caused by the product. To date, there are no internationally agreed upon standards or criteria for assessing causality in individual cases, especially for events that often occur spontaneously (e.g. stroke, pulmonary embolism). Rigorous pharmacoepidemiologic studies, such as case-control studies and cohort studies with long-term follow-up, are usually needed to assess causality in such instances."

The FDA does not recommend any specific categorization of causality, but the categories *probable, possible,* or *unlikely* have been used. The World Health Organization (WHO) uses the following categories: certain, probably/likely, possible, unlikely, conditional/unclassified, and unassessable/unclassifiable. Although the FDA does not advocate a particular categorization system, if a causality assessment is undertaken, the FDA suggests that the causal categories are specified.

In contrast to causality assessment at the individual case level it may be possible to assess the degree of causality between use of a product and an AE when a sponsor gathers and evaluates all available safety data in aggregate, including the following:

1. Spontaneously reported and published case reports
2. Relative risks or odds ratios derived from pharmacoepidemiologic safety studies
3. Biologic effects observed in preclinical studies and pharmacokinetic or pharmacodynamic effects
4. Safety findings from controlled clinical trials
5. General marketing experience with similar products in the class

Finally, in the proposed new safety regulations ("the Tome") of 14 March 2003 "Safety Reporting Requirements for Human Drug and Biological Products—Proposed Rule" (see Web Resource 37-5), the FDA notes the following:

"This proposed revision is consistent with the ICH E2A guidance (60 FR 11286): Causality assessment is required for clinical investigation cases. All cases judged by either the reporting health care professional or the sponsor as having a reasonable suspected causal relationship to the medicinal product qualify as ADR's [adverse drug reactions]."

"FDA is also proposing to amend Sec. 312.32(c)(1)(i) by replacing the phrase 'any adverse experience associated with the use of the drug that is both serious and unexpected' with the phrase 'any SADR that, based on the opinion of the investigator or sponsor, is both serious and unexpected, as soon as possible, but in no case later than 15 calendar days after receipt by the sponsor of the minimum data set for the serious, unexpected SADR.' This proposed amendment would require that the determination of the possibility of causality (attributability) of an SADR to an investigational drug be based on the opinion of either the investigator or sponsor, which is consistent with the ICH E2A guidance (60 FR 11284 at 11286): Causality assessment is required for clinical investigation cases. All cases judged by either the reporting health care professional or the sponsor, as having a reasonable suspected causal relationship to the medicinal product, qualify as ADRs.

"In situations in which a sponsor does not believe that there is a reasonable possibility that an investigational drug caused a response, but an investigator believes that such a possibility exists, the proposed rule would require that the sponsor submit a written IND safety report to FDA for the SADR. In the opposite situation, the same would also be true. These proposed changes would clarify that all spontaneous reports received by manufacturers and applicants that contain a minimum data set (minimum information for a report of a medication error that does not result in SADR) would be reported to FDA (i.e., as an individual case safety report and/or in a summary tabulation). These changes are consistent with the premarketing safety reporting requirements described in section III.B.2.b of this document (i.e., determination of the possibility of causality (attributability) of an SADR to the drug or biological product in a clinical investigation would be based on the opinion of either the applicant/sponsor or investigator). These proposed amendments are also consistent with the ICH E2A guidance (60 CFR 11284 at 11286): Causality assessment is required for clinical investigation cases. All cases judged by either the reporting health care professional or the sponsor, as having a reasonable suspected causal relationship to the medicinal product, qualify as ADRs. For purposes of reporting, adverse event reports associated with marketed drugs (spontaneous reports) usually imply causality."

European Union

The EU position on causality is explained in "Volume 9: Pharmacovigilance—Medicinal Products for Human Use and Veterinary Medicinal Products" (2001). See Web

Resource 37-6. This is far more explicit and categorical than the FDA position. However, this introduces certain reporting issues, discussed below.

"An assessment of causality should be made on each adverse reaction report submitted. Various approaches to assign causality are possible. However, in order to exchange data for European Community purposes four categories of conclusions can be made:

> Category 'A': Probable
>
> Category 'B': Possible
>
> Category 'O': Unclassified (cases where insufficient information was available to draw any conclusion)
>
> Category 'N': Unlikely to be product related (cases where sufficient information was available and where investigation has established this beyond reasonable doubt).

"In assessing causality the following factors should be taken into account:

1. Associative connection, in time which may include dechallenge and rechallenge following repeated administration or in anatomic sites.
2. Pharmacological explanation; blood levels; previous knowledge of the drug.
3. Presence of characteristic clinical or pathological phenomena.
4. Exclusion of other causes.
5. Completeness and reliability of the data in the case reports.
6. Quantitative measurement of the degree of contribution of a product to the development of a reaction (dose-effect relationship).

For inclusion in category 'A' (probable) it is recommended that all the following minimum criteria should be complied with:

1. There should be a reasonable association in time between the administration of the veterinary medicinal product and onset and duration of the reported adverse reaction.
2. The description of the clinical phenomena should be consistent with, or at least plausible, given the known pharmacology and toxicology profiles of the veterinary medicinal product.
3. There should be no other equally plausible explanation(s) of the case. (If such are suggested—are they validated? What is their degree of certainty?).

"In particular, concurrent use of other products, and possible product interactions, or intercurrent disease should be taken into account in the assessment. Where any of the above criteria cannot be satisfied (due to conflicting data or lack of information) then such reports can only be classified as 'B' (possible), 'N' (unlikely) or 'O' (unclassifiable/not assessable). For inclusion in category 'B' (possible), it is recommended that this be applied when drug causality is one of other possible and plausible causes for the described event but where the data does not meet the criteria for inclusion in category 'A.'

"In cases where sufficient information exists to establish beyond reasonable doubt that product causality was not likely to be the cause of the event then such reports should be classified as 'N' (unlikely). Where reliable data concerning an SAR is unavailable or is insufficient to make an assessment or causality then such reports should be classified as 'O' (unclassifiable/not assessable). The causality assessment made by the Competent Authority may differ from that of the Marketing Authorisation Holder. If this is the case, the competent authority should, when possible, communicate its conclusion and the reason(s)for the decision to the Marketing Authorisation Holder."

■ CIOMS I

See also Chapter 25.

Assessment of Causality

"It should be emphasized that manufacturers should not separate out those spontaneous reports they receive into those that seem to themselves to be causally related to drug exposure and those they consider not causally related. A physician in making a spontaneous report to a manufacturer is indicating that the observed event may be due to the drug, i.e. the physician suspects that the event is a reaction. In such a case it would be inappropriate for a manufacturer to impute to the reporting physician an assessment of causality. Thus all spontaneous reports of serious unlabelled reactions made by medical professionals should be considered as CIOMS reports.

However, submission of such a report does not necessarily constitute an acceptance of causality by a manufacturer."

Others

The Uppsala Monitoring Centre uses six categories: certain, probably/likely, possible, unlikely, conditional/unclassified, unassessable/unclassifiable. They note that these categories are the most widely used, although not everyone uses all of them. See Web Resource 37-7. For causality of AEs that occur after immunization, see the WHO aide-memoire at Web Resource 37-8, which uses a similar system.

The French government has used for many years an "imputabilité" decision table based on a combination of a "bibliographic" score (from never reported to well known), chronological criteria (timing, dechallenge rechallenge), and clinical criteria (specific laboratory findings, suggestive clinical picture, other explanations likely), leading to a five-degree global score (0, unrelated; 1, doubtful; 2, possible; 3, probable; 4, definite) (Begaud, *Drug Inform J* 1984;18:275). It is not used outside of France.

Algorithms

Over 30 algorithms have been developed for both manual and computerized causality assessment of individual cases in pharmacovigilance. One of the earlier used algorithms was developed by Prof. J. Venulet in 1980 and updated in 1986 (Venulet, Ciucci, and Berneker, *Int J Clin Pharmacol Ther Toxicol* 1986;24:559).

In a study done to evaluate agreement between various algorithms and those obtained from an expert panel using the WHO method, 200 reports were studied. The rates of concordance between assessments made using the algorithms and the expert panel were 45% for "certain," 61% for "probable," 46% for "possible," and 17% for drug-unrelated terms. Correcting for confounding variables did not significantly improve the results. The authors concluded that full agreement with global introspection was not found for any level of causality assessment (Macedo, Marques, Ribeiro, et al., *J Clin Pharm Ther* 2003;28:137).

Global Introspection

These criteria should be used by a drug safety expert to evaluate case causality:

Reasons to suspect the AE was caused by the drug.

- The AE occurred in the expected time frame (as a function of the drug's pharmacologic or clinical half-life)
- No problems or symptoms before exposure
- No other medical conditions that could cause this AE
- No concomitant medications that could cause this AE
- A positive dechallenge and (better) a positive rechallenge
- The AE is consistent with the established mechanism of action of product ("biologic plausibility")
- A known class effect
- Lack of alternative explanation
- A dose response
- A "typical" adverse drug reaction (e.g., low background rate) such as a fixed drug reaction which would not generally be seen except when due to a drug
- A "clean subject" (e.g., a child)
- Consistency of time to onset (e.g., early for immediate hypersensitivity or long term for tumorigenesis)
- Similar findings in toxicity studies
- Positive in vitro test (e.g., immunoglobulin E antibodies to allergen and elevated serum tryptase in anaphylaxis)
- Positive in vivo test (e.g., intradermal or prick test for immediate hypersensitivity or patch test for delayed hypersensitivity)
- Identified subset at risk or predisposing factor
- Lack of protopathic bias: a drug given to treat early symptoms may appear temporally associated with the subsequent illness, particularly if the drug's efficacy is low

Adapted from the Report of CIOMS Working Group III, Guidelines for Preparing Core Clinical Safety Information on Drugs 1995 (see Chapter 25).

Over-the-Counter Drugs

There are certain safety reporting requirements for over-the-counter (OTC) drugs. To understand what is required, it is necessary to understand how OTC drugs get to market in the US.

The first is the classic way in which a company prepares an NDA or abbreviated NDA that is submitted to the FDA with safety and efficacy data (plus data covering manufacturing, animal, pharmacology, toxicity, etc.). The FDA reviews this dossier and, if acceptable, approves the drug for marketing in the United States. The company may request and the FDA may approve the product for prescription (Rx) or OTC marketing. If after a certain amount of time (usually at least 5 years) and if the safety profile is acceptable, the company or others may apply to the FDA to move the product from Rx to OTC status. This has happened with many products, including loratadine, ibuprofen, and others. This is known as an "Rx to OTC switch." Thus the product is on the market as an OTC product under an NDA or abbreviated NDA.

The second way is to market a product without an NDA or abbreviated NDA. This is permitted for products that fall under one of the "monographs." The monographs are sections of the code of federal regulations 21CFR330. These are products that are "generally recognized as safe and effective." To market a product under the monograph, the company must follow the "recipe" in the monograph and manufacture the product under Good Manufacturing Practices. No safety or efficacy data need to be submitted.

In regard to reporting AEs for OTC drugs, one must know whether the product has an NDA or not. If there is an NDA, then all the safety requirements that the regulations require must be followed. Such drugs must have 15-day reports, NDA periodic reports, and so on just as if they were Rx drugs in terms of safety. If a drug is a monograph product, there is no requirement for safety reporting at all, although the FDA notes that there is no prohibition against reporting AEs.

For an excellent review of the safety situation and OTC products, see Soller (*DIA J* 2004 at http://www.findarticles.com/p/articles/mi_qa3899/is_200401/ai_n9349329).

38

Coding of Adverse Events: MedDRA and Coding Conventions, Conventions and Arbitrary Usage, Drug Dictionaries and Drug-Naming Problems, and Different Drug Names in Different Countries

As pharmacovigilance becomes more and more mechanized and computerized, the need for standard terminologies, formats, dictionaries, narratives, and abbreviations grows. The first two major areas that have been standardized are the medical coding of adverse events (AEs) and medical history and the coding of drug names. Medical coding has become standardized in the world of pharmacovigilance with the use of the *Medical Dictionary for Regulatory Activities* (MedDRA®). There are several other coding systems that have been used. Two of the more prominent ones are COSTART, which the US Food and Drug Administration (FDA) used for AE coding until moving to MedDRA, and WHO-ART from the Uppsala Monitoring Centre. See Web Resource 38-1 for further information. Some still use WHO-ART, although MedDRA is now becoming the accepted standard from the International Conference on Harmonization (ICH).

Coding is done so that companies, regulators, and others are able to communicate with each other using the same medical language. AEs are coded so that similar cases are described (coded) in the same consistent way and so that they can easily be retrieved, analyzed, and compared. It is invaluable for signal detection and analysis.

MedDRA was developed by the ICH based on earlier work done by the United Kingdom health authority. It is owned by the International Federation of Pharmaceutical Manufacturers and Associations, acting as trustee for the ICH steering committee. A service organization known as the Maintenance and Support Services Organization (MSSO) serves as the repository, maintainer, and distributor of MedDRA as well as the source for information on MedDRA. Detailed information is available from the MedDRA website (Web Resource 38-2).

MedDRA is a terminology developed for drugs and devices used for standardized coding of medical issues, including AEs and medical history. It is hierarchical, which means that it has multiple levels (five) ranging from the most general to very specific. It is available in English with some or all of it also available in Dutch, French, German, Italian, Portuguese, Spanish, and Japanese. It has "more or less" been mandated by the FDA for use in AE reporting. The FDA published a rule mandating its use in 2002, and its use is required in the proposed regulations of March 2003. However, these rules are not in force yet. Nonetheless, MedDRA is used and expected in AE reporting. It is also used in Japan, Canada, the European Union (EU), and other countries where it is either mandated or where it is the usual practice. See the MSSO's website page on regulatory status (Web Resource 38-3). It has replaced COSTART, WHO-ART, HARTS, JART, ICD-9, and other older drug coding systems.

MedDRA is updated twice yearly (April and October), and, in general, users update their own computer systems within 60 days of receipt of the upgrade. This too is not fully mandated everywhere but is the common practice. Users may request the addition of new codes to future versions of MedDRA by applying to the MSSO, which then reviews each request. Codes also may be moved, deleted, changed, demoted, and promoted by the MSSO in the updates. Version 9.1 was released in October 2006.

MedDRA terms cover diseases, diagnoses, signs and symptoms, therapeutic indications, medical and surgical procedures, and medical, social, and family histories. MedDRA does *not* cover drug and device names, study design, patient demographic terms, device failure, population qualifiers (e.g., rare, frequent), and descriptions of severity or numbers. It does not give definitions of AEs.

Originally, MedDRA was developed for postmarketing AEs, but it is now used widely for clinical trial AEs also. This has produced complex issues in regard to long trials that might run a year or more and go through one or more MedDRA upgrades. The issue of when and how to update the codes in an ongoing trial is complex and has multiple solutions.

MedDRA now has over 81,000 terms arranged into five hierarchical categories:

1. System organ classes (SOCs): 226
2. Higher level group terms (HLGTs): 332
3. Higher level terms (HLTs): 1,683
4. Preferred terms (PTs): 16,976
5. Lowest level terms (LLTs): 62,950

Because there are so many terms, it is necessary to search for a needed term by computer rather than reading through a written version of the terminology. For this, the MSSO and other companies have developed software, called "browsers," to allow a user to find the terms he or she needs. See the MSSO site for a sample of MedDRA and a downloadable browser (Web Resource 38-4).

Browsers

A browser is software that allows one to find the appropriate term in the dictionary. One or more words (e.g., pain in the leg) are typed in, and the browser determines whether or not there is a direct word-for-word match at one or more of the hierarchical levels. If so, it gives the direct "hit" along with the hierarchical tree; that is, if the direct hit is an LLT, it will display the PT, HLT, HLGT, and SOC (both primary and secondary if more than one exists). If not, most browsers suggest choices for the user to pick from. Some browsers do autoencoding where one may type in a narrative (prose paragraphs) and the browser will extract and code all medical-sounding terms for the user to examine and accept or reject. There are several MedDRA browsers available. The MSSO has one, as do various other companies.

Coding

The actual coding of AEs is a very complex subject and cannot be fully covered here, but some general thoughts and issues on coding are addressed.

The goal of coding is to create one or more AE codes that capture the essence of the adverse experiences that the patient experienced. There should not be too many or too few terms but just enough. Defining "just enough," however, is difficult. There are many complexities that one encounters when coding:

- Should one be "a lumper or a splitter"? That is, should one code "flu-like syndrome" (the lumper) or "fever," "malaise," "fatigue," "muscle aches," "headache," "chills," and "runny nose" (the splitter)? This may be evident to the reader for a term such as "flu-like syndrome" but less clear for the "Hermansky-Pudlak syndrome" (albinism, visual problems, platelet defects with bleeding, lung disease, and often kidney and gastrointestinal disease).

- Should one code "cascade" or "secondary" effects? For example, if a patient becomes dizzy and falls, breaking his or her shoulder and abrading his or her skin, the primary event is dizziness (and should be coded) but should the other terms—the fall, shoulder fracture, skin abrasions—also be coded and thus considered as AEs associated with the drug in question in the database and future labeling?

- Should signs (hepatomegaly) and symptoms (abdominal pain) be coded or only diseases and diagnoses?

- Should provisional or "rule out" diagnoses be coded?
- How specific should one be? Should one code "skin rash on face and neck" or just "rash"?
- Should one code "low blood glucose" or "hypoglycemia"?
- Coding may be done at a less specific level, coding "edema" instead of "facial edema" or "lung disease NOS (not otherwise specified)" instead of a more specific diagnosis (e.g., pneumococcal pneumonia).
- Coding consistency and variability is often a problem, especially when there are multiple coders or coding is done over time (e.g., in a long clinical trial). One might see "elevated liver enzymes," "abnormal liver enzymes," "elevated SGOT," "elevated SGPT," "elevated ALT," or "elevated AST," all of which are capturing the same condition in different patients. This poses problems when one is attempting to retrieve all the cases of liver problems to do safety signaling.
- Having too many codes for a particular case makes it hard to understand what the primary or major issues were. In practice, many users try to limit the number of codes in each case to six or eight at most.
- Cultural differences may affect coding across countries or regions. In addition, language issues may alter coding, especially if people are coding in a language (English) that is not their primary language.

There is, in many cases, no single correct answer to a coding question. Rather it is necessary that people doing coding agree on certain standards or "conventions" that define (sometimes arbitrarily) how to code. The MSSO has published several versions of its coding suggestions entitled "MedDRA® Term Selection: Points to Consider. ICH-Endorsed Guide for MedDRA® Users" (Web Resource 38-5).

The FDA in its "Guidance for Industry Premarketing Risk Assessment" of March 2005 (Web Resource 38-6) has commented on coding:

"Sponsors should explore the accuracy of the coding process with respect to both investigators and the persons who code adverse events.

- Investigators may sometimes choose verbatim terms that do not accurately communicate the adverse event that occurred.
- The severity or magnitude of an event may be inappropriately exaggerated (e.g., if an investigator terms a case of isolated elevated transaminases *acute liver failure* despite the absence of evidence of associated hyperbilirubinemia, coagulopathy, or encephalopathy, which are components of the standard definition of acute liver failure).
- Conversely, the significance or existence of an event may be masked (e.g., if an investigator uses a term that is nonspecific and possibly unimportant to describe a subject's discontinuation from a study when the discontinuation is due to a serious adverse event).

Sponsors should strive to identify obvious coding mistakes as well as any instances when a potentially serious verbatim term may have been inappropriately mapped to a more benign coding term, thus minimizing the potential severity of an adverse event. One example is coding the verbatim term *facial edema* (suggesting an allergic reaction) as the nonspecific term *edema*; another is coding the verbatim term *suicidal ideation* as the more benign term *emotional lability*.

- Prior to analyzing a product's safety database, sponsors should ensure that adverse events were coded with minimal variability across studies and individual coders."

To limit variability, many companies establish a central coding group that either does all AE coding itself or checks and verifies that all coding done by others is done in a consistent and correct manner.

In summary then, a safety department (or, better, the regulatory authority or company) needs to establish detailed coding standards, preferably using accepted (MSSO/ICH) conventions, and train the staff on their use. Because employees come and go and because MedDRA is updated twice yearly, coding training is usually an ongoing process. The MSSO and many vendors provide basic training courses in MedDRA coding, usually running from ½ day to 2 days.

Drug Codes

Another requirement in the pharmacovigilance world is a consistent and up-to-date drug dictionary. Ideally, such a dictionary would have all the names of the drugs sold throughout the world. Unfortunately, this is not a simple task. It is far harder than developing an AE dictionary:

- Each drug may have multiple names (see below).
- Drug names change.
- A drug with the same trade name may have different formulations in different countries.

- Spelling varies, and some languages do not use our alphabet.
- Combination drugs have multiple names.
- Drugs may be very similar, varying only in the salt. They may have the same names or totally different names.

Multiple Names

In January 2006 the FDA issued a warning to consumers against filling US prescriptions abroad because drugs with same or similar names may contain different active ingredients from those sold in the United States and may thus pose health risks. See Web Resource 38-7. They gave two examples:

> "For example, in the United States, 'Flomax' is a brand name for tamsulosin, a treatment for an enlarged prostate, while in Italy, the active ingredient in the product called 'Flomax' is morniflumate, an anti-inflammatory drug. In the United States, 'Norpramin' is the brand name for an antidepression drug containing desipramine but, in Spain, the same brand name, 'Norpramin,' is used for a drug that contains omeprazole, a treatment for stomach ulcers."

A drug, even a simple drug, has multiple names. For example, here is a list of some of the names for the drug cimetidine that are used around the world:

Eureceptor, Gastromet, SKF 92334, Tagamet, Tametin, Tratul, Ulcedine, Ulcimet, Ulcomet, Acibilin, Acinil, Cimal, Cimetag, Cimetum, Dyspamet, Edalene, Peptol, Ulcedin, Ulcerfen, Ulcofalk, Ulcomedina, Ulhys, *N*-cyano-*N*'-methyl-*N*''-((E)-2-([(5-methyl-1H-imidazol-4-yl)methyl]sulfanyl)ethyl)guanidine, 1-cyano-2-methyl-3-(2-(((5-methyl-4-imidazolyl)methyl)thio)ethyl)guanidine, 2-cyano-1-methyl-3-(2-(((5-methylimidazol-4-yl)methyl)thio)ethyl)guanidine, Acibilin, Acinil, Cimetag, Cimetum, Dyspamet, Edalene, Eureceptor, Gastromet, Metracin, and Brumetidina.

Name Changes

As noted above, names may change. Omeprazole was originally sold in the United States as Losec®, but the name was changed to Prilosec® at the request of the FDA because of the possibility of confusion with Lasix®. See Web Resource 38-8.

In the United States, the US Adopted Names Council (USAN) (Web Resource 38-9), which is officially sponsored by the American Medical Association, the US Pharmacopeial Convention, and the American Pharmacists Association, assigns generic names that are unique and nonproprietary. The USAN works closely with the International Nonproprietary Name (INN) Program of the World Health Organization (WHO) (Web Resource 38-10), which assigns international "generic" names.

This is obviously a very complex situation. So, in the example above, cimetidine is the "generic" (and also the INN and USAN, see below) name of the compound that has a chemical name of *N*''-cyano-*N*-methyl-*N*'-[2-[[(5-methyl-1H-imidazol-4-yl) methyl]thio]ethyl]guanidine, which has the trade name of Tagamet®, Peptol®, Nu-Cimet®, Apo-Cimetidine®, Novo-Cimetidine®, and others.

See the website of the Institute for Safe Medication Practices (Web Resource 38-11) for an excellent discussion of all aspects of medication prescribing and medication errors, including name issues. They publish a list of Confused Drug Names (Web Resource 38-12).

World Health Organization (WHO) Drug Dictionary

In the drug safety world, during the preparation of individual case safety reports and aggregate reports (Periodic Safety Update Reports [PSURs], New Drug Application periodic reports etc.), comedications are frequently encountered that have not been seen before. Because comedications can play a major role in safety reports, it is critical to know what medications (both prescription, over the counter, nutraceuticals, etc.) a patient has taken. Often, however, a strange name is encountered and much time is spent tracking it down to understand what it is chemically. It is far more practical to maintain a drug dictionary with all drug names and formulations that one can refer to as needed.

As with an AE dictionary, it is critical to enter data in a correct and consistent fashion to retrieve it properly. Inconsistent coding produces incomplete searches during signaling or preparation of PSURs and other reports.

Creating and maintaining a drug dictionary, unlike an AE dictionary, is far harder and more complex. With an AE dictionary, the vocabulary is controlled and relatively finite. Few "new" medical terms or diseases occur. Many of the changes to MedDRA represent refinements to the current terms. It is expected that within a few years the MedDRA changes will decrease as the dictionary reaches maturity and "steady state."

Drug dictionaries are quite different. New drugs are developed almost weekly. New drugs, line extensions, "rebranding," new formulations, and new trade names are developed, approved, and launched somewhere in the world every day and old drugs are withdrawn. To track the names, formulations, and formulas of all these products in over 100 countries is an impossible task. Whereas MedDRA is updated twice yearly, a drug dictionary, if it is meant to be complete, would need to be updated daily to weekly to remain current. For this and other reasons, ICH has avoided moving into the field of drug dictionaries.

The most useful drug dictionary available is the WHO Drug Dictionary, which is a product of the Uppsala Monitoring Centre. See the website (Web Resource 38-13) for further information.

This dictionary contains 80,107 unique trade names and 266,109 different medicinal products as of September 2005. It is updated quarterly. It contains products registered by the FDA and the European Medicines Agency (EMEA). Most of the drugs are prescription products, but it does contain some over-the-counter products. The dictionary is hierarchical, using system organ classes and the chemical, pharmacologic, and therapeutic properties of each drug. A numerical code is also assigned to each drug. See in particular the monograph on the "WHO Drug Dictionary Enhanced" (Web Resource 38-14).

Companies and other users have handled the dictionary in various ways. Some simply subscribe to the dictionary and use the updates as issued by the Uppsala Monitoring Centre as is. Other companies use the WHO Drug Dictionary as a base and add on to it as new drugs are encountered in individual case safety reports. This dictionary may then "grow" separately from the WHO Drug Dictionary into a proprietary company dictionary. This would pose reconciliation problems when the new update of the WHO dictionary is issued, and thus some companies may choose not to use the WHO upgrades but rather maintain their own home-grown version. The logic behind this is reasonable in the sense that companies often sell limited lines of drugs and may only rarely encounter certain drugs or classes of drugs. A company that makes primarily diabetic drugs needs to have the latest information on all diabetic comedications arriving on the market but may be less concerned about oncology and asthma drugs, for example. They thus have their dictionary group focus on the drugs they encounter more frequently. The downside to this is that companies have drug dictionaries that are significantly different and cannot easily communicate with each other and with health authorities. From the safety officer's point of view, it is necessary to know what drug dictionary is being used and how coding is done, especially in complicated situations and foreign cases.

■ EudraVigilance Medicinal Product Dictionary

One other initiative is worth noting and that is the newly created EudraVigilance Medicinal Product Dictionary by the EMEA. This has been developed for (obligatory) use in certain submissions to the EMEA. See Web Resource 38-15. Those companies actively submitting cases to the EMEA and EU member states need to be familiar with this (free) dictionary. Detailed information is available at the website.

Investigational New Drug Application Reports: 7- and 15-Day Reports and Annual Reports

There are multiple different safety reports that pharmaceutical companies and other sponsors must submit to health authorities. This chapter reviews the reports required now by the US Food and Drug Administration (FDA) and other authorities and summarizes briefly the proposed new reports in the FDA's March 2003 proposed new regulations.

■ Investigational New Drug Application (IND) Reports

The IND obligations are found in 21CFR312. An IND is usually opened and held by a pharmaceutical company, but academics, universities, and individuals may also do so. The term that the FDA uses for the IND holder is generally "the sponsor."

The sponsor is obliged to "review and evaluate the evidence relating to the safety and effectiveness of the drug as it is obtained from the investigator" (21CFR312.56(c)).

This includes 7- and 15-day expedited reports (21CFR312.32) and annual reports (21CFR312.33).

Expedited IND Reports (Alert Reports, 7- and 15-Day IND Reports)

This section describes the reports that are sent to an IND at the FDA for serious, unexpected (unlabeled/unlisted), possibly associated adverse events (AEs) from clinical trials or animal tests that show a significant risk for humans. Each report identifies all similar reports sent to the FDA, and the sponsor analyzes their significance.

The report must be made no later than 15 calendar days after the sponsor's initial receipt of the information. This is the "clock start date." It begins when there is sufficient information that the three criteria are met (serious, unexpected, associated) for an expedited report and that the report has the four criteria (reporter, patient, AE, drug) to be valid.

If the case has a serious outcome of fatal or life-threatening (i.e., serious, unexpected, associated, and fatal or life-threatening), the case is to be reported as a telephone or fax report within 7 calendar days of the first receipt. All 7-day reports are automatically 15-day reports and must then be processed and submitted as an expedited report by day 15.

The events should be submitted on a MedWatch form (3500A). Animal reports and other nonindividual case reports (e.g., epidemiologic studies) are usually submitted as narratives rather than on MedWatch forms. Most companies do not want to put animal data into their clinical safety database. Non-US cases may be submitted on MedWatch or CIOMS I forms. The reports are submitted to the appropriate new drug review division at the FDA.

The sponsor must also notify all participating investigators of these reports. The investigators in turn notify the investigational review boards (21CFR312.32(c)(i and ii)).

The sponsor is also required to report information to the FDA from any source, foreign or domestic; clinical, animal, or epidemiologic investigations; commercial marketing experience; literature reports; unpublished papers; and foreign regulatory authorities (21CFR312.32(b)). The FDA retains the right to change the format and frequency of the reports. For marketed drugs, reporting to the IND is not required unless that case is from the IND clinical trial itself.

Follow-up is required on all safety information received by the sponsor and submitted as a follow-up to the original (initial) 15-day report. Follow-up information shall be handled with the same 15-calendar-day clock. If a case is received and does not meet the criteria of a 15-day report (e.g., reported as a nonserious case initially) and only later does the receipt of follow-up information show the case to meet the reportability criteria, the clock starts when the follow-up information is received.

Other information that the sponsor receives that does not quite fall into these categories but which the sponsor wishes to report should be reported as an information amendment or in the annual report. The FDA notes that reporting of a case by the sponsor does not mean that the FDA or the sponsor believes that the report was necessarily due to the drug. This point may prove to be very important in any potential litigation in which the sponsor might become involved (21CFR312.32(c)(3, 4)). Postmarketing trials should be submitted to the IND (whether conducted under an IND or not) only if the case meets the three criteria (serious, unexpected, possibly related) as determined by the sponsor.

In summary, the sponsor (whether an individual, institution, or company) must submit to the FDA as a 15-day expedited report all clinical trial AEs that are serious, unexpected (not in the investigator brochure or package insert, depending on which one is used: investigator brochure for nonmarketed drugs or new indications of marketed drugs and the package insert for marketed drugs and postmarketing studies), and associated (possibly, probably, likely, definitely, remotely etc. related) with the study drug. If the case is a death or is life-threatening, a 7-day report (phone or fax) must also be made in addition to the 15-day report.

IND Annual Reports

In addition to the 7- and 15-day safety reports, the IND holder must also submit annual reports (21CFR312.33). Within 60 days of the anniversary date of the IND, a brief report of the progress of the investigation must be submitted that includes the following:

Individual study information: A brief summary of the status of each study in progress and each study completed during the previous year:

- The title and number of the study, its purpose, a brief statement identifying the patient population, and a statement as to whether the study is completed.
- The total number of subjects initially planned for inclusion in the study; the number entered into the study to date, tabulated by age group, gender, and race; the number whose participation in the study was completed as planned; and the number who dropped out of the study for any reason.
- If the study has been completed, or if interim results are known, a brief description of any available study results.

Summary information obtained during the previous year's clinical and nonclinical investigations:

- A narrative or tabular summary showing the most frequent and most serious adverse experiences by body system.
- A summary of all IND 15-day safety reports submitted during the past year.
- A list of subjects who died during the investigation, with the cause of death for each subject.
- A list of subjects who dropped out during the investigation in association with any adverse experience, whether or not thought to be drug related.
- A brief description of what, if anything, was obtained that is pertinent to an understanding of the drug's actions, including, for example, information about dose response, information

from controlled trails, and information about bioavailability.

- A list of the preclinical studies (including animal studies) completed or in progress during the past year and a summary of the major preclinical findings.
- A summary of any significant manufacturing or microbiologic changes made during the past year.
- A description of the general investigational plan for the coming year to replace that submitted 1 year earlier.
- If the investigator brochure has been revised, a description of the revision and a copy of the new brochure.
- A description of any significant phase I protocol modifications made during the previous year and not previously reported to the IND in a protocol amendment.
- A brief summary of significant foreign marketing developments with the drug during the past year, such as approval of marketing in any country or withdrawal or suspension from marketing in any country.

Note that if the sponsor wishes, it may transfer some or all duties for clinical trials (including safety) to a third party such as another company or a clinical research organization. In that case the transfer of obligations must be described in detail and in writing to the FDA (21CFR312.52(a)).

Other Clinical Trial (IND) Reporting Issues

Reporting the same 15-day alert case to the IND and the New Drug Application (NDA):

This issue arises when there is an open IND and an approved NDA for the same drug. Normally in simple situations, before NDA approval and while the IND is open, all 15-day reports are sent to the IND. After the NDA is approved, reporting should now, in general, be to the NDA. There is one situation where there must be reporting to both the IND and the NDA.

Double reporting is required if the serious AE meets the three IND reporting criteria (serious, unexpected, possibly related) and is from an IND study. In this case the 15-day report must be sent to both the IND and the NDA. If the serious AE report is from a non-IND study, then it is reported to the NDA only.

Reporting serious AEs to comparator drugs and placebos:

The FDA is largely silent on this issue. International Conference on Harmonization (ICH) E2A III.E.1 proposes that the sponsor decide whether to submit the comparator 15-day case to the health authority or to the manufacturer.

Some countries have been requiring the reporting of placebo and comparator serious AEs. In the United States, placebo cases usually do not meet the four element criteria (patient, reporter, drug, AE) because there is no "drug" and so are usually not reported. One may note, however, that placebos usually do have excipients and often "benign" products such as lactose that can produce AEs. In addition, in any placebo-controlled trial there are usually large numbers of AEs seen with placebos. These are reported at the end of the study in the final study report.

The sponsor of the trial, especially if the trial is a multinational trial, must ensure that all regulatory reporting requirements in each country where there is a clinical trial site are met. These requirements are often different from US/EU/ICH requirements and may also require local language reporting for certain serious AEs.

Blinding and unblinding 7- and 15-day alert reports:

The question of opening the blind on a patient who has a serious AE that is a 15-day report (serious, unexpected, possibly related) but for which the study drug is still blinded (study drug, comparator, placebo) was discussed by the FDA in its final rule amendment of October 7, 1997 (62FR52237) in a commentary section on page 52245. See Web Resource 39-1.

The FDA states that "sponsors should only break the blind for the subject in question. Sponsors should consult with the FDA review division responsible for their IND in situations in which the sponsor believes that breaking the blind would compromise their study (e.g. when a fatal or other serious outcome is the primary efficacy endpoint in a clinical investigation)."

The EU and the member states generally require that cases be unblinded before submission. For example, for postmarketing studies, see Volume 9, section 1.2.2.3, which references ICH E2A's criteria for unblinding.

E2A, which the FDA also references and wishes to follow, notes that when possible and appropriate, the blind should be maintained for those persons, such as biometrics (statistics) personnel. In large companies this often turns out to be difficult to do in practice. Although statisticians may be blinded, in most instances when the blind is broken a MedWatch/CIOMS I form is created, in which case it is noted to be the study drug or control. Usually, serious AE reports are routinely widely dispersed: to the clinical trial physicians, monitors, others in the company, the investigators and the investigational review boards, subsidiaries, clinical research organizations, and data safety monitoring boards. "Leaks" occur and the code is inadvertently revealed to those who are attempting to remain blinded.

Note: Some companies, especially those making ophthalmology products, do not like to use the word "blinded" and prefer to use the word "masked."

Serious AE reporting after the end of the trial:

There are no clear rules in the United States for the duration of time that serious AEs should be collected and reported in the study report and to the FDA as expedited reports after a trial ends. Many use an arbitrary 30-day period after the patient's last dose. This may come from the long-standing clinical medicine tradition of ascribing postoperative deaths to the surgery itself if the death occurred within 30 days of the operation. Clearly, if a drug has a very short or very long terminal half-life (e.g., depot formulations), one may use a different time period.

Survival studies (where all patients are followed until death, such as in cancer trials) present different issues. Here again, many use a 30-day limit after the last dose for collection of serious AEs. All deaths, however, should be collected by the sponsor and, if believed to meet the criteria for a 7- or 15-day report, reported. The issue here in survival studies is that when doing periodic follow-up to see whether the patients are still alive, one often has serious AEs reported "in passing." What to do with these is the issue. There is no consensus on this. Some companies collect and report them. Others do not.

When to Start Collecting Serious AEs in Trials

In general, safety data collection starts as soon as the informed consent is signed and includes the waiting period or washout period (if there is one) when no study drug is administered. This concept was particularly noteworthy in France where any safety issue that occurred during the "biomedical research" was reportable. This included placebo AEs, complications of medical procedures, auto accidents on the way to the hospital, and so forth. The idea is that the AEs occurred in regard to the study itself and not just the study drug.

In regard to FDA reporting, a serious AE that occurred before the drug was administered is generally not related to the study drug and thus does not qualify as a 15-day report. There is at least one situation, however, where this might not always be the case. Anticipatory nausea and vomiting before cancer chemotherapy in patients who have already had therapy is rather common, with an approximate 29% and 11% incidence, respectively. See the National Cancer Institute review of this phenomenon at its website (Web Resource 39-2). Thus one may consider that these serious AEs, which may be due to classic Pavlovian conditioning, are possibly related to the study or treatment drug even though it has not yet been taken.

New Drug Application Reports: 15-Day Alert Reports

The regulations governing postmarketing adverse event (AE) reporting are complex and scattered, with various updates and guidances in force. Some can be found at Web Resource 40-1, Web Resource 40-2, and Web Resource 40-3.

Although postmarketing New Drug Application (NDA) AE reports are conceptually quite similar to premarketing Investigational New Drug Application (IND) AE reports, there are significant differences. The sources and reporters of the events are quite varied (not just from clinical trials and not just from clinical investigators). The handling and reporting to the US Food and Drug Administration (FDA) are also somewhat different. These are explained below.

■ Expedited NDA Reports (Alert Reports, 15-Day NDA Reports) (21CFR314.80)

As with IND safety reporting, there is an obligation for safety reporting after marketing a drug—after approval of the NDA. In clinical trials AEs are reported by inves-

tigators who are health professionals and usually have a relationship with the company (e.g., sponsored trials). Thus cooperation and complete medical reports from a health care professional are usually ensured. Reporting is obligatory under federal regulations for the investigator and the sponsor.

The postmarketing period, however, is quite different. Reports may come from many sources, including patients, families of patients, health care professionals, sales representatives, literature reports, news reports, the FDA, foreign health authorities, and other pharmaceutical companies. Reporting is purely voluntary for everyone except pharmaceutical companies and rests on the good will of the caller. However, sometimes the patients reporting the AE are upset that the AE happened at all. They may take the approach that drugs are safe and this should not have happened. At least in the United States, they often want their money back and, in fact, did not call to report the AE but rather to get a refund.

Health care professionals often call or write to the FDA or the pharmaceutical company to report an AE and are not quite aware that the company, obliged to follow-up and report the case to the FDA, will do extensive follow-up and request copies of reports both from the physician's office and the hospital, laboratory, and even the ambulance service. The busy pharmacists, nurses, or physicians often do not realize what they are getting into when they simply called to do their duty by making a "quick" report of an AE. They did not want to get burdened down with pulling records from perhaps multiple sources and sending them to the company. Yet it is this spontaneous voluntary reporting that is the backbone of the system in place now to collect postmarketing AEs. The quality of these reports is quite variable, especially when reported by nonmedical people. Consumer reports are usually followed up with the treating physician where possible.

In the United States, the NDA holder has an obligation to promptly review all adverse drug experience information received from any source, "foreign or domestic including information derived from commercial marketing experience, post marketing clinical investigations, post marketing epidemiological/surveillance studies, reports in the scientific literature, and unpublished scientific papers" (21CFR314.80(b)). Companies do not have to resubmit to the FDA reports received from the FDA.

The four elements or criteria for a valid 15-day safety report (sometimes called the minimal data set for reportability) are

1. An identifiable patient
2. An identifiable reporter
3. A suspect drug(s)
4. An AE (or fatal outcome if no AE is reported other than "found dead")

See the FDA's 1997 guidance at Web Resource 40-4.

If these four elements are present, then the case is considered reportable to the FDA. If they are not, the company should make due diligence efforts to obtain the missing data. The data should be stored in an electronic database.

An identifiable patient usually means one or more identifiers are present: age, sex, initials, name, and so on. Vague reports such as "I heard there was a patient or two upstate who took drug X and had a stroke" or "a few people had strokes" are not specific enough to meet the criteria for identifiable patient. "A man" or "a young girl" or "six men had strokes" are sufficient to be considered identifiable.

An identifiable reporter is usually clearer. It may be the patient or a family member. As a rule of thumb, an identifiable reporter should be one who can be contacted. Thus an e-mail AE report where there is no other information on the sender than the e-mail address would be a valid reporter because one can respond to the e-mail and get follow-up. (In fact, the response should simply state that the company needs to get follow-up but would prefer not to do it over the internet—neither secure nor private—and to please contact the company by phone, mail, or fax or supply a phone number or postal address for contact.)

The suspect drug is also usually not a problem. However, issues do occur:

- Occasionally someone will send in an AE report and make the comment, "I don't think this is due to your drug but thought I should report it anyway, just in case." This should still be considered the suspect drug (unless another one is noted) and the reporter's comment noted in the narrative. If the product is clearly that manufactured by the company, then this case needs to be processed in the usual manner.

- If it is clear that the drug is the product of another company (e.g., same chemical entity but different manufacturer, whether branded or generic), the case should be sent within 5 days to that manufacturer or company. If, however, it is unclear whether it is the company's product or that of another manufacturer, then the company must process it as if it were clearly its product. The lack of clear "ownership" and product identification should be noted in the report.

- If it is a foreign originated report with the same active ingredient (moiety), then the case should be entered into the database and reported if the reporting criteria are met.

  - The FDA's 2001 postmarketing AE draft guidance states the following for foreign literature: "Reports of serious, unexpected adverse experiences described in the scientific literature should be submitted for products that have the same active moiety as a product marketed in the United States. This is true even if the excipient, dosage forms, strengths, routes of administration, and indications vary."

  - In regard to what the definition of an active moiety is: "An active moiety means the molecule or ion, excluding those appended portions of the molecule that cause the drug to be an ester, salt (including a salt with hydrogen or coordination bonds), or other noncovalent derivative (such as a complex, chelate, or clathrate) of the molecule, responsible for the physiological or pharmacological action of the drug substance." From the FDA's "Frequently Asked Questions for New Drug Product Exclusivity" at its website (Web Resource 40-5).

- Different formulations of the same active moiety must be entered into the database and reported, if appropriate, unless the product is clearly found to be from another company. Thus a topical version of a company's product made by another company (but unclear which one) needs to be reported.

- Combination products that contain the active moiety should also be reported.

The identifiable AE is also usually clear and relates to any "bad thing." The AE should include signs and/or laboratory abnormalities and/or symptoms and/or diseases. More general terms like "experienced unspecified injury" or "irreparable damages" should be excluded. Fatal outcome with no AE should be considered reportable ("found dead in bed"). This is the only instance where an outcome is considered an AE.

One should also be sure to distinguish medication errors and product quality issues. Sometimes two or more things may occur in the same report ("The tablet was blue instead of green and smelled funny; I took two instead of one and then had a bad headache. And I want my money back."). The product quality, medication error, AE and refund issues should each be handled by the appropriate personnel in the company.

The company ("applicant," as used by the FDA in these regulations referring to the NDA) must report each AE that is serious and unexpected (not in the approved labeling = US package insert) whether from the United States or abroad within 15 calendar days of initial receipt of the information.

Note that this is different from the criteria used for IND alert reporting. IND reporting requires three criteria (serious, unexpected, possibly related to the drug). NDA reporting only requires two (serious, unexpected). This is because it is believed that spontaneous reports have "implied" causality or suspicion. The reporter would not have contacted the FDA or the company to report the case if he or she did not believe there was some level of causal relationship between the drug and the AE.

The company must promptly investigate all serious AEs that produced 15-day alert reports and must submit follow-up reports within 15 calendar days of receipt of new information or as requested by the FDA. If additional information is not obtainable, records should be maintained of the unsuccessful steps taken to seek additional information.

The company selling or making the drug is not the only one obliged to report serious AEs. This requirement also applies to any person or entity whose name appears on the label of an approved drug product as a manufacturer, packer, or distributor.

If a company holds more than one NDA for the same chemical entity, the 15-day report should be addressed to the oldest (original) approved NDA if the actual product or formulation is not known or specified. If a company has more than one of its products listed in the report, the case should be sent to the NDA for the first listed product on the report, which is usually the "more" or "most" suspect drug.

Solicited safety information (e.g., from patient outreach or support programs) should be handled as if this was a postmarketing trial and the three (IND) criteria are applied: serious, unexpected, possibly related. That is, the criteria are not those of the NDA (serious, unexpected) but of the IND. There are no 7-day reports to an NDA.

Feeder Groups

Postmarketing AEs may come from many sources: sales representatives; the regulatory, quality, compliance, or telephone operator departments and other company employees (such as the chief executive officer's secretary); lawyers and lawsuits; individual patients, consumers and family; pharmacists; nurses; physicians and other health care professionals; the FDA; company subsidiaries; associated business partners (not part of the company); websites; e-mail; newspapers; the medical literature; TV and radio. The company must set up the appropriate internal procedures (standard operating procedures) to ensure that AEs arriving anywhere in the company reach the drug safety group in a timely manner (usually no more than 1–2 working days).

Unlike IND reports where the reporters are usually clinical investigators or their staff, many postmarketing reports arrive by telephone from unhappy patients or harried medical professionals. The company needs to establish a careful triage of calls to identify those that are product-related and ensure they are sent to a medical professional quickly after the operator answers so that AEs and other product issues are not missed. It is not wise to bounce the call to multiple departments until the right one is found. Voice response systems may fail to elicit the problem ("Press one to get your money back. Press two to report an AE....").

A rather special skill set on the part of the medical professionals in the company who field these calls is required. The caller, especially if a patient, usually wants something (money or replacement drug) and may be angry and hostile. The medical professional must be cool and calm and obtain the needed medical and demographic information while maintaining empathy and sympathy.

Often the caller has contacted the company with a question ("Can drug X cause heart attacks?"), not realizing that the medical professional will explore to see whether there is an AE there. Thus the call is, to a degree, transformed from a request for information to a supplying of information that may anger the caller. The medical professional should write down (on paper or directly into a database) the caller's information, using direct quotes where possible without admitting that the drug necessarily caused any AEs or produced problems. When the call is from a consumer, an attempt should always be made to obtain the contact information of the patient's physician to "medically validate" the report. If follow-up is needed with the caller (e.g., after obtaining medical records), another contact should be arranged.

Literature and Publications

Formal and frequent searches of the published literature using a computerized system (commercial services) that searches large numbers of publications and databases for publications on the company's products (both by trade name and generic name) is required. If the search reveals a citation, article, or abstract that contains a case report or clinical trial with information that meets the four criteria, a 15-day NDA alert report must be sent to the FDA along with a copy of the article (in English). This is handled like any other 15-day report with follow-up sought. If an article describes multiple cases, then a separate MedWatch report should be filed for each (21CFR31.480(d)(1,2)). Note that such literature searches are required for drugs marketed in the European Union and are included in Periodic Safety Update Reports.

The issue of translation arises periodically. If a publication title suggests that the article contains reportable safety information and if the article and the abstract are in a language that no one on staff is able to read (or even minimally decipher), then the article should be translated to determine whether there is a case. This may be very costly for certain languages. Fortunately, most cases are published in English or one of the other major medical languages. The regulatory reporting clock starts when the four elements of a valid case are identifiable. This may mean the clock starts only when the translation is received.

For multinational companies with offices around the world, the issue of who searches which journals should be addressed early on and up front to avoid duplication of labor. The international offices are usually very useful for obtaining follow-up from faraway reporters and non-English speakers. However, it is usually not productive to have each international office search its country's journals for AEs. This is best done through the central database search.

MedWatch to Manufacturer Program: Reports Received from the FDA

The FDA established the MedWatch to Manufacturer Program in which serious spontaneous AEs reported directly to the FDA are sent to the manufacturer as MedWatch forms. See Web Resource 40-6. The reports contain the reporter's name and address, permitting the manufacturer to do follow-up. The reporter must consent to this. The original MedWatch received from the FDA should not be re-sent to the FDA (see 21CFR3.14.80(b)), but any follow-up information should be. Other reports may be received from the FDA under the Drug Quality Reporting System that the FDA established for the reporting and receipt of quality issues on products analogous to the MedWatch Program. See the FDA website (Web Resource 40-7).

Reports Received from the FDA via the Freedom of Information Act (FOIA)

This is a system that allows anyone to obtain information from the US government that is not classified or proprietary (commercial secrets). For a nominal fee, it is possible to obtain from the FDA MedWatch reports on any drug (one's own or competitors). It is a one- or two-step process. The initial request produces a standardized printout or diskette with a line listing of AEs. Any specific AE (the MedWatch form) may be obtained by then requesting the case using its identification number (accession number). The cases received are anonymous in regard to the patient and reporter, thus preventing follow-up. Unfortunately, some follow-up reports are not tied or referenced to the initial reports.

If one does this, the request itself is public information and can be found out (by a company's competitors, for example). Thus there are commercial ventures that perform the search for a company and make the search anonymous. One such company is FOI Services. Their website is listed in Web Resource 40-8.

There are reasons both for and against obtaining cases on one's own drugs:

- Pros
  - The company will know what the FDA knows and will have as complete a data set as possible.

▩ The company will be better able to look for signals and perform signal analysis (including data mining) with a complete database.

■ Cons

▩ No follow-up is possible on a case. What you have is what you have.

▩ It may not always be possible to determine whether a case is a duplicate (e.g., it was reported to the FDA in addition to the company, perhaps by a different reporter). As the reporter and patient identifiers are removed, it may be hard to ascertain whether the case is a duplicate.

▩ Coding and case handling (e.g., narrative style and content) may be different. At this point a decision on whether to recode must be made.

▩ In some cases (less so now) one may not recognize one's own cases if they are rewritten or recoded in the FDA database.

Approximately 80% of cases reported to the FDA come through the company and 20% are direct reports. Thus the company would theoretically increase its database by about 25% by obtaining these reports for its own drug.

Some companies obtain competitor safety information in this way. Such data, however, are not permitted to be used in marketing or sales.

Similar FOI systems exist already or are developing in other countries (notably Canada). Again, issues arise such as duplication, consistency, language, and follow-up when obtaining case reports. Many multinational companies have their local offices obtain these cases where possible.

■ Collection of Reports

Periodically, certain large organizations (such as poison control centers and teratology centers) publish summary or review articles detailing dozens to thousands of reports of AEs with drug names associated. Often there is insufficient information to create individual cases, but occasionally there is a minimal data set (patient identifier, reporter being the poison control center, a drug, and an AE). This may pose a problem in regard to reporting. Usually, follow-up is impossible or impractical. In such cases, a communication to the FDA on the best way to handle this is worth doing. The FDA does not want to receive 5,000 MedWatch forms each with minimal data any more than the company wants to generate them. A summary letter or a single report covering multiple patients may be acceptable.

■ Parent–Child/Fetus Reports

The following is from the FDA's instructions on filling out MedWatch forms (Web Resource 40-9):

"Parent–child/fetus report(s) are those cases in which either a fetus/breast-feeding infant or the mother, or both, sustain an adverse event that the initial reporter considers possibly associated with a product administered to the mother during pregnancy. Several general principles are used for filing these reports:

▩ If there has been no event affecting the child/fetus, report only on the parent.

▩ For those cases describing fetal death, miscarriage or abortion, only a parent report is applicable.

▩ When ONLY the child/fetus has an adverse reaction/event (other than fetal death, miscarriage or abortion), the information provided in section A applies to the child/fetus, and characteristics concerning the parent who was the source of exposure to the product is to be provided in section C.

▩ When a newborn baby is found to have a congenital anomaly/birth defect that the initial reporter considers possibly associated with a product administered to the mother during pregnancy, the patient is the newborn baby.

▩ If both the parent and the child/fetus sustain adverse events, two reports should be provided and linked using the narrative."

■ Follow-up

Follow-up on all serious AEs should be done. There are no absolute rules on what is sufficient in terms of due diligence, but a common rule of thumb in the industry is two follow-up requests (registered letters, voice mail messages left, or contacts with physician's nurse) for "routine" serious AEs are sufficient. New, dramatic, unexpected, fatal, or life-threatening serious AEs may require many more attempts to obtain adequate data to make sense of the case (the true goal of all these efforts). Many in the industry have "war stories" of flying to far-off sites or doing various maneuvers to try to obtain follow-up information on critical cases.

Follow-up on nonserious expected cases is often not done or expected by regulatory agencies. Follow-up on nonserious unexpected cases is, however, generally a good idea and is obligatory in some countries.

■ Instructions on Filling Out the MedWatch Form

There are very detailed instructions on the FDA's MedWatch website (Web Resource 40-10) on how to fill out the MedWatch form (3500A form for manufacturers) and for health care professionals (3500 form for all others) at Web Resource 40-11. Companies should review the instructions (most recently updated in October 2005) and put them into place.

NDA Reports: Periodic Reports

In addition to the 15-day alert reports, the US Food and Drug Administration (FDA) requires the submission of New Drug Application (NDA), Abbreviated NDA, and Biologic License Application (BLA) periodic reports. The regulations covering this are found in 21CFR314.80(c)(2)(I,II).

■ NDA Periodic Reports

As with Investigational New Drug application regulations, there are updates scattered in various other FDA documents:

■ Postmarketing Reporting of Adverse Drug Experiences (March 1992)

■ Guideline for Adverse Experience Reporting for Licensed Biological Products (October 1993)

■ Postmarketing Adverse Experience Reporting for Human Drug and Licensed Biological Products: Clarification of What to Report (August 27, 1997)

■ Guidance for Industry: Post-marketing Safety Reporting for Human Drugs and Biological Products Including Vaccines (March 2001)

The basic regulations state the following (21CFR314.80 (c)(2)(I,II)):

All "adverse drug experiences" not submitted as 15-day alert reports must be submitted in the periodic report. A periodic report for each NDA must be submitted quarterly (every 3 months) for the first 3 years after the approval of the NDA. After the 3-year period is over, the reporting frequency is then yearly unless the FDA requests otherwise.

Each report must be submitted 30 days after the close of the quarter for quarterly reports and 60 days after the close of the anniversary date for yearly reports. Thus the company has 30 or 60 days to prepare the report. The FDA may alter this schedule if they wish to continue quarterly reporting after the 3-year period is over.

Each periodic report is required to contain the following:

■ A narrative summary and analysis of the information in the report and an analysis of the 15-day alert reports submitted during the reporting interval (all 15-day alert reports being appropriately referenced by the applicant's patient identification number, adverse reaction term(s), and date of submission to the FDA).

- A MedWatch form (3500A) for each adverse drug experience not reported as a 15-day expedited report (with an index consisting of a line listing of the applicant's patient identification number and adverse reaction term(s)).

- A history of actions taken since the last report because of adverse drug experiences (e.g., labeling changes or studies initiated).

- Periodic reporting, except for information regarding 15-day alert reports, does not apply to adverse drug experience information obtained from postmarketing studies (whether or not conducted under an investigational new drug application), from reports in the scientific literature, and from foreign marketing experience.

- Follow-up information to adverse drug experiences submitted in a periodic report may be submitted in the next periodic report.

In August 1997 the FDA published a guidance encouraging NDA holders to submit requests to waive the requirements to submit MedWatch forms for nonserious labeled AEs. The March 2001 guidance at Web Resource 41-1 markedly expanded the instructions for a periodic report and is now the up-to-date requirement document.

■ Postmarketing Period Report

The information contained within a postmarketing periodic report should be divided into four sections in the order described below and should be clearly separated by an identifying tab. If information for one of these sections is not included, the applicant should explain why the information is not provided.

Section 1: Narrative Summary and Analysis

A narrative summary and analysis of the information in the postmarketing periodic report and an analysis of the 15-day reports (i.e., serious, unexpected, adverse experiences) submitted during the reporting period must be provided and should include the following:

- The number of non–15-day initial adverse experience reports and the number of non–15-day follow-up reports contained in this periodic report and the time period covered by the periodic report.

- A line listing of the 15-day reports submitted during the reporting period. This line listing should include the manufacturer report number, adverse experience term(s), and the date the 15-day report was sent to the FDA.

- A summary tabulation by body system (e.g., cardiovascular, central nervous system, endocrine, renal) of all adverse experience terms and counts of occurrences submitted during the reporting period. The information should be taken from
  - 15-day reports submitted to the FDA
  - Non–15-day reports submitted in the periodic report
  - Reports forwarded to the applicant by the FDA
  - Any nonserious, expected, adverse experiences not submitted to the FDA but maintained on file by the applicant

For the adverse experience term "product interaction," the interacting products should be identified in the tabulation.

- A summary listing of the adverse experience reports in which the drug or biologic product was listed as one of the suspect products but the report was filed to another NDA, Abbreviated NDA, or BLA held by the applicant.

- A narrative discussion of the clinical significance of the 15-day reports submitted during the reporting period and of any increased reporting frequency of serious, expected, adverse experiences when, in the judgment of the applicant, it is believed the data reflect a clinically meaningful change in adverse experience occurrence.

This narrative should assess clinical significance by type of adverse experience, body system, and overall product safety relating the new information received during this reporting period to what was already known about the product.

The narrative should also state what further actions, if any, the applicant plans to undertake based on the information gained during the reporting period and include the time period for completing the actions (i.e., when the applicant plans to start and finish the action and submit the information to the Agency).

- The narrative discussion should indicate, based on the information learned during the reporting period, whether the applicant believes either that (1) no change in the product's current approved labeling is warranted or (2) there are safety-related issues that need to be addressed in the approved product labeling. If changes in the approved product labeling are under consideration by the FDA, the applicant should state in the narrative the date and number of the supplemental application submitted to address the labeling changes.

Section 2: Narrative Discussion of Actions Taken

A narrative discussion of actions taken must be provided, including any labeling changes and studies initiated since the last periodic report. This section should include

- A copy of current US product labeling
- A list of any labeling changes made during the reporting period
- A list of studies initiated
- A summary of important foreign regulatory actions (e.g., new warnings, limitations in the indications and use of the product)
- Any communication of new safety information (e.g., a Dear Doctor letter)

Section 3: Index Line Listing

An index line listing of FDA Form 3500As or Vaccine Adverse Event Reporting System (VAERS) forms included in section 4 of the periodic report must be provided. The line listing for each FDA Form 3500A or VAERS form submitted should include

- Manufacturer report number
- Adverse experience term(s)
- Page number of FDA Form 3500A or VAERS form as located in the periodic report
- Identification of interacting products for any product interaction listed as an adverse experience

Section 4: FDA Form 3500As or VAERS Forms

FDA Form 3500As or VAERS forms must be provided for the following spontaneously reported adverse experiences that occurred in the United States during the reporting period:

- Serious and expected
- Nonserious and unexpected
- Nonserious and expected

Applicants are encouraged to request a waiver of the requirement to submit individual case safety reports of nonserious, expected, adverse experiences for drugs and certain biologic products as described below. Adverse experiences due to a failure to produce the expected pharmacologic action (i.e., lack of effect) should be included in this section.

For individual case safety reports of serious, expected, adverse experiences, the FDA encourages applicants to include relevant hospital discharge summaries and autopsy reports/death certificates as well as lists of other relevant documents as described for 15-day reports of serious, unexpected, adverse experiences.

Initial non–15-day reports should be included in the periodic report in a separate section from non–15-day follow-up reports. All initial and follow-up information obtained for an adverse experience with a given periodic reporting period should be combined and submitted in the periodic report as one initial non–15-day report (i.e., an initial non–15-day report and a non–15-day follow-up report describing the same adverse experience should not be submitted in the same periodic report). An FDA Form 3500A or VAERS form for a serious, unexpected, adverse experience should not be included in a periodic report because this adverse experience should have been previously submitted to the FDA as a 15-day report.

If no adverse experiences were identified for the human drug or biologic product for the time period involved and no regulatory actions concerning safety were taken anywhere in the world where the product is marketed, the periodic report should simply state this and be submitted to the FDA along with a copy of the current US labeling. The FDA has encouraged the use of Periodic Safety Update Reports in place of periodic reports.

■ Other Reports

The FDA requires other reports for "NDA maintenance":

- Distribution reports (21CFR600.810): This is a 6-month report requiring the submission of all information about the quantity of product distributed under licensing agreements. It does not touch drug safety.
- Annual reports (21CFR314.81(b)(2)): This is a yearly report requiring the submission of information from the previous year that might affect safety, efficacy, or labeling as well as information on labeling changes, distribution, chemistry, manufacturing and controls changes, nonclinical laboratory studies, clinical trial data, and pediatric data.

The Tome: The US Food and Drug Administration's Proposed 2003 Regulations

In March 2003, the US Food and Drug Administration (FDA) published its long-awaited proposed new safety rules. See Web Resource 42-1. The document ran over 90 pages in the *Federal Register*. The rules make extensive and complex changes to the current Investigational New Drug Application (IND) and New Drug Application (NDA) safety regulations. Major new obligations on the part of the pharmaceutical industry were introduced.

The FDA invited comments and received many thousands. As of this writing (August 2006) the FDA has not finalized the rules nor is there any clear indication if or when the FDA will finalize some or all the proposed changes. The changes are summarized briefly here. Some companies have already adopted various aspects of the new rules where they are not in contradiction to current regulations and where it is believed they add value (e.g., always expedited reports [AERs], see below) or decrease workload and harmonize with the International Conference on Harmonization (ICH)

and the European Union (e.g., Periodic Safety Update Reports [PSURs]).

The FDA notes that these changes are in response to ICH/Council for International Organizations of Medical Sciences (CIOMS) and to the Risk Management initiative in Prescription Drug User Fee Act III (The act of Congress that allowed the FDA to collect fees from industry. See Web Resource 42-2). There is an extensive section (prepared by outside consultants) reviewing the benefits to the country and public health and the costs (in terms of dollars and time for the industry).

Some of the changes and new requirements follow.

Definitions

- Individual Case Safety Report (ICSR): a MedWatch or CIOMS I form (or an E2B electronic transmission of a case)

- *Suspected Adverse Drug Reaction (SADR):* The FDA is creating a new concept known as "suspected adverse drug reactions" (SADRs) which is to replace the concepts of "adverse event" (AE) and "adverse drug reaction" in the regulations. An SADR is defined as follows:

"A noxious and unintended response to any dose of a drug/biological product for which there is a reasonable possibility that the product caused the response. In this definition, the phrase 'a reasonable possibility' means that the relationship cannot be ruled out (p. 12,417). Classifying a case as 'probably related,' 'possibly related,' 'remotely related,' or 'unlikely related' to the drug or biological product would signify that a causal relationship between the product and an AE could not be ruled out and thus, the AE would be considered an SADR."

This means that all AEs are possibly related to the drug (and are thus SADRs) unless one can clearly state they are unrelated to the drug. This is now the working concept for clinical trial and postmarketing AEs. Thus the term "adverse event" as now used in the clinical trial and postmarketing regulations will be replaced with the term SADR. The FDA's concept is not entirely in harmony with the ICH, and the FDA (p. 12,417) asked for public comments. There is an extensive discussion on this new concept.

- *The FDA notes that the SADR reports are required to be submitted based on a suspected, not established, causal relationship between an AE and a drug.* Some comments to the FDA expressed a fear that this might be an admission of liability by the company. The FDA is proposing a disclaimer but asked for public comment on whether it should prohibit use of SADR reports in liability actions.

- The FDA now notes that there *are three types of SADRs: (1) serious, (2) nonserious, and (3) outcome unknown* (the last being new and defined as an "SADR that cannot be classified, after active query, as either serious or non-serious"). Note that "active query" is also a new concept discussed below. The three classes of SADRs are important in terms of reporting time frames as discussed below.

- Contractor: A new definition referring to "e.g., a packer, distributor whether or not its name appears on the label of the product; licensee, CRO." The change here is that the name does not need to appear on the label (p. 12,419). In addition, it is clarified that contractors are subject to these regulations.

- Life-threatening: This is now changed slightly to add the sponsor to the definition of who can define a case as life-threatening. Previously it was only the investigator (p. 12,419).

- *Minimal data set for an Individual Case Safety Report (ICSR)*: A minimal data set is an identifiable patient, an identifiable reporter, a suspect drug or biologic, and an SADR. The change here is the replacement of "adverse event" with "SADR."

- The minimal data set is the bare minimum information that must be present to make a case reportable. This is not new. What is new is that (1) serious AEs now need "active query" follow-up to obtain the "full data set" (see below) but (2) for nonserious postmarketing AEs only a minimal data set is needed. No follow-up on these cases needs to be done.

- *Full data set for an ICSR*: A full data set is "completion of all the applicable elements" on the FDA form 3500A (or a CIOMS I form for foreign SADRs) and includes a narrative ("an accurate summary of the relevant data and information pertaining to an SADR or medication error" [ME]).

- The FDA now requires a full data set for postmarketing ICSRs of serious AEs, "always expedited reports" (see below), and medication errors (MEs). This is new and noteworthy.

- *Active query*: "Active query" is "direct verbal contact (i.e., in person or by telephone or other interactive means such as a videoconference) with the initial reporter of an SADR or ME by a health care professional (e.g., physician, PA, pharmacist, dentist, nurse any individual with some form of health care training) representing the manufacturer...Active query entails, at a minimum, a focused line of questioning designed to capture clinically relevant information associated with the product and the SADR, including, but not limited to, information such as baseline data, patient history, physical exam, diagnostic results and supportive lab results."

- Active query is to be used (1) to determine whether an SADR is serious or nonserious if this is not known immediately; (2) to obtain at least the minimum data set for all SADRs and the minimum information for MEs that do not result in an SADR; (3) to obtain a full data set for ICSRs of serious SADRs, "always expedited reports" and MEs; and (4) to obtain supporting documentation for a report of a death or hospitalization (the FDA is now making it obligatory that an autopsy report and/or hospital discharge summary or, failing that, a death certificate be obtained for all deaths). The FDA formally states (p. 12,421): "The agency does not believe that it is sufficient for manufacturers and applicants just to send a letter to reporters of SADRs and MEs requesting further information."

- Spontaneous report: This is "a communication from an individual (e.g., health care professional, consumer) to a company or regulatory authority that describes an SADR or ME. It does not include cases identified from information solicited by the manufacturer or contractor...such as ICSRs or findings derived from a study, company-sponsored patient support program, disease management program patient registry, including pregnancy registries or any organized data collection scheme...." The FDA notes that solicited reports are to be considered "study" information and are to be handled according to the postmarketing safety reporting requirements for a study.

- ME: This is "any preventable event that may cause or lead to inappropriate medication use or patient harm while the medication is in the control of the health care professional, patient or consumer...related to professional practice, health care practice, health care products, procedures and systems including prescribing, order communication, product labeling, packaging and nomenclature, compounding, dispensing, distribution, administration, education, monitoring and use."

- An *"actual ME"* is one that involves an identifiable patient whether the error was prevented before administration of the product or, if the product was administered, whether the error results in a serious SADR, nonserious SADR, or no SADR.

- A *"potential ME"* is "an ICSR of information or complaint about product name, labeling, or packaging similarities that does not involve a patient."

- The FDA notes that an overdose is not an ME, because it is not considered preventable.

- Listed/unlisted: This is defined, per ICH definitions, as whether an SADR is included in the company core safety information (CCSI). The determination of listedness is made by examining the "nature, specificity, severity or outcome" of the SADR. The CCSI is per substance not product/formulation. The CCSI is used for PSUR determination whereas "labeled/unlabeled" (whether an SADR is in the US labeling) is used for US expedited reports (p. 12,422). Thus for PSURs use the CCSI for "listedness," and for expedited reporting use the local labeling for "labeledness."

■ IND Safety Reports

- The FDA restates the current IND definitions using SADR and the other new terms noted above. It clarifies that foreign postmarketing cases for drugs marketed in the United States with an open IND do not have to be reported to the IND (but may have to be reported to an open NDA if it exists).

- No SADR is to be submitted to the FDA that does not have at least the minimal data set. If such data are not available, the sponsor must maintain records of any information received along with a record of its efforts to obtain a minimum data set.

- *The FDA notes that the E2A definition of causality is now used.* This clarifies the issue that if either the sponsor or the investigator believes a case is "possibly related," then the case is considered possibly related and able to be submitted.

- Serious unexpected SADRs that have the minimum data set are expedited (15-day reports). "FDA expects sponsors to use due diligence to acquire immediately the minimum data set for a report and to determine the outcome (serious or nonserious) and expectedness of an SADR upon initial receipt.... Sponsors should include in any written IND safety reports subsequently filed with FDA a chronological history of their efforts to acquire this information if there is a delay....It is not necessary to include the chronological history in IND safety reports sent to investigators."

- *"Information sufficient to consider product administration changes."* This is discussed and defined as follows: "The sponsor must also notify FDA and all participating investigators (in 15 calendar days) in a written IND safety report of information that...might materially influence the benefit-risk assessment of an investigational drug or that would be sufficient to consider changes in either product administration or in the overall conduct of a clinical investigation." Examples include "any significant unanticipated safety finding or data in the aggregate from an in vitro, animal, epidemiological or clinical study...." These findings should be reported in narrative form and not on a 3500A form.

- *Sponsors must monitor to see whether there is an increase in the rate of occurrence of expected serious SADRs and report this in the IND annual report.* It is noted specifically that, in contrast to ICH rules in which this increased frequency rule applies only to postmarketing situations, the FDA has decided to use it in premarketing situations too. They state somewhat unclearly: "FDA has decided to apply this rule to its requirements for premarketing expedited safety reports because of the limited reliability of increased frequency reports."

- The FDA notes that "the sponsor of a clinical study (p. 12,425) under an IND for a drug marketed in the US is only required to submit IND safety reports for SADRs from the clinical study itself whether from domestic or foreign study sites of the IND." Sponsor must also submit such safety information to the NDA under the postmarketing safety rules.

- The FDA notes that "An investigator must report to the sponsor any serious SADR immediately and any other SADR promptly unless the protocol or IB specifies a different timetable."

In summary, the major change here is the use of the SADR concept, which means that all serious study AEs are presumed possibly related unless it can be clearly shown they are not related to the study drug. It also makes clear that a full data set is expected for each SADR.

Postmarketing Reporting

- SADRs received from the FDA should not be resubmitted to the FDA as expedited reports but should be included in periodic reports (PSURs, etc.).

- For expedited reports, two copies must be submitted and for the 6-month ICSR, PSUR, Interim Periodic Safety Report (IPSR), or Traditional Periodic Safety Report (TPSR) submissions, one copy. See below for definitions.

- For combination products, the international birth date is the date of the product that was most recently approved for marketing.

- For combination products also marketed individually, a separate PSUR may be used or the data may be submitted in the PSUR for either of the products (p. 12,444).

Expedited Reports

Expedited reporting has now become much more complicated. It is summarized as follows:

- Serious and unexpected SADRs: Submit ICSR in 15 calendar days.
- Information sufficient to consider product administration changes: Submit narrative in 15 calendar days.

- *(NEW) Unexpected SADRs with outcome unknown even after due diligence*: Submit ICSR in 45 calendar days. Follow up after that in 15 days.

- *(NEW) Always expedited reports:* The FDA specified AEs whether expected or not: submit ICSR in 15 calendar days.

- *MEs:* All US MEs whether actual or potential: 15 calendar days.

- *(NEW) 30-day follow-up*: Follow up for initial serious and unexpected SADR reports, AERs, and MEs that do not have a full data set: 30 calendar days. Follow up after that in 15 days.

- *(CHANGE) 15-day follow-up*: New information for expedited or follow-up reports including follow-up received after the 30-day follow-up is submitted: 15 calendar days.

- SADR reports to manufacturer or applicant: 5 calendar days

Further details on these requirements are as follows:

- Companies may request waivers to change these requirements.

- Data sets: Upon receipt of SADRs and MEs, the company must determine the outcome (serious versus nonserious) and whether the minimum data set is present (identifiable patient, identifiable reporter, suspect drug/biologic, SADR).

- If it is not possible to know whether the case is serious or not, the company must use active query to determine the outcome and report this to the FDA in 30 calendar days. Thus unknown outcomes should not automatically be classified as nonserious.

- If there is not a minimal data set, the case should not be submitted to the FDA but records kept of due diligence attempts made.

- However, MEs that do not have an SADR and do not have a minimum data set do have to be submitted to the FDA (in contrast to SADRs without the minimum data set). That is, all MEs (with or without the minimum data set must be submitted).

- *All serious SADRs, AERs, and MEs must have a full data set*. If such data are not available initially, active query must be done. If after active query there is still not a full data set, the data on hand must be submitted and the reasons for the inability to acquire a full data set must be supplied as well as documentation of the efforts made to obtain the data ("i.e. description of unsuccessful steps taken to obtain this information," p. 12,430).

- For serious SADRs from consumers, the company must contact the health care professional and do active query to get a full data set. If this fails, full details of the steps taken (as above) must be described.

- For nonserious SADRs with a minimum data set, no follow-up is required.

- Thus all MEs and all SADRs with minimum data sets must be reported to the FDA either as expedited reports or in periodic reports/summary tabulations.

- *Lack of efficacy (LOE)* cases are no longer to be reported as expedited reports or ICSRs. Rather, they would be submitted as an aggregate report if the information is sufficient to consider a change in product administration. In addition, frequency analysis must be done to compare expected LOE from premarketing clinical trials with what is seen in the postmarketing setting. An analysis of medically relevant LOE must be done in periodic reports.

- The term "alert reports" is now replaced with ICH-approved terminology, "expedited reports."

- The clock starts when a minimum data set for an SADR is first obtained.

- A serious unexpected SADR with a minimum data set but without a full data set must be submitted in 15 calendar days. Active query must be done and the full data set submitted 30 calendar days later (p. 12,431). The FDA stresses the need for complete case information for serious SADRs.

- The new concept of "information sufficient to consider product administration changes" is a new expedited report based on data from in vitro, animal, epidemiologic, or clinical trials whether under an IND suggesting a significant human risk must be submitted in 15 calendar days.

- Unexpected SADRs without an outcome (i.e., not known if serious or nonserious). The FDA expects there to be few of these cases. Companies must do due diligence and obtain an outcome within 45 calendar days. Failure to get this information must be explained.

- *(NEW) Always Expedited Reports*: This new category requires submission in 15 calendar days of the minimum data set whether expected or unexpected. These are cases the FDA wants to know about in 15 days whether in the labeling or not:

  - Congenital anomalies, acute respiratory failure, ventricular fibrillation, torsades de pointe, malignant hypertension, seizures, agranulocytosis, aplastic anemia, toxic epidermal necrolysis, liver necrosis, acute liver failure, anaphylaxis, acute renal failure, sclerosing syndromes, pulmonary hypertension, pulmonary fibrosis, transmission of an infectious agent by a marketed drug/biologic, endotoxin shock, any other medically significant SADR that the FDA requests (in writing).

  As above, if only a minimal data set is available, active query must be done to get the full data set with submission 30 calendar days later. Further follow-up data would be submitted 15 calendar days after receipt.

- 15-day follow-up submission is done for the following cases: serious and unexpected SADRs that contain a full data set; information sufficient to consider product administration changes; unexpected SADRs with unknown outcomes; AERs with a full data set; actual and potential MEs with a full data set; 30-day follow-up reports for the full data set and 15-day follow-up reports beyond that.

- SADRs that are first submitted as serious/expected or nonserious/unexpected and for which new data show the case to be serious and unexpected must be submitted as 15-day follow-up reports rather than as a new serious and unexpected SADR.

- *Supporting documentation on deaths*: For deaths, companies must submit a copy of the autopsy report. If not done or not available, a death certificate must be submitted. If an autopsy report later becomes available, it must be submitted even if a death certificate has already been submitted. If the patient was hospitalized, the hospital discharge summary must be submitted. All such documents must be translated into English if the original is not in English. Each report would be a 15-calendar-day follow-up report. Companies have 3 months to get these data. If not obtained in 3 months, the FDA assumes active query was done and full documentation of efforts made to obtain it must be kept (but not submitted).

- *Supporting documentation*: Other: Every expedited report must contain, *in the narrative*, a list of relevant documents (e.g., medical records, laboratory results, data from studies) regarding the reports that are maintained by the manufacturer. Copies of such documents must be submitted in 5 calendar days upon FDA request.

- Scientific literature: No significant changes. It is stated that a copy of the article must be included in expedited reports, but it is not stated that it must be in English or translated into English.

Contractors and Shared Manufacturers

- *SADRs and MEs from contractors and shared manufacturers* have 5 calendar days to send the data to the manufacturer, who has the follow-up and reporting responsibilities.

Prescription Drugs Marketed without an Approved Application

- Expedited reports are required. A list of the current addresses where all safety data are kept must accompany such reports.

SADRs from Class Action Lawsuits

- SADRs from class action lawsuits should not be submitted as expedited reports because the FDA believes they would have been received from other sources.

Blood Products

- There are extensive changes here. They have been omitted from this discussion. Please see the document itself.

Postmarketing Periodic Safety Reports

(NEW) The FDA is requiring for all drugs a semiannual report of ICSRs as well as a choice (depending on age of the drug) of either traditional NDA periodic reports or PSURs/IPSRs. That is, each product will have two reports submitted:

- A semiannual report with MedWatch forms
- A PSUR or a TPSR ("Traditional Periodic Safety Report" a new name for the old "NDA periodic report")

Semiannual Reports

- If TPSRs are used: The company must submit the individual case reports (MedWatch or CIOMS I) for all serious unexpected SADRs (US and ex-US) and nonserious unexpected US SADRs if TPSRs are submitted.

- If PSURs are used: The company must submit the individual case reports for all serious listed SADRs (US and ex-US) and nonserious unlisted US SADRs if PSURs/IPSRs are submitted.

- ICSRs for serious listed SADRs that were previously submitted to the FDA as serious unexpected SADRs in expedited reports are not submitted.

- There is an extensive discussion of the rationale for this reporting on pages 12,442–12,443. These reports are used to monitor frequency changes, and the FDA is requesting comment on this.

- Follow-up done on serious expected SADRs should be submitted in the next semiannual report unless the case becomes unexpected. No follow-up is reported or done for nonserious SADRs. No LOE reports should be submitted (rather they are noted in the PSURs or TPSRs).

Old Drugs (Before 1/1/98): Traditional NDA Periodic Reports (Now Called TPSRs)

- For older products (before 1/1/98), the company may continue to use classic "NDA Periodic Reports" now called "Traditional Periodic Safety Reports" (TPSRs). These reports must be submitted at 5, 7.5, 10, 12.5, 15, 20, 25, 30, and so on years after approval. By definition these drugs are all over 5 years old already so the question of what is submitted before 5 years is moot.

- These reports have narrative summaries and analyses of ICSRs of serious expected SADRs and nonserious unexpected US SADRs; now excluded are nonserious expected SADRs; discussion of increased frequency reports of serious expected SADRs and LOE reports, safety-related actions to be taken, location of safety records, and contact person (a licensed medical doctor) information. Note that ICSRs that had not been submitted to the FDA are no longer submitted here because they are now submitted in the ICSR semiannual report.

Summary tabulations (lists and counts) of all SADRs broken down as serious expected SADRs, nonserious unexpected SADRs, nonserious expected SADRs and expected SADRs with unknown outcome in the United States, plus other tabulations. MEs must also be submitted (p. 12,437).

■ Alternatively, companies may do PSURs (as below) instead of TPSRs.

New Drugs (After 1/1/98): PSURs

■ *New drugs must have PSURs.* This is the ICH-approved "core PSUR" plus appendices unique to the United States.

■ Core document: introduction, worldwide marketing status, actions taken for safety reasons, changes to CCSI, worldwide patient exposure, summary tabulations, safety studies, other information, overall safety evaluation, and conclusion.

■ *US appendices*: US labeling, spontaneous reports from consumers, SADRs with unknown outcome, SADRs from class action lawsuits, LOE reports, information on resistance to antimicrobial drug products, MEs, US patient exposure, location of safety records, and contact person.

■ The PSURs must be submitted every 6 months after US approval of the application for 2 years and then annually for 3 years and then every 5 years.

■ *The international birth date (IBD) is used only to set the data lock point, not the periodicity.* For example, if the US approval is on July 1, 2003 for a drug already on the market in Europe with an IBD of April 1, 1996 (and subject only to 5-year PSURs in Europe on April 1, 2001, April 1, 2006, etc.), the US PSUR can use either July 1 or April 1 for data lock point. Thus the first US 6-month report could be either January 1, 2004 (using the July 1 birth date) or October 1, 2003 (using the April 1 birth date). Even though the drug is on a 5-year schedule in the European Union, it must begin a 6-month schedule in the United States.

■ The FDA is silent on the E2C PSUR changes recommended by ICH and signed off by the FDA in February 2003. This should be raised as a comment. These changes allow bridging reports, executive summaries, and so on.

■ Further notes on the core PSUR.

■ The FDA does not require line listings in the core PSUR (that is, the PSUR without the US-specific sections) because it receives the cases in the ICSR

semiannual reports. However, the FDA accepts them if the company wishes.

■ The summary tabulations in the core PSUR must include all serious SADRs for studies as defined above (e.g., registries, disease management programs, etc.).

Further notes on the US appendices of the PSUR.

■ The CCSI in effect at the beginning of the period covered by the PSUR must be included.

■ A copy of the current approved US labeling must be included. Any safety information that is included in the CCSI but not in the US labeling must be identified and the discrepancy explained. Any safety-related changes to the US label made during the PSUR period must be described with supplement numbers and submission dates. *Any suggested changes in US labeling should also be described.*

■ Consumer SADRs: This appendix contains summary tabulations (e.g., serious unlisted SADRs, serious listed SADRs, nonserious unlisted SADRs, nonserious listed SADRs) for US nonserious reports and worldwide serious reports. For SADRs that are serious and unlisted, cumulative data (all cases reported to date by consumers) must be provided *and the impact of all the spontaneous reports discussed.* The FDA may request MedWatch forms for all cases that must be supplied within 5 calendar days.

■ SADRs with unknown outcome: This appendix has summary tabulations for unlisted and listed SADRs with unknown outcome from all spontaneous sources. *The overall impact must be discussed.* The FDA may request MedWatch forms for all cases that must be supplied within 5 calendar days.

■ Class action lawsuits: *This appendix contains summary tabulations for all SADRs from such lawsuits.* See page 12,441 for further detail.

■ LOE reports: This appendix has an assessment of whether the company believes the frequency of LOE reports is greater during the reporting period than would be predicted by the premarketing clinical trials.

■ Include changes in US microbial in vitro susceptibility, the relationship of changes in US microbial in vitro susceptibility and clinical outcomes, therapeutic failure that may possibly be due to resistance to the antimicrobial drug product, and whether the US labeling should be revised due to this information.

■ *MEs*: This appendix contains summary tabulations for all US reports of MEs. For actual MEs, summary tabulations for serious SADRs, nonserious SADRs, and no SADRs must be reported. For serious SADRs cumulative data must also be provided. For potential MEs the number of reports for specific efforts is provided. If an SADR occurs, summary tables must be included. *The impact of the MEs must be discussed.*

- *US patient exposure*: This appendix contains an estimate of US patient exposure with the method used described.

- *Location of safety records*: This appendix lists the address where the data are maintained.

- *Contact person*: This appendix contains the name, e-mail, and fax and phone number of the *licensed medical doctor*(s) responsible for the content and medical interpretation of the data. Note the definition of "licensed" is not given.

Interim Periodic Safety Reports

- The FDA did not accept the 5-year interval for PSURs and thus requires an abbreviated *"Interim Periodic Safety Report"* (IPSR) at 7.5 and 15 years after US approval. (Note that the European Union no longer accepts the 5-year term and has lowered it to 3 years.)

- This is similar to a PSUR but excludes summary tabulations, new information after the data lock point, summary tabulations of spontaneous consumer SADRs, summary tabulations for SADRs with unknown outcomes, summary tabulations for reports from class action lawsuits, and summary tabulations for US MEs.

Medical Dictionary for Regulatory Activities (MedDRA)

- There is an extensive discussion of MedDRA aimed mainly at small companies and individual investi-

gators/reporters. Details on this are omitted here (see p. 12,445).

- The preferred term (PT) is to be used in reporting to the FDA of individual cases.

Forms

- The *licensed physician* responsible for the content of each MedWatch form should be noted in box G1 of the FDA's standard form. Companies can design their own MedWatch forms as they do now (p. 12,445).

Recordkeeping

- Records and documents should be kept for 10 years.

Abbreviated NDAs

- All these rules apply to Abbreviated NDAs too.

Annual Report

- All marketed drug products have an annual report submitted. The safety sections of these reports are to be omitted (p. 12,447).

In Vivo Bioavailability and Bioequivalence Studies

- *Formerly exempt bioavailability and bioequivalence studies are no longer exempt from these rules. Approved labeling and not the investigator brochure is to be used (p. 12,448). The FDA requests comments on this proposal.*

Periodic Safety Update Reports

Periodic Safety Update Reports (PSURs) were proposed by the International Conference on Harmonization (ICH) in E2C over a decade ago and have been in use in Europe since 1995 and in many other countries, including Japan and Canada. In the United States, the ICH E2C document was published in November 1996 (Web Resource 43-1), and their use was described in the proposed new rules by the US Food and Drug Administration (FDA) in March 2003 (Web Resource 43-2). A formal program was set up by which manufacturers may send PSURs instead of New Drug Application (NDA) periodic reports. In February 2004 the FDA published the ICH addendum to E2C on PSURs (see Web Resource 43-3).

In the March 2001 guidance (Web Resource 43-4), the FDA described the mechanism available to obtain a waiver to submit PSURs in place of NDA periodic reports. The FDA indicated the E2C document may be used and also recommended the following:

- "If all dosage forms and formulations for the active substance, as well as indications, are combined in one PSUR, this information should be separated into specific sections of the report when such separation is appropriate to accurately portray the safety profile of the specific dosage forms. For example, one should not combine information from ophthalmic drop dosage forms and solid oral dosage forms. One copy of the PSUR should be submitted for each approved NDA or ANDA whose product is covered in the PSUR as well as an additional copy for review by the postmarketing pharmacovigilance office.

- "Copies of the FDA Form 3500A or VAERS form that are required by the regulations must be included. These forms should be included with the PSUR as an appendix. You can request a waiver for submission of certain nonserious, expected adverse experiences on an FDA Form 3500A as described in the previous section.

- "A summary tabulation should be included as an appendix listing all spontaneously reported U.S. individual case safety reports from consumers if such cases are not already included in the PSUR. Summary tabulations should be presented by body system of all adverse experience terms and counts of occurrences and be segregated by type (i.e., serious/unexpected; serious/expected; nonserious/unexpected; and nonserious/expected).

- "A narrative should be included as an appendix that references the changes, if any, to the approved U.S. labeling for the dosage forms covered by the PSUR based on new information in the PSUR. A copy of the most recently approved U.S. labeling for the product(s) covered by the PSUR should be included.

- "Applicants can request a waiver to submit PSURs to the FDA based on the month and day of the international birth date of the product instead of the month and day of the anniversary date of U.S. approval of the product. The waiver request should specify that these PSURs would be submitted to the FDA within 60 calendar days of the data lock point (i.e., month and day of the international birth date of the product or any other day agreed on by the applicant and the FDA).

- "Applicants can also request a waiver to submit PSURs to the FDA at a frequency other than those required under §§ 314.80(c)(2)(i) and 600.80(c)(2)(i)."

A summary of the contents and format of a PSUR are found in Chapter 26.

To summarize, the FDA has indicated that it will allow the use of the ICH-accepted E2C PSUR in place of NDA periodic reports with additional US-specific sections. Under the Tome (the proposed new regulations), the PSUR will ultimately replace all NDA periodic reports.

Business Partners and Exchange of Safety Data: Due Diligence

Development costs for a new chemical entity from creation to marketing range from $400 million to $800 million (depending on how one calculates these costs) (Frank, *J Health Econ* 2003;325:330; see Web Resource 44-1). In addition, patents are now being challenged and generics are proliferating. One of the responses to these phenomena includes the development and marketing of a product by multiple partner companies. No matter which side of the argument one is on regarding the appropriateness of some drug development, these costs and risks are very high and companies look for ways to protect themselves from the risks of failure.

One response is partnerships. The goal is to speed up development, share costs, and use the additive or synergistic strengths of each partner. Codevelopment often is limited to two partners, but combinations of three or more partners are not uncommon, especially when expanding into areas (e.g., Japan, China) where language, laws, and customs are often a challenge for US and European Union (EU) companies. The current trend in the pharmaceutical world is for codevelopment and copromotion/marketing of products as expenses skyrocket and simultaneous rather than sequential international development occurs.

Whenever two or more companies join forces, for whatever reason, a written contract is developed between or among them. Normally these contracts are developed by the "business development" or "licensing group" with input from the legal department and other groups on a "need to know" basis. Often they are developed under great secrecy (for competitive reasons), and others in the company are not informed of the situation until the last minute when their input and or approval is requested, often with a minimal amount of lead time ("The CEO wants to sign this contract tomorrow morning. Please approve your section now.").

The safety group (unless involved in due diligence, see below) may be one of those groups learning of the agreement at the last minute and asked to review a document with a minimal or even nonexistent safety section. Sometimes when the safety section is present, it is incorrect and would not keep the company in compliance with US Food and Drug Administration (FDA) and other health authority regulations or help protect the company from litigation and other pitfalls.

When such a situation occurs, the immediate acute step is to ask that the safety section, if inadequate, be removed and replaced with one of two things:

1. A "generic" or "one size fits all" safety section (see below).

2. A statement that a safety section is needed and will be developed by the safety groups of the respective signatory companies to cover safety data issues within, say, 90 days. It will be appended to the agreement or will act as a stand-alone agreement (whichever the lawyers prefer). This time frame may need to be shortened if the sales or studies start in a shorter time. Often, however, studies or sales will not begin for several months, giving all parties sufficient time to develop a safety section.

Why a Written Safety Exchange Agreement Is Needed

There are multiple reasons:

- To remain in compliance with FDA requirements (e.g., 21CFR314.80(b)) as well as those of other countries

- To give guidance and instructions to all involved parties with regard to their responsibilities for drug safety

- To ensure that all parties receive the safety documents that they need to remain in full compliance with all regulatory and legal requirements in their jurisdictions of sale or study

- To ensure that adequate signaling is done and that a benefit-to-risk analysis incorporates as complete a database as possible

- To produce the best product labeling possible to protect the public health

- To have data ready for a corporate or health authority audit or inspection

- To have data available for litigation should that situation arise, particularly in the United States

The need for such agreements is now well recognized and accepted in most companies. The author and colleagues published a review of the necessary contents of a safety exchange agreement a decade ago. Though out of date in some respects (mainly new obligations now required), it remains worth reviewing (Fieldstad, Kuryatkin, Cobert, *Drug Inform J* 1996;30:965–971).

Telling the Safety Department about a New Contract

The safety department should be informed of any agreement being negotiated early on in the process to review the document and determine what is needed in regard to safety. This should be included in all standard operating procedures that exist on the negotiation of agreements with other parties where drug products (either finished products or components) are involved. Agreements for non–product-related items do not need to be included (e.g., raw chemical products, supplying the vending machines or ordering furniture).

There are many types of arrangements that must have safety agreements. They include but are not limited to agreements on licensing-in or licensing-out, manufacturing, comarketing, codevelopment including preclinical and/or clinical development, advertising, clinical study research, consultants, contract sales forces, distribution, disease management programs, patient support programs, promotion and copromotion, speakers bureau consultants, master vendors, other vendors, and other services.

The Generic or Boilerplate or Template Agreement

Even before any agreement is on the table, the drug safety and the legal groups (at least) should develop a "boilerplate," "generic," or template agreement that is approved by management and that is general enough to be inserted into almost any type of contract either in the body of the contract or as an appendix until a customized agreement is made to replace it. The agreement should, at the very least, specify the following:

- Exchange between the parties of all serious adverse events (AEs) from clinical trials, spontaneous reporting, solicited reporting, literature, and health authorities. Cases should be exchanged as either MedWatch/CIOMS I forms or E2B files within a specified time frame from first receipt by anyone in the companies. They should be exchanged in sufficient time to meet expedited reporting rules (usually 15 calendar days) so that exchange should be no later than 10 or so calendar days. Deaths and life-threatening serious AEs (SAEs) from trials should be exchanged in time to meet 7-day reporting requirements (e.g., 5 calendar days).

- All regulatory submissions (Periodic Safety Update Reports [PSURs], Investigational New Drug Application [IND] annual reports, New Drug Application [NDA] periodic reports, and their local equivalents) should be exchanged between the parties within a specified time (e.g., 1 week) after submission to the health authorities.

- A formal and detailed safety agreement will be completed by the two drug safety groups within, say, 90 days of the signing of the contract.

The above generic agreement should suffice in almost all cases until the formal safety document is created. Additions, of course, may be added to the generic agreement if the specific case warrants it and if there is sufficient time to get agreement internally and from the other contractual partner. This could include exchange of communications with the health authorities, including safety reviews of PSURs, literature searches, and a data dump (e.g., a paper printout or an electronic file of all AEs in the safety database) from the partner holding the safety database.

Developing a Safety Agreement with the Safety Department

As soon as the type of contract is determined and the safety department is brought into the discussions, the area of involvement should be ascertained: geographic territories (United States only, United States and elsewhere, only outside the United States, etc.), regulatory and marketing status (IND or equivalent, NDA or equivalent, and in which territories—marketed in some and in trials in others; controlled substance, etc.), and labeling, if available, to get an idea of indications and uses. This allows the tailoring of the specific agreement to ensure that all needs are met.

At this point the safety department will be able to determine what is needed. If the drug has never been marketed, for example, there will not be an issue of postmarketing spontaneous SAE reports, and this does not need to be included in the agreement (though a clause indicating that the agreement will be revised, say, 60 days before a marketing request is submitted anywhere in the world does). If more than one other partner is involved, this also allows the signatories to determine various responsibilities and negotiate any new or altered requirements.

Again, there is no "one size fits all" safety agreement that can simply be dropped into a contract to take care of everything. Each agreement must be negotiated individually. Usually, face-to-face contacts between the two safety departments facilitate the successful preparation of a safety agreement. As always, contrary to the saying, business is personal, and it is always easier to develop a successful working relationship of trust and confidence if personal contact has been established rather than relying only on e-mails, video conferences, and telephone calls. A meeting should be set up at the earliest reasonable time after preliminary negotiations are started to hammer out the final document. The safety department needs to be given sufficient authority to negotiate such an agreement (pending, of course, final management and legal approval on both sides).

The Safety Agreement Database

For companies that make many agreements worldwide, it is imperative that a database containing the key points of the safety agreements (and if possible the imaged agreements themselves) be maintained. Multinational companies may have tens of thousands of such agreements, in multiple countries, sometimes in multiple languages, often with differing durations, responsibilities, and territories. The agreements will become out of date rapidly as new terms are made, new products launched, new formulations made, and new partners (or distributors or sales forces, etc.) brought in. A database will help track this. The database may start as a spreadsheet, but it may be necessary to develop (with the informatics department) or purchase a database to track and report on agreements. As always, the database must have the appropriate security, testing, validation, and change control.

Historically, the legal and new business departments will not keep sufficiently detailed records to ensure regulatory compliance regarding safety matters (a sad fact of life). Thus it falls on the drug safety department to do its best to ensure that all revisions to agreements are transmitted to the central (or designated) safety department. A dedicated person is needed to track and revise such agreements and changes to them. Any new conditions (new INDs, NDAs, marketing authorizations, new products, new regulations, new PSUR dates, etc.) must be transmitted to the drug safety groups involved (e.g., the processing group, the PSUR group, etc.).

Periodic reports of contracts in force, dates of expiration (where they exist), and obligations should be issued to the parties who need them.

■ The Safety Agreement Contents

Ideally, all agreements should be in English. This is not always the case. If not, they should be translated into English for all parties involved to be able to know and adhere to their obligations. The contents should cover the following.

The Regulatory Status

A table by country with approval date, license holder, companies marketing the product, and name should be included. A copy of the regulatory table in a PSUR is usually acceptable. It should contain

- IND or equivalents
- NDAs, marketing authorizations, or equivalents (in the EU, type of approval: central, mutual recognition, etc.)
- Other: compassionate use, restrictions on use

The Regulatory Responsibilities

It should be clarified what regulatory responsibilities are to be held by each party and in what country (if multiple countries are involved). Particular attention should be paid to assignment of regulatory responsibilities in countries where each contractual party has a regulatory office. The actual names and contact information for the responsible parties should be listed in an appendix (allowing easy updating of changes in personnel, phone numbers, etc.).

It should be clarified who does reporting in each country, who makes contact with health authorities, and who answers questions (and if consultation with the other party is obtained or not within X number of days, etc.). The qualified person(s) in the EU should be clearly stated. A mechanism should be outlined for the obtaining of any waivers or changes to routine procedures that may be desired by the clinical teams such as reporting certain SAEs monthly or quarterly rather than as expedited reports.

Regulatory Documents

The owner and maintainer of documents should be specified for the Investigator Brochure, the Summary of Product Characteristics, the package insert, the product monograph, the investigational and clinical core safety documents, and protocols. Any consultation and approval for each should be specified. The timing and format of exchange should be spelled out for all documents.

Health Authority Queries and Requests

It should be stated clearly how health authority requests and queries are to be handled. Usually, the company in the country where the request is made must do the physical answering (in the local language) but the content of the response needs to be done by agreed-on methods, particularly if it is a critical medical question involving stopping of studies, drug withdrawal, or labeling change. Case-specific questions of minor import may usually be answered locally, but anything more important should be resolved by the appropriate groups in each company (usually via a joint operating committee). A method of dispute resolution must be specified so that senior management can make the final determination in the appropriate time frame. This usually involves the regulatory and safety departments as well as the clinical research groups in each company.

Regulatory Submissions

It should be clearly noted who submits which documents in which countries. This includes individual cases (7- and 15-day cases) whether by paper, electronically, or E2B. It should be stated whether copies of submissions should be exchanged (even though the identical MedWatch or CIOMS I form has already been exchanged by the drug safety groups already). This might be necessary if the other party wishes to know the serial number (in IND submissions) or date of submission.

Similarly, all other regulatory submissions (investigator brochures, labeling changes, NDA periodic reports, IND annual reports, information amendments, desk copies, etc.) should be spelled out and exchange methodology noted. It is critical to specify whether the other parties have review and approval privileges or are merely given information copies of such documents.

Investigator and Investigational Review Board /Ethics Committee Notifications: Blinding and Unblinding

The mechanism and responsibilities for the preparation of the investigator notification—also called the investigator letter (including the similar case analysis for the US IND)—as well as the sending of it (in local languages if need be and on local letterheads) need to be detailed. In addition, in those countries where the sponsor must inform the ethics committees/investigational review boards, this should be spelled out. It should be clarified whether the same exact letter is to be used worldwide, and if so, a mechanism for its preparation (within the same 15 calendar day time frame required for the alert report itself) must be specified.

Most regulatory agencies prefer or require that all expedited reports be submitted unblinded (the code broken). If this is done, the companies must agree on a mechanism for unblinding and the transmission of the unblinded cases (or just the unblinding code) to the other party(ies). This can be very difficult if companies want to keep the clinical research team and statisticians blinded.

Databases

It should be agreed who maintains what in their respective databases. It should be agreed by all parties that one party (often the largest company or the originating company) maintains the "official" database that will be used as the definite one for the preparation of all regulatory reports.

It is nearly impossible, if not totally impossible, to maintain duplicate databases when each party does data entry. Logistical and technical difficulties prevent "mirror databases" from being developed. These include different commercial databases, different drug dictionaries, different ways of handling data (laboratory data not in the narrative), different coding conventions, different narrative writing styles, and so on.

All parties should "agree to disagree" and accept that each will maintain a database but that one agreed-on database will be the "official" one. In the EU, a qualified person must be physically present with direct access to the database (see Volume 9). Most regulatory agencies understand the impossibility of maintaining exact duplicate databases.

As an alternative, only one database is maintained by one company with access to the data for the drug in question by the other companies. This has been problematic for security reasons to date, but new technology may permit this more easily in the future. It has also been difficult because corporate standard operating procedures usually require all safety data to be collected and maintained by each company.

Definitions

Either in the body of the agreement itself or as an appendix, the parties should agree on the definitions of terms used, including serious, nonserious, medically significant (important), expedited, expected, unexpected, labeled, unlabeled, listed, unlisted, and causality (relatedness). This may be a contentious issue because there are no international standards and the parties need to agree on definitions, particularly for ambiguous terms such as "unlikely related," the four criteria for the minimal data set, clock start date, and so on. The language of exchange should be specified as well, and how documents not in English will be handled (full translations or not).

The Clock Start Date

This is an area of some controversy. The regulations in the United States and EU have been unclear about when the regulatory clock starts. If company A receives the case on February 5 and sends the case to company B on February 10, when does the regulatory clock start for company B? Many interpret the current requirements to say that the clock starts when the first person of any of the contractual partners receives a valid case. Thus, under this view the clock starts for company B on February 5. Others say the clock starts for company B when company B received the case: February 10. FDA regulations are not explicit but various warning letters suggest that the clock starts when the first company anywhere receives the case (February 5 in the above example).

In the EU the wording of Volume 9 is somewhat hazy but the wording in Volume 9A, Page 45, Section 4.2 on Reporting Time Frames is clearer:

> "In general, where the Marketing Authorisation Holder has set up contractual arrangements with a person or organisation for e.g. the marketing of or research on the suspected product, the clock starts as soon as any personnel of the Marketing Authorisation Holder or the person/organisation receives the minimum information. Explicit procedures and detailed agreements should exist between the Marketing Authorisation Holder and the person/organisation to ensure that the Marketing Authorisation Holder can comply with his reporting obligations."

In addition CIOMS V is very clear and states on page 203 Licensor-Licensee Arrangements:

> "The time frame for expedited regulatory reporting should normally be no longer than 15 calendar days from the first receipt of a valid case by any of the partners."

Many companies and others feel that these requirements are too strict, not enforceable, and not practical. However, many companies do successfully use the stricter interpretation.

Data and Mechanisms of Data Exchange

The physical exchange method must be specified:

- "Push versus pull," that is does party A send ("push") data to party B or does party B go onto a website or portal to obtain ("pull") it.
- Fax, e-mail with attached pdf files
- E2B (and any import/export issues related to E2B)
- Paper copies
- Documents where a signature copy is needed to be maintained on file

A method of verification of receipt of faxes or e-mails should be determined so that no SAEs (and potential expedited reports) are missed. E2B transmissions usually verify automatically, but fax or e-mail transmissions may require a positive response acknowledging receipt.

The documents to be exchanged must be specified. This is particularly critical for individual case reports. Will MedWatch forms, CIOMS I forms, an SAE data collection form, or source documents be exchanged? If CIOMS I or MedWatch forms, will they be complete or draft and on what day after clock start? If source documents, will finalized MedWatch or CIOMS I forms also be exchanged? Is it acceptable that each party creates its own narrative and coding, realizing that there will be differences between the two (or more) parties? If reconciliation is desired, how can this be done rapidly so that 7- and 15-day reports are consistent?

- In practice, it is not uncommon that the party that receives the case handles the full processing of the case (including follow-up) and sends a completed MedWatch or CIOMS I form to the other partner(s) by a particular calendar day (usually 8 to 10). This will allow the other parties to enter the data into their database (unchanged) and transmit any expedited cases to the health authority. This will also allow them time to check the case against local labeling if the product is marketed with different labeling in the recipient company's territories.
- Once a sufficient volume of cases is attained (suggesting success in the clinical trial or marketing), a "well-oiled machine" must exist to process and transmit SAEs. Reconciliation and "discussions" over particular cases must be the exception and not the rule if on-time regulatory reporting is to be maintained. Keep in mind that submission of a case as an expedited report does not admit that the drug caused the event.

- Seven-day expedited reports from clinical trials must be handled in a much more rapid time frame (usually 4–5 calendar days) to ensure regulatory compliance.
- Companies should reach agreement that the most conservative call on seriousness, expectedness, and causality carries the day for SAEs. That is, if one company believes a case is unlabeled or possibly related and the other does not, the case is considered unlabeled or possibly related. This may force a company to submit a case as an expedited report that it does not believe to be one because the other company does.
- If clinical research organizations are involved, the agreement must account for them in terms of timing and exchange method. Written agreements with the clinical research organizations are, of course, required. For IND studies, the FDA must be notified in writing of the duties devolved onto the clinical research organization.

Follow-ups are done by the party receiving the original SAE (or non-serious AE if follow-ups are done for these). The other parties may pose questions for the company doing the follow-up but usually follow-up is left to their discretion and medical expertise. It should be specified when it is done and how frequently. All follow-up information is handled in the same manner as initial information. For serious cases, there is data exchange within 8–10 calendar days on a CIOMS I or MedWatch form.

It should be stated clearly who reviews the worldwide literature for SAEs and how they are handled when found.

A method used by many companies is as follows:

- All SAEs are exchanged as CIOMS I (or MedWatch) forms by calendar day 10 after clock start anywhere in the world at the first company (or agent) and used as is without changes to coding or narrative. Much less commonly, the SAE data collection form (from clinical trials and spontaneous cases) is exchanged by calendar day 5. In this case, each company writes its own narrative and does its own coding based on this "source document" to create a MedWatch or CIOMS I form. Because these reports are created by each company on their own, they differ.
- All clinical trial deaths or life-threatening SAEs are exchanged within 4 to 5 calendar days. Sometimes this is limited to the subset of unlabeled (unexpected) cases only; this requires that the receiving company trust the judgment of the

sending company on labeledness. This covers 7-day expedited cases.

- All nonserious spontaneous cases are exchanged on a monthly basis (or twice monthly if the volume is very large). Line listings or MedWatch/CIOMS I forms may be used.

- Nonserious clinical trial cases are not exchanged and are kept only in the clinical trial database.

- Follow-up is done for all SAEs with at least two contacts attempted for spontaneous cases (more if a critical case such as an alert report) and whatever is necessary for clinical trial cases (where the investigator should be accessible to give complete follow-up).

Signaling and Safety Reviews

The agreement should specify whether signaling is done by one or more parties and, if so, how disputes are resolved. It is common to form a safety review committee that meets periodically, usually by telephone or video conference, to review the logistics and operational issues of safety handling as well as any SAEs and safety signals that arise. Usually, the logistics and operations dominate the initial meetings until all glitches are resolved. At that point, with operational issues minimal and with more SAEs arriving, the signal reviewers predominate. Meetings may be weekly to biweekly initially and then at a monthly or quarterly frequency if no safety or signaling issues arrive. Ad hoc meetings should be held, as needed, for urgent issues.

Other Issues

If not noted elsewhere, mechanisms for dispute resolution should be described in detail:

- Other product-specific issues relating to devices, vaccines, biologics, and nutraceuticals.

- Any specific regulatory requests (e.g., special reporting of certain SAEs) should be mentioned.

- An agreed-on time to review the safety exchange agreement should be specified. It is usually yearly but may be more or less frequent if circumstances warrant. Any change in regulatory status (e.g., a new IND being opened or an NDA approval) should trigger a review of the safety agreement.

Appendices

The appendices should contain information that may change frequently, including names, addresses, contact information, territories in question, product names, and registration numbers.

CHAPTER 45

Audits and Inspections

The US Food and Drug Administration (FDA), the European Medicines Agency (EMEA), the United Kingdom's (UK's) Medicines and Healthcare Products Regulatory Agency (MHRA), and many other national health authorities are permitted or required by law to perform inspections (audits) of companies to ensure that they are in compliance with the adverse event (AE) reporting regulations.

■ FDA Inspections

In the United States the FDA does two types of safety inspections: routine surveillance inspections and "for cause" or "directed" inspections. The selection criteria include simple routine surveillance, looking at all companies on a periodic (e.g., every 1–2 years) basis, or some sort of trigger at FDA, such as a history of violations (late expedited reports or periodic reports, significant recalls, etc.) or the recent launch of a major new chemical entity. Inspections may be done in the United States or abroad, and all drugs marketed in the United States are "fair game."

If the inspection is for cause, the inspectors have specific information, including MedWatch forms or other information they may or may not reveal to the company under inspection. The inspector may have reviewed previous FDA audits of the company as well as AE lists from the FDA database (Adverse Event Reporting System) and periodic reports.

The inspectors (usually one or two per audit) are often from the local FDA office and are sometimes accompanied by inspectors from other offices who might have a particular specialty or from the main office. They are guided by an inspection manual (Web Resource 45-1) that summarizes what the inspectors should examine. Obviously, it behooves the company to review this document and to ensure that the areas scrutinized in an FDA inspection are handled correctly.

The goals of the inspection set at a high level are to ensure that the company is adhering to all appropriate federal regulations in regard to safety data collection, analysis and storage (both paper and electronic), reporting to the FDA, and product labeling and that drug risks are recognized rapidly and handled in an appropriate manner to protect the public health. Areas inspected include AEs, medical errors, and product quality complaints. In general, FDA examiners may examine all company records except those relating to finance and budgets. Although they can be reviewed by the inspectors, internal audits are generally not examined to protect the integrity of the internal audit process. It is argued by companies that if internal audits are so examined, there will be a tendency to be less frank and forthcoming in such audits. To date this has been followed by the FDA, although EMEA auditors have asked for and received internal audits.

The inspections are usually unannounced, and the FDA inspector or inspectors simply arrive at the offices of the company for the inspection. They present their credentials and documentation for the company to sign, acknowledging their arrival and the review of credentials. Applicants, manufacturers, packers, and distributors are subject to AE audits.

The auditors will likely ask for the following:

- Organizational charts to ascertain the personnel involved in handling AEs, complaints, and safety data
- All safety standard operating procedures (SOPs) (or a listing of them)
- All correspondence, meeting minutes, and notes relating to AE handling
- A list of all products marketed in the United States along with their approved current package inserts (product labeling)
- A list of all collection sites, processing sites, and reporting units that handle cases liable for submission to the FDA
- Copies of all contracts or safety agreements covering the receipt, handling, evaluation, and reporting of AEs to the FDA, including non-US agreements

They may then ask for safety information on specific drug products (from the inspectors' manual):

- Drugs most likely to have unexpected serious adverse experiences
- Drugs that could cause serious medical problems if they fail to produce their expected pharmacologic actions
- Drugs most likely to have unexpected adverse experiences are those meeting the following criteria:
  - Approved within the last 3 years, focusing on lack of effect (efficacy) reports
  - New molecular entities
  - Known or suspected bioavailability or bioequivalence problems

They will then select specific cases (again from the inspectors' manual) and request the approved product labeling in force at the time of receipt of the cases:

- Serious unlabeled adverse drug experiences (ADEs), particularly those involving death or hospitalization
- Incomplete, serious, unexpected ADE reports or reports with unlabeled ADEs and no outcome reported
- Periodic reports that include serious unexpected ADEs that should have been submitted as 15-day reports

They examine the cases for completeness and accuracy to ensure that all serious and unexpected spontaneous reports were submitted to the FDA within 15 calendar days:

- Was information on the form available at the time of submission?
- Was all relevant information included on the form?
- Was the initial receiving date supplied to the agency (Form 3500A Item G.4) the same date as the initial receipt of information by the manufacturer?
- Was new information obtained by the firm during their follow-up investigation and was this information submitted to the agency?
- Where feasible, particularly when hospitalization, permanent disability, or death occurred, did the firm obtain important follow-up information to enable complete evaluation of the report?

Periodic reports are examined to ensure that all US reports not submitted as expedited reports were submitted in a timely manner.

The FDA will request to meet with the appropriate people (both managers and staff) to go through the documents received. The company needs to make preparations (see below) to handle these requests. Questions may include the following:

- How does each type of AE come into the company and how are they handled?
- Are AEs being missed? Are all possible routes of entry into the company covered to ensure that cases are not missed?
- How are cases numbered and tracked?
- Case-handling specifics: How are mail and phone calls triaged and handled? How are AEs or potential AEs and complaints logged in?
- Are medical evaluations performed for each case and by whom and when?
- How and when is follow-up done?

- Who assesses seriousness and labeledness? Is the correct label used?

- Who determines if a case is a 15-day alert report or is to be included in the New Drug Application periodic report?

- Who sends the expedited reports and periodic reports to the FDA? Where are these documents stored or archived?

- Are safety meetings held? How often? Topics covered? Attendance?

- How is labeling handled and how does the company ensure that the labeling reflects the safety status of the drug?

- Is the database sufficient in terms of validation, change control, security, electronic signature (21CFR11), and audit trails?

Historically, the FDA's major findings have been

- Failure to submit or late expedited and periodic reports

- Inaccurate or incomplete reports to the FDA

- Failure to do follow-up for serious and unexpected AEs

- Lack of or inadequate written SOPs

- Failure by the company to follow its own SOPs

- Database issues, including inadequate validation and security

The FDA cites specific deviations they find on a document known as the "FDA-483 form." The manual states, "Clear deviations such as, failure to submit ADE reports, failure to promptly investigate an ADE event, inaccurate information, incomplete disclosure of available information, lack of written procedures or failing to adhere to reporting requirements, should be cited on the FDA-483 issued to management. Questions on medical judgment or evaluation on the part of the firm's management should be discussed with the firm and included in the narrative report but should not be cited on the FDA-483." This form is left with the company at the end of the inspection after the FDA inspectors' close-out meeting with the company. In addition, the FDA also issues an "Establishment Report" sometime after the inspection (even if no issues were found) describing what was inspected.

If serious deviations are found, the FDA may also issue a Warning Letter if any of the following are found (from the inspectors' manual):

- Failure to submit reports for serious and unexpected AEs (alert reports)

- Fifteen-day alert reports submitted as part of a periodic report but not otherwise submitted under separate cover as 15-day alert reports (also applies to foreign and domestic AE information from scientific literature, postmarketing studies, and spontaneous reports)

- Fifteen-day alert reports that are inaccurate and/or not complete

- Fifteen-day alert reports that are not submitted on time

- The repeated or deliberate failure to maintain or submit periodic reports in accordance with the reporting requirements

- Failure to conduct a prompt and adequate follow-up investigation of the outcome of AEs that are serious and unexpected

- Failure to maintain AE records for marketed prescription drugs or to have written procedures for investigating AEs for marketed prescription drugs without approved applications

- Failure to have written procedures for the surveillance, receipt, evaluation, and reporting of postmarketing ADEs to the FDA for marketed prescription drugs

- Failure to submit 15-day reports derived from a postmarketing study where there is a reasonable possibility that the drug caused the AE

The receipt of a Warning Letter is a very serious issue. It is addressed to senior management (sometimes the chief executive officer of the corporation) and requires a detailed written response within a short time (usually 15 working days) indicating the corrective actions to be done. The letters are also public information and are published on the FDA's website. See Web Resource 45-2.

The FDA retains the right to go to more extreme penalties if the 483 and Warning Letter methods do not work. These include product seizure, withdrawal of the New Drug Application, injunctions, consent decrees, and criminal and/or civil prosecution.

■ **EMEA Inspections**

Council Regulation 2309/93 created the EMEA, setting out its core tasks. The EMEA's Inspections Sector (Web Resource 45-3) handles Good Clinical Practice, Good Manufacturing Practice, and Good Laboratory Practice inspections including pharmacovigilance (Web Resource

45-4). See the UK's MHRA website on pharmacovigilance inspections for a more detailed idea of what is involved in inspections (Web Resource 45-5).

Unlike the United States, the EMEA charges for each inspection: 17,400 euros (about $21,000) plus expenses paid by the company being inspected. Inspections may be done by a team of three to five inspectors from the EMEA or from health authorities in the individual member states. Inspections may be done outside of the European Union. Usually, advance notice is given of the audit, but not always. The inspectors may specify in advance the documents they wish to examine and request that the company send them on a CD or DVD well before the audit. To get an idea of what will be requested and what the inspection will cover, it is highly advisable to study the Summary of PV Systems document that the MHRA requires of companies to be inspected (Web Resource 45-6).

Inspections may have a wider scope than those done by the FDA and may focus on both pre- and postmarketing safety issues, computer systems, validation, and quality issues. The inspectors, who are often specialized pharmacovigilance inspectors, may forward an agenda in advance, although they may change it or add to it during the inspection. It is not uncommon for the inspectors to interview many people at all levels of responsibility and function, with or without their manager present. The company's qualified person plays a major role in the inspection.

At the end of the inspection there is usually a close-out meeting, but a written report may not be supplied on the spot. It is sent several weeks later. The inspectors give an idea of the findings, which are grouped as follows (from the MHRA website):

- Critical: a deficiency in pharmacovigilance systems, practices, or processes that adversely affects the rights, safety, or well-being of patients or that poses a potential risk to public health or that represents a serious violation of applicable legislation and guidelines
- Major: a deficiency in pharmacovigilance systems, practices, or processes that could potentially adversely affect the rights, safety, or well-being of patients or that could potentially pose a risk to public health or that represents a violation of applicable legislation and guidelines
- Other: a deficiency in pharmacovigilance systems, practices, or processes that would not be expected to adversely affect the rights, safety, or well-being of patients

■ Internal Inspections

It is highly recommended that companies set up within their quality or compliance groups a regular schedule for inspections of the company's pharmacovigilance functions covering pre- and postmarketing situations and paralleling the type of audit done by the FDA and the EMEA. These should be done at least yearly, especially if the company's products (new or old) have significant safety issues.

■ Company Inspection Procedures

Every company should have an SOP in place on how to handle outside audits. It should cover the following:

- A procedure should be in place to alert the receptionist at all company sites on what to do if the FDA shows up. Who to call (immediately) to greet the inspectors and then who will handle all logistics during the inspection.
- An "escort" or "host" or "facilitator" should be designated who will accompany all FDA inspectors at all times. The host handles all the logistics and ensures that meeting rooms, refreshments (usually limited to no more than coffee and cake), and the appropriate company representatives are available to meet with the FDA. If there is more than one inspector, the company should ensure that there are sufficient hosts to accompany all inspectors should they split up. These are often company representatives from the quality, compliance, or regulatory sections. It is generally believed not to be wise to have company attorneys present unless the FDA also has attorneys present.
- A minute taker ("scribe") must be present at all meetings to record all issues brought up, to note all promises made by the company, and to ensure that all promised deliverables are delivered. The minute taker should write up the minutes of the meeting (including listing all documents delivered) at the end of each day's audit.
- A system to have copies made of documents that are requested by the FDA must be in place. Copies should be done on special paper marked "confidential" or the equivalent. Duplicates of everything handed to the FDA should be retained in the company's inspection files.
- The meeting room should be separate from the drug safety section. It is generally not wise to have

the auditor wandering around the section being inspected unless this is arranged in advance or officially requested. Obviously, the drug safety section should ensure that all documents are in their appropriate places and that the staff is aware the FDA is present.

■ Never lie. Always tell the truth. Answer the questions posed. Do not volunteer information. Do not guess. If you do not know the answer to a question, say so. Try to find (with the help of the facilitator) someone who can answer it. If you do not understand a question, ask for it to be repeated or clarified.

■ The people being interviewed by the inspectors should have a supply of their business cards with them.

■ Avoid internal abbreviations and terms that outsiders would not be expected to understand. If the inspectors are non-native English speakers from abroad, use simple English sentences. Avoid references (e.g., sports analogies) that visitors from abroad would not be expected to know.

Ethical Issues and Conflicts of Interest

➥ **NOTE:** The comments in this chapter represent those of the author and not of the organizations of which he is or has been a member or employee.

The ethical issues of business and medicine have become complex and difficult. Years ago, before medicine was thought of as "big business," the ethics of medicine were somewhat cleaner (at least on paper). Physicians adhered to the Hippocratic Oath that said, in regard to drugs, "I will neither give a deadly drug to anybody who asked for it, nor will I make a suggestion to this effect." It is not so simple now that we know almost all drugs can be deadly. See "The Hippocratic Oath Today: Meaningless Relic or Invaluable Moral Guide?" at Web Resource 46-1.

The physician's obligations for most of the years since Hippocrates were primarily to the individual patient. The physician had little in his or her armamentarium that was effective in diagnosis or treatment. Diagnosis relied on the physician's brain without laboratory tests or other investigations. Real medications were few, often useless, adulterated, or impure. Clinical research dates only to the 19th century, and surgery was, at least until anesthesia was developed also in the 19th century, crude and painful at best and fatal at worst. The physician comforted and predicted and often did little else.

How that has changed! Physicians (plus nurses, physician assistants, nurse practitioners, midwives, and many other health care providers) now have an extraordinary array of diagnostic and therapeutic choices available. There are far more choices than the practitioner is able to keep up with and use appropriately.

But the cost of this great improvement in diagnosis and therapeutics has been the introduction of complexity and conflicting agendas as health care professionals now have obligations to society, employers, governments, insurance companies, partners, and hospitals. The days when the patient paid his or her $5 cash for an office visit (and $8 for a home visit) are long gone. The world of big business has now caught up with big medicine. Costs of physician and other health care provider services, procedures, surgeries, laboratory tests, medications, and devices have skyrocketed. The entire dynamics of medicine and health care have changed.

The question of what is a pharmaceutical company's (whether private or public) responsibility should be addressed. There are, broadly speaking, two schools of thought on this. The first is the one of "fiduciary responsibility," which states roughly that a company's role is to maximize profitability and shareholder/stockholder value while staying within the law. The second view holds that companies have additional moral obligations to their "stakeholders" above and beyond simply making as much money as possible for the stockholders (owners) of the company. The stakeholders include the employees, the communities where the company is located, the public at large, and vendors. America and other parts of the world have shifted from the first view toward the second one or some combination thereof. There is currently a major and ongoing debate on corporate ethics and responsibilities, with one side saying that "corporate ethics" is a contradiction in terms and the other that we are moving to a new view of corporate behavior. This debate then tempers the view one takes regarding the behavior of companies and their individual employees, regulators, customers, bystanders, and others.

Accompanying the changes in the structure of medicine have been changes in the roles and obligations of physicians and other health care providers. For example, the physician's role in clinical research is ambiguous. By doing clinical research, the physician is experimenting on patients (or even normal subjects) with new medications that may not help the individual patient but that may help humankind (if the new product represents a real breakthrough) and definitely will help the drug company involved. This is a concept not envisioned in Hippocrates' time. An attempt to define the physician's ethical obligations was spelled out in an American Medical Association position paper in 2004. See Web Resource 46-2. In particular, it notes the conflict between the research and the individual patient's needs: "Recognize that considerations relating to the well-being of individual participants in research take precedence over the interests of science or society."

The specific ethical obligations and considerations in regard to the pharmaceutical industry is a topic of lively discussion, and many websites offer opinions. A Google search on "ethics" and "pharmaceuticals" produced 1.57 million hits, and a search on "ethics" and "drug safety" produced 181,000 hits (December 27, 2005), including

- Pharmacoethics.com at Web Resource 46-3: "Dedicated to the exploration of ethical issues related to the development, promotion, sales, prescription, and use of pharmaceuticals."

- The American Society for Bioethics and Humanities at Web Resource 46-4 "promotes the exchange of ideas and fosters multidisciplinary, interdisciplinary, and interprofessional scholarship, research, teaching, policy development, professional development, and collegiality among people engaged in clinical and academic bioethics and the medical humanities."

- The Centre for Professional Ethics at the University of Central Lancashire (United Kingdom) at Web Resource 46-5.

- The Canadian Bioethics Society at Web Resource 46-6 is "interested in sharing ideas relating to bioethics and in finding solutions to bioethical problems."

- Academy of Pharmaceutical Physicians and Investigators is a "non-profit association dedicated to providing global leadership for the clinical research profession by promoting and advancing the highest ethical standards and practices." They have produced a code of ethics (Web Resource 46-7) that specifically includes postmarketing product safety surveillance in its preamble.

For an excellent review of the ethical issues in the pharmaceutical world, see M.D.B. Stephens' superb section entitled, "Ethical Issues In Drug Safety" (in Stephens' *Detection of New Adverse Drug Reactions*, 5th ed., Wiley, 2004, pp. 591–648). This article covers clinical trials, the use of placebo, ethics committees, conflicts of interest, informed consent, patient protection, publications, symposia, advertising and promotion, labeling, and relations with government.

Companies are set up, as noted above, to make money. They do so by selling drug products, products that have known faults or defects listed in the labeling as adverse events (AEs), warnings, and precautions. For all new products, the complete risk profile is not completely known until well after marketing begins and exposure to much larger and heterogenous populations than during clinical trials occurs.

For just about all drugs, the safety of use in pregnancy has not been studied. The company has invested enormous amounts of money in the development and then promotion of the products that have a finite (financial) life span due to patent expiration. When a drug is approved, it is judged by health authorities to have a benefit profile greater than its risk profile that is translated by the public into the shorthand of "safe and effective," although it really means "relatively safe and relatively effective."

Companies will do everything within their power to promote and protect their products. The drug safety group (along with the product quality department if separate) is the department that receives only bad news about product use. This department must determine, in very short time frames, whether the serious or fatal problems reported are due to the drug or not. Some of the cases must be reported to the government within a week or 2 and others tallied up in summary reports as signals for internal corporate review and, sometimes, submission to the health authorities.

The role of the drug safety group is to protect the public health as its primary duty. A secondary duty is to protect the company's products only insofar as this does not conflict with the primary protection of the public health. It is always interesting to read the introduction to the corporate standard operating procedure or mission statement for the drug safety group to see whether this distinction is respected.

The next sections address some of the areas of controversy that touch drug safety.

■ Dynamics at Play in Regard to Drug Safety and Companies

- Corporations are rarely run by physicians or clinicians and more often by nonmedically trained marketers, sales personnel, lawyers, and accountants. Such managers, who work their way up the corporate ladder, usually do not do a stint in the drug safety department. It is thus understandable that the senior corporate view on drug safety is sometimes vague and often ill-defined.

- The rules governing drug safety are arcane, highly technical, and very difficult to understand (even for those in the business). Management rarely wants details but rather prefers "executive summaries" of data that may not capture the nuances of the clinical judgment involved in drug safety decisions. In addition, there is legal discouragement about writing down real or potential "bad things" about the drug products in e-mail or memos. Management may work on the MEGO ("my eyes glaze over") or MITIN ("more information than I need") principles regarding drug safety.

- The drug safety group is a "cost center" and not a profit center. Pharmacovigilance professionals often argue that their approach saves the company money and shame by preventing safety problems from becoming safety crises resulting in crisis management procedures, patient harm, litigation, restrictions on use, or even withdrawal from the market. This argu-

ment, of theoretical dollars saved by the safety department, usually carries little weight.

- The drug safety function is not glamorous and usually not well funded—at least not as well funded as the clinical research and sales organizations. The same holds true, by the way, in most drug regulatory authorities: There is more staff studying dossiers in view of approving new products than staff studying adverse drug reaction reports. And in medical schools, pharmacovigilance is not even part of the curriculum. As the saying goes, drug safety is the "poor stepchild."

- In many companies, the drug safety group is scattered at several sites around the United States or the world and often away from the main campus or headquarters of the company ("out of sight, out of mind").

- Delivering bad news up the corporate ladder is, in the best of times, accepted but not welcomed. In the worst of times, it is actively discouraged and punished. It is hard to "speak the truth to power." The messengers are indeed sometimes "killed." The mechanism of reporting on signals that could drastically reduce sales, if confirmed or made known, is often convoluted, requiring the safety message to work its way up the corporate chain before it reaches someone with decision-making power.

- Delivering bad news is generally not as well paid as delivering good news (completing clinical trials, selling more drug, etc.) in companies. No one is compensated more for sending in additional 15-day alert reports.

- Rightly or wrongly, the reputation for honesty of drug companies (including their drug safety groups) is not high in the eyes of health authorities, regulators, consumer groups, and the public. This tends to produce a mentality within the companies of "circling the wagons." Companies, again rightly or wrongly, put little trust or credence into AE reports from certain groups such as consumer groups, disease groups, and attorneys and react defensively.

- The drug safety group is usually grudgingly accepted as a "necessary evil" by other groups in the company ("the sales prevention department").

- Business negotiations for in-licensing new products often do not think of drug safety or bring it into play at the very last minute.

- It is often very difficult to convince sales and marketing departments of the need to train both new and current sales people on AE reporting ("The job of the sales force is to sell."). Training is often relegated to giving out reading material, or if an actual physical presentation is permitted, it is often done at 4:30 pm on the last day of training.

- Drug safety often reports into the medical research department. Less commonly it reports into the legal or regulatory departments. It should never report to a marketing or sales function. The drug safety organization may report to a nonempowered, low-level, relatively junior employee with little organizational voice or influence.

- There are few ways for management to measure drug safety performance. Clearly, measuring the on-time reporting performance for 15-day, Periodic Safety Update Reports, New Drug Application periodic reports, and Investigational New Drug Application annual reports is the most common metric used, but this simply captures mechanical performance and not the medical protection and risk management aspects of pharmacovigilance. Softer measures such as "FDA's satisfaction with our performance" are nearly impossible to measure.

- Pharmaceutical companies are asked to present statistically significant efficacy data to prove that a drug should be approved by the health authorities to market a product. Thus many in senior management assume that safety data work the same way. They do not.

- Management often takes the view that a serious safety issue must be proven with hard data. There must be clear causality associated with the drug and no alternate explanations for the problem. Thus some managers will not accept drug safety physicians' views that a particular serious and severe medical problem is probably or possibly due to the drug and that a change in the product labeling is warranted. Clear proof in several or many patients is demanded.

- Alternative explanations are often presumed to be the cause of the problem. "This patient smokes, drinks, is hypertensive and both parents have heart disease. How can you say our drug caused this patient's heart attack?" (See also the fialuridine story in Chapter 47.)

- The problem may be reduced to a more simple question: Is the drug innocent until proven guilty of a safety problem or is the drug guilty of a safety problem until proven innocent? In the past, the American "innocent until proven guilty" view pre-

dominated. Now, the pendulum seems to be swinging toward early notification of the public of potential safety issues even if events are not clearly due to the drug. Whether this will prove to be good for the public health (moving people off dangerous drugs) or bad for the public health (moving people to other more toxic or costly alternatives) remains to be seen.

- The "level playing field" argument is often made by nonmedical personnel in regard to reporting and acting on safety issues. The argument for this runs roughly as follows: "If we as a company have to report that our drug X seems to be causing ventricular fibrillation, then our competitors' products, which also cause ventricular fibrillation (as evidenced by Freedom of Information or medical literature reports), should also be obliged to change their labeling." This then puts pressure on the drug safety department to either not report or to minimize such events until they are "proven." Companies thus try to make deals ("We'll change our label if you make our competitors also change theirs" or "This should be class labeling").

- Interestingly, physicians are now found more and more commonly in marketing departments where they tend to take on the coloration of marketers and lose the coloration of physicians. They then may take on an adversary ("devil's advocate") role in relation to the drug safety physicians.

- In a similar vein, physicians working in the medical research department (phases II and III) often become quite "protective and possessive" about the drugs they are studying and may take a doubting view that "their" drug could produce such serious AEs and that these serious AEs are "unrelated" to the study drug. This is one of the reasons why the final determination of causality, labeling, and reportability should rest in the drug safety group.

- Physicians and, to a lesser degree, other health care professionals working in industry (including drug safety) are/were often looked down on by the physicians and health care workers "out in the real world." Some consider pharmaceutical professionals to have "sold out."

- There are no formal training programs in the United States for drug safety personnel either in medical, nursing, or pharmacy school. There are courses lasting from a day to a week or 2 (usually by nonacademic institutions) on drug safety, and there is a scarcity of textbooks. Training tends to be similar to an apprenticeship.

- Sometimes there is a perception in the industry that the US Food and Drug Administration (FDA) is not taking the stand. For example, the FDA issuing nonbinding guidances or draft regulations often puts the industry in a difficult position. It is hard to convince company management to fund expensive initiatives that may never become regulations (e.g., the 2003 Tome is still, at this writing, not final). It is always easier for the drug safety unit to ask for and receive new funding or resources if the FDA forces it by law or regulation.

- Drug safety officers, unless they worked previously at the FDA, really do not have a good feel for how the FDA works (and vice versa). Although there are contacts between industry and the FDA through the International Conference on Harmonization, Council for International Organizations of Medical Sciences, and other venues, such contact is usually at a distance and defensive due to perceived conflicts of interest.

- Drug safety personnel, as with any other company personnel, may own stock or receive stock options. Hence, pay is tied to company performance as well as the individual's work.

- Drug safety units are under continued scrutiny by the FDA (particularly in the form of inspections) and, in wise companies, by internal auditors.

- There are significant pressures on drug safety personnel in regard to work volume and time allocated to complete tasks (especially those time frames regulated by law), difficulty in finding experienced safety officers, and difficulty in training safety officers.

- The upward corporate career mobility for personnel in drug safety groups is limited usually to that group. Rarely do employees move high up in the corporate hierarchy unless they leave the drug safety unit.

There are clear and obvious potential conflicts evident in such a "self-policing" situation. The drug safety personnel are paid by the company and will, in general, receive better pay and more rewards if the company does well and sells more drugs. On the other hand, enlightened companies have tended to realize more and more that they cannot "play games" with the drug safety units. Drug safety personnel tend to be somewhat defensive and "paranoid," lacing their world view with dark humor. Whether

the job produces such character traits or rather attracts people with such traits from the beginning is unclear.

■ Dynamics at Play in Regard to Drug Safety and Health Agencies

- The health workers in the FDA and other agencies are not involved in the fiduciary aspects of profit-making companies. Their job is more clearly that of protecting the health of the public.

- In the United States, the FDA and the personnel in the FDA have multiple masters to answer to (either formally in the organization structure or informally), including the senior management of the FDA, the cabinet department to which they report (Health and Human Services), the President, Congress, and various other overseers including the Justice Department and the Public Health Service. Funding is not always dispersed at a level perceived to be necessary for adequate functioning.

- The FDA is heavily scrutinized by the press and the media, more so than safety departments in pharmaceutical companies.

- Employees at the FDA tend to make less money than corresponding personnel in pharmaceutical companies.

- The FDA tends to be underfunded and understaffed compared with the resources in pharmaceutical companies if one looks at the number of AEs received and the drugs under scrutiny. Some multinational companies' drug safety departments are bigger than FDA's.

- The perception is that the FDA is not expected or "allowed" to make mistakes. Bad outcomes, serious outcomes, and patient deaths are not supposed to occur in drugs approved by the FDA. The FDA approves drugs "too quickly or too slowly" according to one's point of view.

- The perception is that the FDA is going through a turbulent period (short-term commissioners, loss of experienced personnel, reorganizations, the possible removal of the drug safety function from the FDA by Congress, etc.), a sort of mini-crisis.

- Duplicative and, in a sense, competitive pharmacovigilance is done by other major health authorities abroad. If a drug is removed from the market or the labeling changed outside the United States, the

FDA often feels obliged to explain why they do not believe there is a problem for US patients.

- The FDA has limited regulatory powers. For example, there is limited regulatory power to force label changes and regulate neutraceuticals and old over-the-counter products. It is also difficult and time consuming to change the regulations.

- The FDA safety officers, unless they previously worked in industry, often do not have a good feel for how corporate decisions and governance occurs.

- It is not clear how the lower level safety officers are able to get their views brought up the line (see Chapter 50).

- FDA workers may not own stock in drug companies or consult for them.

■ Dynamics at Play in Regard to Drug Safety and Academia and Nonacademic Health Care Facilities

- In the United States, and to a lesser degree in Canada, the role in drug safety training, surveillance, and research by the universities, medical, nursing, and pharmacy schools is minimal. These schools train health care practitioners but not with the goal of drug safety. Courses tend to focus on the concepts of pharmacology and the clinical use of medications.

- Occasionally, industry physicians hold academic positions at medical schools, often in the clinical research units and occasionally in the clinics (seeing patients, though malpractice insurance issues tend to prevent this in the United States). Thus there is little "cross-fertilization" among colleagues.

- In contrast, France, for example, has a very tight relationship between the regulatory agency and the regional University Hospitals in handling drug safety (see Chapter 13).

- There is heavily paid consultation and clinical research performed by academics for the pharmaceutical industry. Physicians and other scientists in academia perform clinical trials and postmarketing trials, give lectures in speakers' bureaus funded by the industry, and so on. They are sometimes referred to as "opinion leaders." They may own stock in pharmaceutical companies.

- Academics may sit on FDA advisory committees. Ideally, they should have no conflicts of interest. If any do exist, they must be declared. It is sometimes hard to find an expert in a drug or disease that has not at some point in his or her career worked with the industry to study new products or uses.

- Academics may sit on hospital formulary committees and have a major say in which products are used (and sold) in that institution, even when they have been paid to study these products.

- Some academic research units receive some funding from industry, and clinical trials done in academic units usually charge industry significant "university overhead" to allow the trials to be done at their institutions. Thus industry becomes a significant source of academic funding at some institutions. In addition, some institutions now make significant money from drug sales for which they hold patents and receive royalties (see Chapter 28 on the Bayh-Dole Act). There are virtually no medical or pharmacy faculties that do not receive grants, awards, scholarships, speakers' fees, unrestricted educational grants, CME expenses, professorships (chairs) etc. from industry. Some companies go so far as to install a pharmaceutical research center or an endowed chair on the campus of prestigious medical faculties.

■ Dynamics at Play in Regard to Drug Safety and Consumer Groups, Disease Groups, and Websites

- These are usually nonprofit organizations created by patients with common diseases or medication use.

- There are occasional organizations or sites set up with other goals in mind. See Web Resource 46-8 that states, "This site provides news and legal information about defective drugs which may cause serious side effects" (accessed December 28, 2005).

- Also see Web Resource 46-9 run by The Public Citizen's Health Research Group.

- A common view is that the industry is monolithic and "bad." The groups often believe (sometimes quite rightly) that the industry regards them as adversaries.

- Sometimes these groups do collect useful information (including safety information) that is made available to the health authorities and industry.

- They often believe industry cannot police itself and do not trust industry drug safety conclusions.

Dynamics at Play in Regard to Drug Safety and Television and the Media

- Drug safety issues sell newspapers and draw eyes to websites and television.

- Such stories do not need to be based on scientific data but may rather rest on accusations or human-interest issues.

- Safe drugs do not make good stories. Dangerous ones or potentially dangerous ones do.

- There is no obligation to present both sides of a story.

- There is little obligation to correct stories that turn out to be incorrect or overblown ("A lie can travel half way around the world while the truth is putting on its shoes." Mark Twain).

- Experienced reporters and television personalities are far more skilled at communications on television than drug safety personnel (even those who have had "media training") and can make a non–media-savvy interviewee look quite silly or foolish.

- Data presented in the media may be "precise" but not "accurate."

Dynamics at Play in Regard to Drug Safety and Lawyers/Litigation

- Drug safety personnel in the industry and government generally do not like to testify in court and try to avoid lawyers and litigation.

- Dealings with lawyers and litigation tend to take enormous amounts of time and offer little in return to the safety personnel involved.

- Law and litigation involve, usually, adversarial procedures and are very different from the collegial, consensual, and scientific approach most safety officers have from training, experience, and affinity. There is no obligation to be even-handed or present both sides of the story.

- Testimony, whether in court or at depositions, is usually highly stressful and time-consuming.

- There are monetary goals involved in addition to the claimed goals of fairness and justice in lawsuits.

Comment and Summary

The entire field of drug safety is chock full of conflicts of interests and personal or institutional agendas, some of which are obvious and some less so. No one owns the truth. Trust but verify. All statements should be questioned and skepticism is a virtue. Safety data are incredibly dynamic and change daily. What is true today may not be so tomorrow. Beware of statements such as those listed below. They may not all be false, but they should be viewed with skepticism until proven otherwise:

- "Of course I've consulted for XX Inc. or received speakers' bureaus fees but they do not influence my judgment in any way."

- "Of course I see drug reps, but they are not my sole source of information and I make independent judgments."

- "I've never received a dime from industry. But I own a lot of their stock. Or my wife or children do."

- "This drug is (perfectly) safe."

- "Our only interest is the public health."

- "I only do what is right for the patient, not the clinical trial or company."

- "This drug has not been shown to produce atrial fibrillation" (or some other serious AE. "The cases we do have are under investigation and all the patients had risk factors."

- "The serious AE was due to the patient's lifestyle and risk factors."

- "We have no reports that this drug caused atrial fibrillation." But someone else might.

But all is not lost nor does cynicism reign everywhere. The current system, which is made up of multiple competing forces pulling in different directions sometimes and in the same directions at other times, has tended to arrive at the truth after all is said and done. It arguably takes too long and some people are hurt and some even die. We have nothing better yet but many people in the FDA, the industry, the European Medicines Agency, the US Congress, the Institute of Medicine, Health Canada, and elsewhere are searching assiduously. The history of science suggests we will get better and better though slowly, asymptotically, and with pain along the way.

Real-World Safety Issues and Controversies: Fialuridine

Fialuridine (FIAU) was a drug used to treat hepatitis B virus (HBV) in the early 1990s. Its use in one clinical trial in particular produced seven cases of severe hepatic toxicity (including five deaths) in 15 patients. This trial produced major fallout in the world of clinical research in the United States. The events are briefly reviewed here, and a few comments are made in regard to the drug safety aspects of the study.

FIAU is a pyrimidine nucleoside analogue that was believed to be a very promising treatment for HBV patients. It had previously been studied in a major cancer hospital against other viral infections, including cytomegalovirus (CMV) and various herpes viruses, with some promising results. Animal studies revealed vomiting, diarrhea, mild cardiac toxicity at high doses, and bone marrow toxicity. No liver toxicity was noted in any of the animal models (rat, mouse, and monkey).

In 1989 a small pharmaceutical company together with the National Institutes of Allergy and Infectious Diseases did a phase I/II dose escalation trial in human immunodeficiency virus (HIV) patients with positive CMV cultures using fiacitabine (FIAU is an active metabolite of fiacitabine). The study of 12 patients did not show an effect on the CMV. Adverse events (AEs) reported were nausea, fatigue, and an increased creatine phosphokinase in one patient. No one died during the study. Follow-up showed four deaths, including one patient who had hepatitis B about 6 months after the end of the study. His death was believed to be due to the underlying hepatitis and other hepatotoxic medications he was taking.

In 1990 a short-term treatment (2 weeks) study of FIAU was done on HIV patients. During the study it became clear that there was a significant effect on HBV but probably little CMV efficacy. The protocol was amended to allow HBV patients to enter also. Investigators at the National Institutes of Health (NIH) joined the study team. Significant decreases in HBV DNA were noted. Some patients also developed doubling or tripling of serum transaminase levels. It was unclear whether the transaminase elevations were AEs due to the drug or due to the so-called flare phenomenon of elevated transaminases seen when HBV viremia drops with other drug treatment (e.g., interferon).

The positive results from this trial led to the starting in 1991 of a trial of 4 weeks of FIAU therapy. The trial showed excellent results in the groups receiving the highest dosages with major reductions in HBV DNA. No AEs producing dropout or dose modification occurred. "Flares" and HBV DNA rebound were noted in several patients, but three of nine patients had continued suppression of HBV DNA, normal liver tests, and were HBV antigen negative. One patient developed abdominal pain (but with normal liver and pancreas tests) that resolved 4 months after the trial. One patient was diagnosed with cholelithiasis, and another had an episode of peripheral neuropathy. One patient died. He had chronic hepatitis B and had a good result with FIAU in the trial as judged by his HBV DNA level. He had nausea and fatigue during the trial. One month after the last dose of FIAU, his transaminase was noted to be four times normal and he complained of nausea, fatigue, and abdominal pain. A nonstudy physician recommended cholecystectomy, which was done under general anesthesia. Liver biopsy revealed chronic active hepatitis and steatosis. He deteriorated after surgery and died a few months later. An autopsy revealed steatosis. His death was attributed primarily to the anesthesia drugs administered.

Based on these results, the NIH and Eli Lilly, Inc. (now developing the drug) began a study in 1993 of carefully selected hepatitis B patients with a planned treatment period of 6 months of FIAU. Within the first few weeks of the study start, some patients complained of fatigue, nausea, cramps, and diarrhea. Some patients had dose interruption. No abnormal laboratory tests were noted. However, all patients had decreases in HBV DNA, and 6 of 10 became HBV DNA negative. The data were reviewed at about 6 weeks into the trial, and because of the positive results, the investigators opted to continue.

A few days later one patient who had discontinued the drug 2 weeks previously presented to an emergency room with nausea, weakness, and hypotension. The transaminases were normal, but the bilirubin and lactic acid levels were elevated. The patient went on to develop liver and renal failure and, in spite of liver transplantation, died. The autopsy revealed pancreatitis, glomerulonephritis, esophageal varices, and pneumonia. The liver showed micro- and macrovascular steatosis, cholestasis, and chronic active hepatitis.

Within 2 or 3 days of the patient first showing up at the emergency room, the study was stopped and all patients still on FIAU were told to stop the drug. All patients (15) were admitted to the NIH Clinical Center for observation. In spite of stopping the drug, seven patients developed hepatic failure, pancreatitis, neuropathy, and myopathy and were to have liver transplantation. Five died (some after transplantation) and two survived. Eight of the 15 patients had no AEs.

As a result of this disaster, several inquiries were set up. The US Food and Drug Administration (FDA) established an internal task force and issued a report in November 1993. It was believed that there were many episodes of "missed toxicity" and that the AEs were attributed to the disease rather than to the study drug. They also believed the informed consents and the study monitoring and oversight were not adequate. The FDA issued warning letters to the investigators charging, among other things, the failure to immediately report serious AEs to the sponsor and investigational review boards, failure to reduce or terminate dosing in subjects with moderate toxicity, failure to describe all foreseeable risks in the informed consent, failure to follow-up on serious AEs, failure to include complete and accurate safety data in the investigator brochure, and failure to adequately monitor by not ensuring that all AEs were reported in the case report forms.

The NIH did its own investigation and concluded that the rationale for the studies being done was strong, especially in light of the lack of other (oral) therapy for the disease in question. They believed the protocols were "meticulously" prepared and implemented and that the fatal outcomes could not have been predicted from the AEs. They also noted that the AEs were adequately reported. Thus the NIH and the FDA investigations came to opposite conclusions.

Next, an investigation was done by the Institute of Medicine (IOM) (Web Resource 47-1) at the request of the Secretary of Health and Human Services. The IOM is a private, nonprofit, nongovernmental organization that is part of the National Academy of Sciences. Its review largely agreed with that of the NIH. It concluded that there was excellent attention paid to safety monitoring and that there were no significant violations of study conduct or informed consent. They concluded, in fact, that the rapid action to stop the study actually saved lives and prevented an even worse tragedy.

There was much discussion and criticism after these events. Press coverage was vivid and lurid, and a congressional investigation in 1994 occurred with strong charges being thrown about. Further work revealed that the FIAU toxicity was due to mitochondrial damage by the drug.

Much has occurred since then in regard to tightening and harmonization of regulations and clinical trial oversight. It is not the intent to review the issues in clinical trial regulation, oversight, and monitoring or the politics here. Instead the drug safety implications are discussed.

- Serious and nonserious AEs due to (study or marketed) drugs may occur that mimic the disease being treated. The implications of this are major. It is not adequate to attribute serious AEs to the disease or condition being treated, background medical conditions, intercurrent problems, or other non-drug causes without a careful consideration of a drug-related etiology. A very high level of suspicion that the drug produced the serious AE must be kept at all times when evaluating whether a drug has produced a particular AE. The drug is not "innocent until proven guilty."

■ Clinical trial safety oversight by the company (sponsor) and the investigator must be "meticulous." All the regulatory requirements (protocol design, investigator qualification, AE collection, reporting and review, consent forms, investigational review board oversight, safety data review committees, etc.) must be followed strictly and completely.

▪ A data safety plan (risk management, see Chapters 14–16) must be drawn up and in place before the study starts.

▪ Prestudy signals (from animal data or other clinical trials or class drugs) must be followed carefully.

▪ Investigator (and sponsor, monitor) training must be done before the study starts and during the study if new personnel become involved. The training should be of high quality, customized to the study, and done by a training specialist (not simply printed material).

▪ A sponsor physician must be designated as clearly in charge of the ongoing safety review. A decision on whether to unblind him/her or not should be made at the beginning of the trial. If blinding is kept in place for the study physician, another mechanism must be established to follow (unblinded) safety data, such as a safety monitoring committee.

▪ The use of qualified investigational review boards with high-quality experienced personnel who have sufficient time to review safety data must occur. Sponsors and investigators must supply the investigational review boards with easily reviewable data sent at frequent periods.

▪ Companies and institutions doing clinical trials must have a crisis management plan in place to be able to do a preliminary investigation and to take appropriate actions on critical safety issues within a few hours.

▪ Larger political and governmental solutions should also be considered (presumably they are) including full-time dedicated national safety monitoring committees, a separate safety organization within the federal government, involvement of academia in ongoing safety monitoring (as in France), limitation of proprietary secrets, an AE reporting system in a federal database for clinical trial AEs combining the safety efforts put into case report form safety reporting with those for regulatory serious AE reporting (this refers to duplication of reporting in clinical trials: to the drug safety group and in the case report form), continued research into trend analysis and early signaling, and so on.

See an excellent review on the FIAU safety issues:

Nickas J. Clinical trial safety surveillance in the new regulatory and harmonization environment: lessons learned from the "Fialuridine crisis." *Drug Inform J* 1997;31:63–70.

An excellent review of the situation is available:

Saag M. A review of the FIAU tragedy and its effect on clinical research. *J Clin Res Practice* 1999;1:21–32.

Also see the IOM report:

Manning FJ, Swartz M, eds. Review of the Fialuridine (FIAU) clinical trials. Committee to Review the Fialuridine (FIAU/FIAC) Clinical Trials. Division of Health Sciences Policy. Institute of Medicine. Washington, DC: National Academy Press, 1995.

Real-World Safety Issues and Controversies: Fen-Phen

➡ **NOTE:** (Unless otherwise noted the word "drug" or "drug product" should be taken in this book to include "biologics" and "vaccines.")

What is now called the "fen-phen" issue refers to the combination use of fenfluramine and phentermine. Both products had long been approved (1973 and 1959, respectively) by US Food and Drug Administration (FDA) as appetite suppressants.

Reports in the literature of pulmonary hypertension and fenfluramine appeared in the 1980s and 1990s. Reports of headache, insomnia, nervousness, irritability, palpitations, tachycardia, and elevations in blood pressure were seen with phentermine. Few long-term data were available for the use of these drugs at the time.

The combination of fenfluramine and phentermine was never approved by the FDA, and their use was "off label." However, millions of prescriptions for their use were written (Diet pills redux [editorial]. *N Engl J Med* 1997;337:629–630).

After this increased use, reports of toxicity started to appear. One report cited the death of a 29-year-old woman after only 23 days of the combination (Mark, Patalas, Chang, et al., *N Engl J Med* 1997;337:602–606.). Also in 1997 the Mayo Clinic reported 24 women who developed valvular heart disease (mitral, aortic, and tricuspid, sometimes more than one valve) after a mean of 12 months of combination therapy (with one woman using the drugs for only 1 month). One-third had pulmonary hypertension, and several required valve surgery (Connolly, Crary, McGoon, et al., *N Engl J Med* 1997;337:635). Valvular disease with only fenfluramine or only dexfenfluramine was also reported.

By November 1997, the Centers for Disease Control and Prevention reported 144 spontaneous cases of fenfluramine or dexfenfluramine with or without phentermine producing valvular disease. Reports of abnormal echocardiograms done in fen-phen or dexfen-phen patients were received by the FDA. They noted 30% abnormal echocardiograms in 291 asymptomatic screened patients, primarily with aortic regurgitation. Many of the patients were women.

Fenfluramine and dexfenfluramine were withdrawn from the market in late 1997. Phentermine was not withdrawn because no cases were reported to the FDA with this drug alone (as of September 1997).

The FDA noted in its Q&A of September 1997 (Web Resource 48-1) that because valve disease is not usually associated with drug use, it was not screened for in patients and no cases were detected in 500 patients in a 1-year clinical trial. It noted that the link between symptoms and drug use was not "obvious." In addition, there were few animal data to suggest this toxicity, and early on most patients and physicians did not give too much thought to pulmonary toxicity with these drugs.

After this publicity, not surprisingly, many new cases were noted and lawsuits were filed. In October 1999, the manufacturer agreed to a class action settlement of up to $4.75 billion. A trust was established by the manufacturer by order of the US District Court to administer the claims and payments of benefits to registered class members providing for benefits, including refunds for the costs of Pondimin® and Redux™, medical monitoring and some medical treatment or payment for monitoring and treatment, and compensation for specifically defined valvular heart conditions. See the AHP Diet Drug Settlement website at Web Resource 48-2.

Several safety lessons were learned:

- Untested combinations of approved products may be quite dangerous even if the individual products are not—and especially if the individual products are.
- Old products are not always well "known" or studied.
- Old safety lessons or safety clues may be minimized or forgotten.

- Unintended consequences (adverse events [AEs]) may occur at any time (see fialuridine, Chapter 47, and diethylstilbestrol, Chapter 6) in an unexpected organ system or patient.

- Dose matters. But sometimes it does not.

- "Absence of evidence is not evidence of absence." That is, just because there is no finding of a particular AE or disease in clinical trials or patients treated with a drug does not mean that it was sought. And if it was sought, it might not have been sought in the right patients at the right time with the proper diagnostic tools and tests.

- Companies, physicians, and regulators should be very careful about off-label use, and better ways to monitor their effects need to be developed. There are many valid medical reasons for certain off-label uses, especially in oncology, but extreme care must be exercised, particularly when there is no clear clinical or scientific basis for such use.

- Intelligent and clever clinicians can still discover serious drug AEs in the course of their daily practice. Such serious AEs should indeed be reported to the health authority or company.

- Drug usage, when popular and extrapolated to the populations of North America, Europe, Japan, and elsewhere, can produce enormous benefits to individuals, health care practitioners, and society in general. It can also produce major disasters.

Real-World Safety Issues and Controversies: Nomifensine

Nomifensine (Merital®) was first used in Germany in 1976, in the United Kingdom (UK) in 1977, and in the United States in 1985 as an antidepressant. From 1978 to 1985, some 165,000 to 251,000 prescriptions were written each year. Between 1978 and 1979 four reports of hemolytic anemia were received by the manufacturer. A case report was published in the medical literature in 1979. From 1981 to 1982 three more UK cases were reported. From 1979 to 1980 the company did immunologic studies of some 300 patients. In 1981 the UK labeling was changed to indicate that rare cases of hemolytic anemia were reported.

At this time the labeling also stated that rare cases of liver enzyme elevation were noted. In the 1980s the use of nomifensine increased, and by 1986 a total of 296 adverse event (AE) reports were received by the manufacturer, including 16 positive Coombs' tests and 45 hemolytic anemias as well as 27 jaundice, 12 abnormal liver function tests, 6 hepatitis, and 1 hepatic necrosis report. The first UK fatalities were reported in 1985.

Further case reports were published from 1980 to 1985 noting hemolytic anemia (with and without renal failure), thrombocytopenia, hepatitis, fatal alveolitis, a systemic lupus erythematosus–like fatal reaction, and fatal immune hemolysis. By June 1985 the estimated incidence of hemolytic anemia was 1 in 20,000. Further reports were received, and by November the estimated rate was 1 in 4,000.

Dear Doctor letters were sent out in 1985 in the United Kingdom, and the drug was withdrawn from all worldwide markets in January 1986 (Stonier, *Pharmacoepidemiol Drug Safety* 1:177–185, 2002; Stonier, Edwards, Nomifensine and haemolytic anemia, in *Pharmacovigilance*, Wiley, 2002).

It should be noted that during this time (late 1970s to the 1980s) the state of drug safety and pharmacovigilance reporting was markedly different from today. The International Conference on Harmonization, EMEA, and MedWatch were not yet in existence, and many countries had disparate or nonrigorous AE reporting systems.

The drug was approved by the US Food and Drug Administration (FDA) in 1984 (after some 6 years reviewing the dossier), and marketing began in the United States in July 1985. It was estimated that up to 10,000,000 patients were exposed to the drug by then. As noted above, the drug was withdrawn from all markets (including the United States) in January 1986.

The question then arose in the United States of how the FDA could have approved the product and then permitted marketing while the crescendo of cases was building up, especially in 1984–1985. Hearings in the US House of Representatives (Congress) were held in early 1986, and an investigation was launched by the FDA in August 1986.

A summary report was issued by the FDA (Kurtzweil, *FDA Consumer*, September 1991, p. 42, see Web Resource 49-1), the FDA investigation revealed that two deaths, an Italian in 1980 and a French woman in 1984 (before the approval in the United States), were known to the company but not reported to the FDA until 1986, months after the drug was withdrawn from the market. Nine other deaths, including three in the United States, also occurred. As the FDA notes in its report: "The investigation, which lasted a year and a half, was lengthy because officials of the US company refused to allow personnel who had been directly involved in analyzing and reporting adverse drug reactions to speak to FDA investigators. In addition, months often passed before they provided written answers to investigators' questions."

The FDA was able to gather evidence showing that the company, Hoechst AG in Germany, and a former medical director of the clinical research division "had been aware of the deaths of the two European women shortly after they had occurred but had failed to report them to FDA as required." The FDA found no evidence that the US division of the company (Hoechst-Roussel) had withheld information from the FDA. In December 1990 the US Federal Attorney in New Jersey charged Hoechst AG and the medical director by name with failing to report the two European deaths. No charges were filed against Hoechst-Roussel. In April 1991, Hoechst AG and the medical director pleaded guilty to the charges and were fined the maximum amount allowed by law. The nomifensine became something of a worldwide "cause célèbre."

Several safety lessons were learned:

- Always do the right thing.
- Do not withhold safety data from the FDA and other health authorities.
- The company should speak with one voice and say the same (correct) thing to all health authorities at the same time.
- Report all data in a proper and timely manner and document it with meticulously kept records.
- Proper written procedures must be in place to ensure that all safety data are reported to all branches of the company (especially multinational companies) that need these data. The company should perform periodic internal audits to ensure that this is happening. Any deficiencies should be remedied immediately, and data that should have been reported must be reported to the health authorities as soon as the issue is discovered (painful though this may be).
- Cooperate with all health authority investigations.
- The senior officers of the company must understand the significance of the drug safety function and put their full weight, support, and resources into ensuring that safety is done correctly.
- Maintain a high index of suspicion that AEs may be due to the drug and not to other causes.
- Physicians and those in positions of senior responsibility in the company should be aware that they may be held personally liable (criminally and civilly) if they do not do their safety duties.
- Ensure that safety information is reported to the FDA and health authorities as required before, during, and after Investigational New Drug and New Drug Application submission and review with particular attention paid to the period that the New Drug Application is under review.

Real-World Safety Issues and Controversies: Vioxx® and Dr. Graham

The last 25 years or so have produced watershed changes in drug safety. The first was in the 1970s when the regulations for adverse event reporting were tightened in the United States. In 1989 the International Conference on Harmonization was created. In 1995 the European Medicines Evaluation Agency was created. In the beginning of the 21st century, fen-phen, Vioxx®, clinical trial deaths, proposed new US Food and Drug Administration (FDA) regulations (the Tome), and Dr. David Graham's revelations marked additional turning points in drug safety. One could say that the 21st century started with seismic changes in the drug safety world, the fallout from which is still playing out.

On November 18, 2004, Dr. David J. Graham, MD, MPH, Associate Director for Science and Medicine in the FDA's office of Drug Safety, testified before a Congressional Committee in Washington, DC. See Web Resource 50-1. Dr. Graham noted that during his career he "made a real

difference for the cause of patient safety," indicating that his efforts at the FDA led to the withdrawal from the US market of Omniflox® (an antibiotic causing hemolytic anemia), Rezulin® (a diabetes drug producing liver failure), fen-phen and Redux® (weight loss drugs causing cardiac valve injury, see Chapter 48), and PPA (a decongestant and weight loss product causing hemorrhagic stroke). He also indicated that his work contributed to the withdrawal of Trovan® (an antibiotic causing liver failure and death), Lotronex® (a gastrointestinal drug causing ischemic colitis), Baycol® (a lipid-lowering drug causing muscle injury, kidney failure, and death), Seldane® (an antihistamine causing cardiac arrhythmias and death), and Propulsid® (a gastrointestinal drug causing cardiac arrhythmias and death). He noted that he recommended the market withdrawal of 12 drugs of which only 2 remain on the market.

He then went on to summarize his views on Vioxx®. It is not the intent to summarize the Vioxx® issues here, many of which are still unfolding. Rather the intent is to review Dr. Graham's views on drug safety. He reviewed several studies of both low- and high-dose Vioxx® and indicated that they showed increased risk for heart attacks in the 1.5- to 7-fold range. He noted that an FDA study reported in August 2004 indicated an increased risk of heart attack and sudden death of 3.7 for high dose and 1.5 for low dose compared with Celebrex®. He indicated that the report estimated that nearly 28,000 excess cases of heart attack of sudden death were caused by Vioxx® and that this was a conservative estimate. He noted that if the risk levels seen in two Merck trials were applied, the figure would range from 88,000 to 139,000 cardiac events with a 30–40% mortality. He also referred to a study from the Cleveland Clinic in which it was estimated that up to 160,000 cases of heart attacks and strokes were due to Vioxx®. These figures, however, have not been accepted by all parties and are still the subject of controversy and discussion.

Dr. Graham then briefly reviewed various drug disasters dating back to the sulfanilamide (a drug tainted with antifreeze) tragedy in the 1937 that killed some 100 children (see Web Resource 50-2) to the thalidomide birth defect issue that produced some 5,000 to 10,000 birth defects (outside the United States). He noted the passing of the Food, Drug and Cosmetic Act "basically creating the FDA" in 1938 and the 1962 amendment requiring toxicity testing and safety information preapproval as well as evidence of efficacy for drug approval.

Yet in spite of this, Dr. Graham indicated that "Today, in 2004, you, we, are faced with what may be the single greatest drug safety catastrophe in the history of this country in the history of the world. We are talking about a catastrophe that I strongly believe could have, should have been largely or completely avoided." Dr. Graham then, using dramatic words, stated that "In my opinion, the FDA has let the American people down, and sadly, betrayed a public trust. I believe there are at least 3 broad categories of systemic problems that contributed to the Vioxx® catastrophe and to a long line of other drug safety failures in the past 10 years. Briefly, these categories are 1) organizational/structural, 2) cultural and 3) scientific."

He noted in regard to organization that the FDA's Center of Drug Research and Education (CDER) is geared entirely to approving drugs and that "When a CDER new drug reviewing division approves a new drug, it is also saying the drug is 'safe and effective'." When a serious safety issue arises after marketing, the immediate reaction is almost always one of denial, rejection, and heat. They approved the drug so there cannot possibly be anything wrong with it. The same group that approved the drug is also responsible for taking regulatory action against it postmarketing. This is an inherent conflict of interest. At the same time, the Office of Drug Safety has no regulatory power and must first convince the new drug reviewing division that a problem exists before anything beneficial to the public can be done.

He noted in regard to culture that the "culture is dominated by a world-view that believes only randomized clinical trials provide useful and actionable information and that post-marketing safety is an afterthought. This culture also views the pharmaceutical industry it is supposed to regulate as its client, over-values the benefits of the drugs it approves and seriously under-values, disregards and disrespects drug safety."

In regard to science, Dr. Graham noted that "the scientific standards CDER applies to drug safety guarantee that unsafe and deadly drugs will remain on the US market.... The real problem is how CDER applies statistics to post-marketing safety."

As can be imagined, this testimony made headlines in the media. The FDA, at the same congressional hearing, defended itself. Dr. Sandra Kweder presented the FDA's view of the Vioxx® data along with initiatives to strengthen drug safety at the FDA, including a study by the Institute of Medicine due to be completed in 2006 as well as the three Risk Management initiatives subsequently published by the FDA (see Chapters 15–17) and internal changes to address difference of professional opinions within the FDA.

Dr. Steven Galson, Acting Director of CDER, also issued a statement (Web Resource 50-3) indicating that "Dr. Graham's congressional testimony does not reflect the views of the Agency." He noted that the FDA judges each drug individually on a case-by-case basis both before and after marketing approval. He noted that the Office of Drug Safety is separate from the Office of New Drugs (both within CDER) and that the Office of Drug Safety has independent research authority. He noted the FDA is open to new ideas and that the Institute of Medicine study commissioned by the FDA will include recommendations for changes in the Center's organization structure.

The reactions to this controversy from within the FDA covered the spectrum. Some believed Dr. Graham was raising a panic in the minds of patients, that "Big Pharma wants to keep everybody in the dark," and the words "ignorance" and "deceit" were used (Web Resource 50-4). Others noted an increase in "black box" warnings added to drugs, with 58 black box warnings in the period of January to September 2005 compared with 26 in the comparable period in 2004 (Web Resource 50-5).

Controversy continued in 2005 with the resignation of the FDA commissioner after less than 3 months on the job and the transfer of a reviewer in the animal health after alerting her supervisors of an increase in problems with a veterinary drug. The FDA appointed a new drug safety head and proposed a new program, DrugWatch, to bring safety issues to the attention of the public shortly after their identification (Web Resource 50-6).

Congress responded in 2005 with the introduction of bills to require pharmaceutical companies to register clinical trials (Web Resource 50-7) and to create a new office within the FDA called the Center for Post-Market Drug Evaluation and Research that would take over the safety functions of the Office of Drug Safety. Another bill, HR 870, introduced in early 2005 (Web Resource 50-8) would encourage pharmaceutical companies to ensure that all serious adverse events are reported to FDA, stating that

"An individual who violates a provision of [this bill] shall be imprisoned for a term of a minimum of 20 years and a maximum of life, fined not more than $2,000,000, or both, if—(1) the individual is employed as the chief executive officer or a member of the senior executive management group of the manufacturer of a drug; and (2) the violation involves, with respect to such drug, knowing concealment by the individual of evidence of a serious adverse drug experience... .

"...the Secretary [of Health and Human Services] shall require the chief executive officer of the manufacturer of the drug to submit a separate, written attestation on an annual basis—(A) stating that the manufacturer has disclosed to the Secretary all evidence of any serious adverse drug experience related to the drug.

"If the chief executive officer of a manufacturer of a drug for which an approval of an application filed under subsection (b) or (j) is in effect fails to submit a timely attestation for the drug as required by paragraph (1), the Secretary—(A) may issue an order withdrawing approval of the application."

Although it is unclear which if any of these proposals or other proposals will ultimately become law in the United States, there is clearly a debate now ongoing in the government and throughout the country at large on the safety of drugs, in part fueled by the many drug safety lawsuits now working their way through the courts.

It appears that we are now entering a new watershed period that will change pharmacovigilance and will alter the way companies, the FDA, health care practitioners, and patients approve, evaluate, prescribe, market, and use drugs. The Internet is allowing information to propagate at rates unimaginable only a few years ago and is decreasing the time allowed for contemplation and action. Also added to the equation are privacy issues; litigation; actions that occur regarding the same drugs in Europe, Japan, and elsewhere; and the globalization of the pharmaceutical industry with new companies arising in China, India, and elsewhere. On the other side is the perceived need for new drugs to treat the diseases afflicting an aging population as well as the threats of pandemics of influenza and other infectious diseases. How this will play out remains to be seen. Predictions are dangerous, and the only sure thing one can say is that the field of drug safety in 5 or 10 or 20 years will be radically different from what we see today.

URLs by Chapter

Ref.	URL	Notes
3-1	http://www.fda.gov/cder/Offices/ODS/AnnRep2001/annualreport2001.htm	FDA 2001 Annual Report
3-2	http://www.who-umc.org/DynPage.aspx	The Uppsala Monitoring Centre (UMC)
3-3	http://www.umc-products.com/graphics/2489.pdf	UMC Database
4-1	http://www.fda.gov/cder/about/history/Histext.htm	History of the Center for Drug Evaluation and Research
4-2	http://www.accessdata.fda.gov/scripts/cdrh/cfdocs/cfcfr/CFRSearch.cfm	Searchable 21CFR
4-3	http://www.accessdata.fda.gov/scripts/oc/ohrms/index.cfm	Regulation updates
4-4	http://www.fda.gov/opacom/laws/fdcact/fdctoc.htm	Food, Drug & Cosmetic Act
4-5	http://www.fda.gov/cder/regulatory/default.htm	Regulations summary page
4-6	http://www.fda.gov/cder/guidance/index.htm	All CDER regulations
4-7	http://www.fda.gov/cber/aereporting.htm	CBER safety information
4-8	http://www.fda.gov/medwatch/getforms.htm	MedWatch reporting forms
4-9	http://www.fda.gov/medwatch/elist.htm	MedWatch automatic mail service
4-10	http://www.fda.gov/medwatch/safety/ade/t_cder.htm	1992 Guideline
4-11	http://www.fda.gov/cder/guidance/1830fn1.pdf	1997 Guidance
4-12	http://www.fda.gov/cder/guidance/4177dft.pdf	2001 Guidance
4-13	http://www.fda.gov/cder/aers/chapter53.htm	FDA inspectors' guide
4-14	http://www.fda.gov/OHRMS/DOCKETS/98fr/03-5204.pdf	The Tome

Ref.	URL	Notes
4-15	http://eudravigilance.emea.eu.int/human/euPoliciesAndDocs.asp	EU safety documents
4-16	http://eudravigilance.emea.eu.int/human/docs/Vol9en.pdf	EU Volume 9
4-17	http://eudravigilance.emea.eu.int/human/docs/Guidance/cp and guidance SUSARs 23 04 04.pdf	EU Guidance on trial ADRs
4-18	http://eudravigilance.emea.eu.int/human/docs/Guidance/cp and guidance database SUSARs16 April 2004.pdf	Guidance on the EU Database
4-19	http://eudravigilance.emea.eu.int/human/docs/2309-93_2codified_.pdf	EU 1995 document
4-20	http://eudravigilance.emea.eu.int/human/docs/reg95-540en.pdf	EU 1995 regulation
4-21	http://eudravigilance.emea.eu.int/human/docs/Regulations/Reg_2004_726_20040430_EN.pdf	EU 2004 regulation
4-22	http://eudravigilance.emea.eu.int/human/docs/Directives/Dir2001-20_en.pdf	EU Clinical Trial Directive
4-23	http://www.fda.gov/cder/reports/rtn/2004/rtn2004-3.htm#AERS	FDA post-marketing reports for 2004
5-1	http://www.fda.gov/medwatch/What.htm	MedWatch
5-2	http://www.ipecamericas.org/	Excipients Council
6-1	http://www.fda.gov/cber/genetherapy/gttrack.htm	Gene therapy
6-2	http://www.fda.gov/cder/guidance/3647fnl.doc	Retroviral drugs
6-3	http://www.desaction.org/	DES Action USA
6-4	http://reprotox.org/samples/1035.html	Bendectin
6-5	www.phac-aspc.gc.ca/csc-ccs/docs/ biology/Pharma-Systematic-Review-English-Final.pdf	Canada
7-1	http://www.fda.gov/medwatch/articles/medcont/postrep.htm	FDA CME on AEs
7-2	http://www.imshealth.com/ims/portal/pages/homeFlash/us/0,2764,6599,00.html	IMS
7-3	http://www.theannals.com	The Annals of Pharmacotherapy
8-1	http://www.tourism.city.osaka.jp/en/search_osaka/search/sights_01.php&s=3201034	Osaka
8-2	http://www.fda.gov/cder/cderorg.htm	CDER Organization Chart
8-3	http://www.fda.gov/cder/audiences/acspage/index.htm	Advisory Committees
8-4	http://www.fda.gov/cder/drugSafety.htm	Drug Safety Oversight Board
8-5	http://www.fda.gov/cder/index.html	CDER main web site
8-6	http://www.fda.gov/cder/pmc/default.htm	Regulatory documents
8-7	http://www.fda.gov/cder/pmc/default.htm	Post-marketing safety commitments
8-8	http://www.fda.gov/cder/foi/index.htm	Freedom of Information
8-9	http://www.fda.gov/cder/drug/default.htm#Drug%20Safety	Miscellaneous section
8-10	http://directory.psc.gov/employee.htm	HHS employee directory
8-11	http://www.fda.gov/cder/cdernew/listserv.html	FDA email updates
8-12	http://www.fda.gov/cder/drug/drugsafety/DrugIndex.htm#I	Drug information
8-13	http://www.fda.gov/medwatch/What.htm	MedWatch—foods, supplements, formulas
8-14	http://www.fda.gov/medwatch/elist.htm	MedWatch E-List
8-15	http://www.fda.gov/medwatch/safety.htm	MedWatch product safety information

Ref.	URL	Notes
8-16	http://www.fda.gov/cder/aers/extract.htm	AERS
8-17	http://www.vaers.org/	VAERS
8-18	http://vm.cfsan.fda.gov/%7Edms/aems.html	Nutritionals
8-19	http://www.fda.gov/cdrh/maude.html	MAUDE
8-20	http://www.fda.gov/medwatch/report/consumer/consumer.htm	MedWatch reporting by consumers
8-21	http://www.fda.gov/medwatch/report/hcp.htm	MedWatch voluntary reporting by health professionals
8-22	https://www.accessdata.fda.gov/scripts/medwatch/	MedWatch electronic submission
8-23	http://www.fda.gov/medwatch/report/hcp.htm	MedWatch vaccine, device and veterinary
8-24	http://www.fda.gov/medwatch/hipaa.htm	HIPAA
8-25	http://www.fda.gov/medwatch/report/mfg.htm	Mandatory manufacturer reporting
8-26	http://www.accessdata.fda.gov/scripts/cdrh/cfdocs/cfcfr/CFRSearch.cfmfr=310.305	21 CFR 310.305
8-27	http://www.accessdata.fda.gov/scripts/cdrh/cfdocs/cfcfr/CFRSearch.cfmfr=312.32	21 CFR 312.32
8-28	http://www.accessdata.fda.gov/scripts/cdrh/cfdocs/cfcfr/CFRSearch.cfmfr=314.80	21 CFR 314.80
8-29	http://www.accessdata.fda.gov/scripts/cdrh/cfdocs/cfcfr/CFRSearch.cfmfr=312.32	21 CFR 312.32
8-30	http://www.accessdata.fda.gov/scripts/cdrh/cfdocs/cfcfr/CFRSearch.cfmfr=600.80	21 CFR 600.80
8-31	http://www.fda.gov/cber/transfer/transfer.htm	CBER
8-32	http://www.fda.gov/cber/pdufa.htm	PDUFA
8-33	http://www.fda.gov/medwatch/report/guide2.htm	Guidance 1997
8-34	http://www.fda.gov/cder/Offices/ODS/AnnRep2001/annualreport2001.htm	FDA Annual Report 2001
8-35	www.fda.gov	FDA home page
8-36	http://www.fda.gov/oc/opacom/hottopics/default.htm	Hot topics
8-37	http://www.fda.gov/medwatch/index.html	MedWatch home page
8-38	http://www.iom.edu/project.aspid=26341	Institute of Medicine
8-39	http://www.fda.gov/cder/drug/infopage/vioxx/vioxxQA.htm	Vioxx
8-40	http://www.fda.gov/cder/news/feninfo.htm	Fen-Phen
8-41	http://www.fda.gov/cder/drug/advisory/mdd.htm	Anti-depressants
9-1	http://www.emea.eu.int/	EMEA
9-2	http://www.eudravigilance.org/human/Q&A.asp	Eudravigilance
9-3	http://www.emea.eu.int/	EMEA
9-4	http://www.eudravigilance.org/human/evMpd01.asp	Eudravigilance medicinal product dictionary
9-5	http://www.ich.org/LOB/media/MEDIA436.pdf	E2A
9-6	http://eudravigilance.emea.eu.int/human/index.asp	Eudravigilance
9-7	http://heads.medagencies.org/heads/docs/HMA_2ndreport_20050511.pdf	EMEA risk management ad hoc group
9-8	http://www.emea.eu.int/pdfs/human/phv/11590605en.pdf	EMEA risk management action plan
9-9	http://heads.medagencies.org/heads/docs/summary.pdf	Establishing a risk management strategy
9-10	http://www.emea.eu.int/exlinks/exlinks.htm	Member states HAs

Ref.	URL	Notes
9-11	http://www.diahome.org/docs/Events/Events_search_results.cfmRegion=2	DIA in Europe
9-12	http://www.ibc-lifesci.com/default.aspsrc=lsi	IBC
9-13	http://www.iir-conferences.com/	IIR
9-14	http://www.melifesciences.com/	Marcus Evans
9-15	http://www.peri.org/	PERI
10-1	http://www.fda.gov/opacom/backgrounders/foiahand.html	Freedom of Information
10-2	http://www.umc-products.com/DynPage.aspxid=4910&mn=1107	UMC Vigibase
10-3	http://www.drugsafety.com/Halo.asp	Galt Halo™
10-4	http://www.druglogic.com/	Lincoln Technologies QScan™
11-1	http://www.who-umc.org/defs.html	Signal definition
12-1	http://www.hhs.gov/ocr/hipaa/	HIPAA at HHS
12-2	http://www.fda.gov/cder/guidance/6359OCC.htm	FDA Guidance Good PV Practices
12-3	http://www.cdt.org/privacy/eudirective/EU_Directive_.html	EU Privacy Directive
12-4	http://www.answers.com/topic/directive-95-46-ec-on-the-protection-of-personal-data	Wikipedia
12-5	http://europa.eu.int/comm/justice_home/fsj/privacy/	EU Data Protection
12-6	http://www.fda.gov/medwatch/articles/medcont/postrep.htm	FDA Confidentiality
13-1	http://www.fda.gov/foi/warning.htm	FDA Warning Letters
13-2	http://www.fda.gov/cder/audiences/acspage/	FDA Advisory Committees
13-3	http://www.phrma.org	PhRMA
13-4	http://www.va.gov/	Veterans Administration
13-5	http://www.nih.gov/	National Institutes of Health (NIH)
13-6	http://www.cdc.gov/	Centers for Disease Control (CDC)
13-7	http://agmed.sante.gouv.fr/	French AFSSAPS
13-8	http://ead.univ-angers.fr/~pharmaco/pharmacovigilance/organisation/afssaps.htm	A French regional pharmacovigilance center
13-9	http://vm.cfsan.fda.gov/~frf/forum00/sa-moo.htm	Bordeaux Regional Center
14-1	http://www.fda.gov/oc/tfrm/1999report.html	FDA Risk Management May 1999
14-2	http://www.fda.gov/cder/guidance/6357fnl.htm	Premarketing Risk Assessment
14-3	http://www.fda.gov/cder/guidance/6358fnl.htm	RiskMAPs
14-4	http://www.fda.gov/cder/guidance/6359OCC.htm	Good PV Practices
15-1	http://www.fda.gov/cder/guidance/6357fnl.htm	Premarketing Risk Assessment
15-2	http://www.annals.org/cgi/content/full/136/6/471	Moerman and Jonas article
16-1	http://www.fda.gov/cder/guidance/6358fnl.htm	Risk Minimization Action Plans
16-2	http://www.fda.gov/medwatch/safety/2005/safety05.htm#Accutane	Isoretinoin
17-1	http://www.fda.gov/cder/guidance/6359OCC.htm	Good Pharmacovigilance Practices
18-1	https://www.pharmacoepi.org/	International Society of Pharmacoepidemiology
18-2	http://www.cdc.gov/nccdphp/drh/epi_gloss.htm	CDC definition
18-3	http://www.aegis.com/pubs/beta/1999/be990414.html	Definitions
18-4	http://www.dehs.umn.edu/homeiaq/glossary_frame.html	Definitions

Ref.	URL	Notes
18-5	http://www.bdid.com/termse.htm	Definitions
18-6	http://www.healthsystem.virginia.edu/internet/cancer/glossary.cfm	Definitions
18-7	http://www.un.org/Pubs/CyberSchoolBus/special/health/glossary/	Definitions
18-8	http://www.pharmacoepi.org/aboutpe.cfm	Definitions
18-9	http://www.jr2.ox.ac.uk/bandolier/band25/b25-6.html	Deeks article
18-10	http://www.jr2.ox.ac.uk/bandolier/index.html	Bandolier
19-1	http://www.fda.gov/foi/warning_letters/g4502d.htm	Kos warning letter
19-2	http://www.fda.gov/opacom/Enforce.html	Recalls
19-3	http://www.fda.gov/bbs/topics/enforce/2005/ENF00915.html	Recalls August 2005
20-1	http://www.marchofdimes.org	March of Dimes
20-2	http://www.fda.gov/cder/guidance/5917dft.htm	FDA Guidance Pharmacokinetics
20-3	http://www.who.int/child-adolescent-health/publications/NUTRITION/BF_MM.htm	WHO essential drugs
20-4	http://www.fda.gov/womens/informat.html#motherhood	FDA women's health
20-5	http://www.fda.gov/fdac/reprints/breastfed.html	Breast milk or formula
20-6	http://www.pegintron.com/peg/application	Rebetol®
20-7	http://www.pegasys.com/about-pegasys/what-is-copegus.aspx	Copegus®
20-8	http://www.perinatology.com/exposures/druglist.htm	Perinatology
20-9	http://www.motherisk.org/	Motherisk
20-10	http://www.motherisk.org/women/mandate.jsp	Motherisk goal
20-11	http://www.motherisk.org/women/drugs.jsp	Motherisk drugs
20-12	http://www.otispregnancy.org/	OTIS
20-13	http://www.entis-org.com/section=home&lang=UK	ENTIS
20-14	http://www.eurocat.ulster.ac.uk/whatis.html#WhatisEUROCAT	EUROCAT
20-15	http://www.sos.se/epc/english/Medical%20Birth%20Registry.htm	Swedish Medical Birth Registry
21-1	http://www.fda.gov/fdac/special/newdrug/kidmed.html	FDA article on testing drugs in children
21-2	http://www.fda.gov/ohrms/dockets/98fr/120298c.pdf	FDA 1998 rule
21-3	http://www.fda.gov/cder/guidance/2891fnl.pdf	FDA 1999 guidance
21-4	http://www.fda.gov/cder/guidance/3756dft.pdf	FDA 2000 draft guidance
21-5	http://www.fda.gov/cder/guidance/4099FNL.PDF	ICH E11 guidance
21-6	http://www.hhs.gov/news/press/2003pres/20030121.html	FDA testing 12 drugs
21-7	http://www.fda.gov/cder/guidance/3636fnl.htm	FDA 2001 geriatric guidance
21-8	http://www.fda.gov/cder/about/whatwedo/testtube-12.pdf	Medications and older adults
21-9	http://www.netwellness.org/healthtopics/aahealth/tuskegee.cfm	Clinical trial diversity
22-1	http://www.fda.gov/cder/consumerinfo/druginteractions.htm	FDA consumer leaflet
22-2	http://www.uspharmacist.com/oldformat.aspurl=newlook/files/feat/mar00druginteractions.htm	U.S. Pharmacist
23-1	http://vm.cfsan.fda.gov/~lrd/cfr1.html	Labeling 21CFR1.3(a)
23-2	http://www.fda.gov/cder/Offices/ODS/labeling.htm	FDA approved patient labeling
23-3	http://www.fda.gov/cber/rules/labelelec.htm	XML format standard
23-4	http://www.fda.gov/cder/regulatory/ersr/SPLFinal2004/frame.htm	FDA presentation

Ref.	URL	Notes
23-5	http://www.fda.gov/cder/guidance/5537fnl.htm	FDA labeling guidance prescription drugs
23-6	http://www.fda.gov/cder/guidance/5534fnl.htm	FDA labeling guidance clinical studies
23-7	http://www.fda.gov/cder/guidance/6005dft.htm	FDA labeling guidance implementation
23-8	http://www.fda.gov/cder/guidance/5538dft.htm	FDA labeling guidance warnings
23-9	http://www.fda.gov/cder/regulatory/physLabel/physLabel_qa.htm	FDA labeling guidance Q&A
23-10	http://www.fda.gov/cder/drug/DrugSafety/DrugIndex.htm	FDA specific drugs
23-11	http://www.pdr.net	PDR
23-12	http://www.vidal.fr/	Vidal
23-13	http://www.rote-liste.de/	Rote Liste
24-1	http://www.fda.gov/opacom/laws/fdcact/fdcact5a.htm	Federal Food, Drug, and Cosmetic Act
24-2	http://www.gpoaccess.gov/fr/	Federal Register
24-3	http://www.gpoaccess.gov/cfr/index.html	Code of Federal Regulations
24-4	http://www.fda.gov/cder/guidance/index.htm	CDER guidance Web site
24-5	http://www.fda.gov/medwatch/report/mfg.htm	FDA pharmacovigilance regulations
24-6	http://www.fda.gov/cder/guidance/index.htm	FDA guidances
24-7	http://europa.eu.int/eur-lex/en/	EU legislation
24-8	http://eudravigilance.emea.eu.int/human/euPoliciesAndDocs.asp	EU legislation and guidance documents
24-9	http://pharmacos.eudra.org/F2/eudralex/vol-1/CONSOL_2004/Human%20Code.pdf	EU directive
25-1	http://www.cioms.ch/	CIOMS Web site
25-2	http://www.unesco.org/	UNESCO Web site
26-1	http://www.ich.org/cache/compo/475-272-1.html	ICH reports
26-2	http://www.fda.gov/cber/gdlns/ichm2ectdqa.htm	M2
26-3	http://www.fda.gov/cder/guidance/index.htm	E2B (M)
26-4	http://www.fda.gov/cder/guidance/6675fnl.pdf	E2B (M) Q&A
26-5	http://www.fda.gov/cder/guidance/1830fn1.pdf	FDA 1997 guidance
27-1	http://www.ppdi.com/	PPD
27-2	http://www.quintiles.com/default.htm	Quintiles
27-3	http://www.sentrx.com/	Sentrx
27-4	http://www.orbisclinical.com	Orbis Clinical
28-1	http://www.cogr.edu/docs/Bayh_Dole.pdf#search='bayhdole%20act	Bayh-Dole
28-2	http://www.emory.edu/EMORY_REPORT/erarchive/2005/August/August%201/drugsale.htm	Emory University
28-3	http://www.mndaily.com/daily/1999/02/10/news/glaxo/	University of Minnesota
28-4	http://www.fda.gov/oc/ohrt/irbs/default.htm	FDA Web site
28-5	http://www.hhs.gov/ohrp/humansubjects/guidance/contrev2002.htm	HHS
28-6	http://www.fda.gov/cber/gdlns/irbclintrial.htm	FDA draft guidance

Ref.	**URL**	**Notes**
28-7	http://www.emea.eu.int/pdfs/human/ich/013595en.pdf	ICH E6E
28-8	http://www.fda.gov/foi/warning_letters/g5667d.pdf	FDA warning letter
28-9	http://www.fda.gov/cber/gdlns/clindatmon.pdf	FDA guidance DSMC
28-10	http://www.emea.eu.int/pdfs/human/ewp/587203en.pdf	EMEA guidance
28-11	http://www.jcrinc.com/subscribers/intlnewsletter.aspdurki=10120&site=49&return=9551#foot	Joint Commission
29-1	http://www.snomed.org/	SNOMED
29-2	http://www.nlm.nih.gov/news/press_releases/paperlesspr03.html	HHS
31-1	http://www.arisglobal.com/products_totalsafety.php	Aris global
31-2	http://www.relsys.net/index.asp	Argus
31-3	http://www.phaseforward.com/products_safety_clintrace.html	Clintrace
31-4	http://www.oracle.com/industries/life_sciences/aers45_datasheet.pdf	AERS by Oracle
32-1	http://www.fda.gov/cder/aers/chapter53.htm	Field Reporting Requirements
33-1	http://www.iso.org/iso/en/ISOOnline.frontpage	ISO
35-1	http://www.fda.gov/cder/Offices/ODS/AnnRep2004/default.htm	FDA annual report 2004
35-2	http://www.fda.gov/cder/aers/chapter53.htm	FDA enforcement
36-1	http://money.cnn.com/2005/11/03/news/fortune500/merck_humeston/	Vioxx®
36-2	http://www.fda.gov/medwatch/report/mmp.htm	MedWatch to manufacturer
36-3	http://www.fda.gov/cber/gdlns/safety031201.pdf	FDA guidance 2001
37-1	http://www.fda.gov/cber/gdlns/safety031201.htm	FDA guidance 2001
37-2	http://www.lareb.nl/documents/njm2005_1993.pdf	Netherlands Journal of Medicine
37-3	http://www.fda.gov/cber/gdlns/safety031201.htm	FDA guidance 2001
37-4	http://www.fda.gov/cber/gdlns/pharmacovig.htm	FDA guidance 2004
37-5	http://www.fda.gov/CBER/rules/safereport.htm	Proposed rules - Tome
37-6	http://pharmacos.eudra.org/F2/eudralex/vol-9/pdf/Vol9en.pdf	Volume 9
37-7	http://www.who-umc.org/DynPage.aspxid=22682	Uppsala Monitoring Centre
37-8	http://www.who.int/vaccines-documents/DocsPDF05/815_new.pdf	WHO aide memoire
38-1	http://www.umc-products.com/DynPage.aspxid=4918&mn=1107	UMC WHO-ART
38-2	http://www.MedDRAmsso.com/NewWeb2003/index.htm	MedDRA
38-3	http://www.meddramsso.com/MSSOWeb/evweb/index.htm	MSSO regulatory page
38-4	http://www.meddramsso.com/MSSOWeb/search/query.asp	MedDRA browser
38-5	http://www.meddramsso.com/NewWeb2003/document_library/PTC_nov_2004_draft_FINAL.pdf	Points to consider
38-6	http://www.fda.gov/cder/guidance/6357fnl.htm#_Toc98731677	FDA guidance
38-7	http://www.fda.gov/bbs/topics/news/2006/NEW01295.html	FDA warning
38-8	http://www.fda.gov/fdac/features/695_prescrip.html	FDA names
38-9	http://www.ama-assn.org/ama/pub/category/2956.html	USAN
38-10	http://www.who.int/medicines/services/inn/en/index.html	WHO INN
38-11	http://www.ismp.org/	Institute for Safe Medication Practices
38-12	http://www.ismp.org/tools/confuseddrugnames.pdf	Confused drug names

Ref.	URL	Notes
38-13	http://www.umc-products.com/DynPage.aspxid=2829&mn=1107&mn2=1139	WHO Drug Dictionary
38-14	http://www.umc-products.com/graphics/2489.pdf	WHO Drug Dictionary Enhanced
38-15	http://eudravigilance.emea.eu.int/human/evMpd01.asp	Eudravigilance
39-1	http://www.fda.gov/medwatch/report/100797.pdf	FDA amendment
39-2	http://www.cancernet.gov/cancertopics/pdq/supportivecare/nausea/HealthProfessional/page4	National Cancer Institute
40-1	http://www.fda.gov/cder/Offices/ODS/regs.htm	FDA regulations
40-2	http://www.fda.gov/cder/guidance/index.htm	FDA guidances 1
40-3	http://www.fda.gov/cder/regulatory/default.htm#Specific%20Regulatory	FDA guidances 2
40-4	http://www.fda.gov/cder/guidance/1830fn1.pdf	FDA 1997 guidance
40-5	http://www.fda.gov/cder/about/smallbiz/exclusivity.htm	FDA FAQ
40-6	http://www.fda.gov/medwatch/report/mmp.htm	MedWatch to Manufacturer
40-7	http://www.fda.gov/cder/Offices/CRMS/DQRS.htm	Drug Quality Reporting System
40-8	http://www.foiservices.com/brochure/drugdocs.cfm	FOI Services
40-9	http://www.fda.gov/medwatch/report/instruc_10-25-05.htm#H1	MedWatch instructions
40-10	http://www.fda.gov/medwatch/report/instruc_10-25-05.htm#H1	MedWatch instructions for manufacturers
40-11	http://www.fda.gov/medwatch/REPORT/CONSUMER/INSTRUCT.HTM	MedWatch instructions for health care professionals
41-1	http://www.fda.gov/cber/gdlns/safety031201.pdf	FDA guidance 2001
42-1	http://www.fda.gov/cber/rules/safereport.pdf	The Tome. Proposed regulations
42-2	http://www.fda.gov/oc/pdufa3/2003plan/default.htm	PDUFA
43-1	http://www.fda.gov/cder/guidance/1351fnl.pdf	ICH E2C
43-2	http://www.fda.gov/cber/rules/safereport.pdf	FDA new rules 2003
43-3	http://www.fda.gov/cber/gdlns/ichclinsafety.htm	ICH E2C addendum
43-4	http://www.fda.gov/cber/gdlns/safety031201.htm#xi	FDA 2001 guidance
44-1	http://www.cptech.org/ip/health/econ/frank2003.pdf	Drug cost estimates
45-1	http://www.fda.gov/cder/aers/chapter53.htm	FDA inspection manual
45-2	http://www.fda.gov/cder/warn/	FDA warning letters
45-3	http://www.emea.eu.int/Inspections/index.html	EMEA inspections sector
45-4	http://www.emea.eu.int/Inspections/GCPgeneral.html	EMEA pharmacovigilance inspections
45-5	http://www.mhra.gov.uk/home/idcplgIdcService=SS_GET_PAGE&nodeId=826	UK MHRA inspections
45-6	http://www.mhra.gov.uk/home/groups/is-insp/documents/websiteresources/con2018030.pdf	Summary of PV systems
46-1	http://www.pbs.org/wgbh/nova/doctors/oath_today.html	Hippocratic oath
46-2	http://www.ama.com.au/web.nsf/doc/WEEN-5WW5YY/$file/090304%20Code%20of%20Ethics%202004%20(final,%20March%202004).pdf	AMA position paper
46-3	http://www.pharmacoethics.com/	PharmacoEthics.com
46-4	http://www.asbh.org/	American Society for Bioethics and Humanities
46-5	http://www.uclan.ac.uk/facs/health/ethics/index.htm	Centre for Professional Ethics

Ref.	**URL**	**Notes**
46-6	http://www.bioethics.ca/mission-ang.html	Canadian Bioethics Society
46-7	http://appinet.org/ethics.php	Academy of Pharmaceutical Physicians and Investigators
46-8	http://www.adrugrecall.com/	Drug recalls
46-9	http://www.worstpills.org/	Worst pills
47-1	http://www.iom.edu/	Institute of Medicine
48-1	http://www.fda.gov/cder/news/feninfo.htm	FDA Q&A
48-2	http://www.settlementdietdrugs.com/index.cfm/fuseaction/sdd.index/index.cfm	AHP diet drug settlement
49-1	http://www.findarticles.com/p/articles/mi_m1370/is_n7_v25/ai_11348640	FDA summary report
50-1	http://finance.senate.gov/hearings/testimony/2004test/111804dgtest.pdf	Testimony of Dr. Graham
50-2	http://www.annals.org/cgi/content/full/122/6/456	Sulfanilamide
50-3	www.fda.gov/bbs/topics/news/2004/NEW01138.html	CDER statement
50-4	www.newstarget.com/z002476.html	Reaction
50-5	http://business.timesonline.co.uk/printFriendly/0,,2020-9073-1921288-12609,00.html	Black box
50-6	http://www.fda.gov/cder/guidance/6657dft.htm	DrugWatch
50-7	http://finance.senate.gov/press/Gpress/2005/prg022805.pdf	Congress
50-8	http://thomas.loc.gov/cgi-bin/bdquery/zd109:h.r.00870:	HR870

Abbreviations

Abbrev.	Meaning
AARP	American Association of Retired Persons
ADE	Adverse Drug Experience
ADME	Absorption, Distribution, Metabolism, and Excretion
ADR	Adverse Drug Reaction
AE	Adverse Event
AERS	Adverse Event Reporting System
AFSSAPS	Agence Française de Sécurité Sanitaire des Produits de Santé
AHA	American Hospital Association
AIDS	Acquired Immune Deficiency Syndrome
ALT	Alanine Transaminase
AMA	American Medical Association
ANDA	Abbreviated New Drug Application
APhA	American Pharmacists Association
AST	Aspartate Aminotransferase
BLA	Biologic License Application
CANDA	Computer Assisted New Drug Application

Abbrev.	Meaning
CBER	Center for Biologics Evaluation and Research
CCA	Clear Cell Adenocarcinoma
CCDS	Company Core Data Sheet
CCSI	Company Core Safety Information
CDC	Center for Disease Control
CDER	Center for Drug Evaluation and Research
CDRH	Center for Devices and Radiological Health
CDS	Core Data Sheet
CEO	Chief Executive Officer
CERTS	Centers for Education & Research on Therapeutics
CFR	Code of Federal Regulations
CHF	Congestive Heart Failure
CHMP	Committee for Medicinal Products for Human Use
CIOMS	Council for International Organizations of Medical Sciences

Abbrev.	Meaning
CMC	Chemistry, Manufacturing Controls
CME	Continuing Medical Education
CNN	Cable News Network
CNS	Central Nervous System
CPK	Creatine Phosphokinase
CPS	Compendium of Pharmaceuticals and Specialties
CRC	Clinical Research Center
CRF	Case Report Form
CRO	1. Clinical Research Organization 2. Contract Research Organization
CRU	Clinical Research Unit
CSI	Core Safety Information
CTC	Clinical Trials Certificate
CTD	Common Technical Document
CTX	Clinical Trials Exemption
DCSI	Development Core Safety Information
DDMAC	Division of Drug Marketing, Advertising, and Communications
DES	Diethylstilbesterol
DIA	Drug Information Association
DMC	Data Monitoring Committee
DNA	Deoxyribonucleic Acid
DQRS	Drug Quality Reporting System
DRMP	Development Risk Management Plan
DSB	Drug Safety Oversight Board
DSMC	Data Safety Monitoring Committee
DSUR	Development Safety Update Report
DTD	Document Type Definition
ECG	Electrocardiogram
EDC	Electronic Data Capture
EDI	Electronic Data Interchange
EEA	European Economic Area
EMA	European Medicines Agency
EMEA	European Medicines Agency formerly known as the European Medicines Evaluation Agency
ENTIS	European Network of Teratology Information Services

Abbrev.	Meaning
ER	Emergency Room
EU	European Union
EUDRACT	European Clinical Trials Database
FAQ	Frequently Asked Questions
FD&C	Food, Drug, and Cosmetic Act
FDA	Food and Drug Administration
FIAU	Fialuridine
FMEA	Failure Mode and Effects Analysis
FOI	Freedom of Information
FTC	Federal Trade Commission
GCP	Good Clinical Practices
GLP	Good Laboratory Practice
GMP	Good Manufacturing Practice
GPVP	Good Pharmacovigilance Practices
GRAS	Generally Recognized as Safe
GRASE	Generally Recognized as Safe and Effective
HA	Health Authority
HBV	Hepatitis B Virus
HCV	Hepatitis C Virus
HHS	Department of Health and Human Services
HIPAA	Health Insurance Portability and Accountability Act
HIV	Human Immunodeficiency Virus
HLGT	Higher Level Group Term
HLT	Higher Level Term
HMO	Health Maintenance Organization
IB	Investigator Brochure
IBD	International Birth Date
ICD	International Classification of Diseases
ICH	International Conference on Harmonization
ICSR	Individual Case Safety Report
ID	Identification
IFPMA	International Federation of Pharmaceutical Manufacturers and Associations

Abbrev.	Meaning
IIS	Investigator-Initiated Study
IIT	Investigator-Initiated Trial
IND	Investigator's New Drug Application
INN	International Normalized Nomenclature
INR	International Normalized Ratio
IPSR	Interim Periodic Safety Report
IRB	Investigational Review Board
ISO	International Organization for Standards
ISPE	International Society of Pharmacoepidemiology
ISS	Integrated Summary of Safety
IT	Information Technology
JCAHO	Joint Commission on Accreditation of Healthcare Organizations
LLT	Lower Level Term
LOE	Lack of Efficacy
LSSS	Large Simple Safety Studies
LVEF	Left Ventricular Ejection Fraction
MA	Marketing Authorization
MAH	Marketing Authorization Holder
MAUDE	Manufacturer and User Facility Device Experience Database
MD	Medical Doctor (Physician)
ME	Medication Error
MedDRA	Medical Dictionary for Regulatory Activities
MHRA	Medicines and Healthcare Products Regulatory Agency
MMWR	Morbidity and Mortality Weekly Report
MSSO	Maintenance and Support Service Organization
NCE	New Chemical Entity
NDA	New Drug Application
NDS	New Drug Submission
NGO	Non-Governmental Organization
NIH	National Institutes of Health
NNH	Number Needed to Harm
NOS	Not Otherwise Specified
NP	National Formulary

Abbrev.	Meaning
NSAE	Non-Serious Adverse Event
NSAID	Non-Steroidal Anti-Inflammatory Drug
NY	New York
ODS	Office of Drug Safety
OTC	Over The Counter
OTIS	Organization of Teratology Information Services
PD	Pharmacodynamics
PDF	Portable Document Format
PDR	Physicians' Desk Reference®
PDUFA	Prescription Drug User Fee Act
PERI	Pharmaceutical Education and Research Institute
PharmD	Doctor of Pharmacy
PhD	Doctor of Philosophy
PhRMA	Pharmaceutical Research Manufacturers of America
PI	Package Insert
PIL	Patient Information Leaflet
PK	Pharmacokinetics
PPA	Phenylpropanolamine
PRR	Proportional Reporting Ratio
PSUR	Periodic Safety Update Report
PT	Preferred Term
PV	Pharmacovigilance
PVWP	Pharmacovigilance Working Party
QA	Quality Assessment
QC	Quality Control
QP	Qualified Person
RCT	Randomized Clinical Trial
RiskMAP	Risk Minimization Plan
RN	Registered Nurse
RNA	Ribonucleic Acid
RR	Risk Ratio
RSI	Reference Safety Information
Rx	Prescription
SADR	Suspected Adverse Drug Reaction
SAE	Serious Adverse Event
SAR	Serious Adverse Reaction

Abbrev.	Meaning	Abbrev.	Meaning
SEC	Securities and Exchange Commission	SSRI	Selective Serotonin Reuptake Inhibitor
SESAR	Suspected, Expected Serious, Adverse Reaction	SUSAR	Suspected, Unexpected, Serious Adverse Reaction
SGML	Standard Generalized Markup Language	TPSR	Traditional Periodic Safety Report
SGOT	Serum Glutamic Oxaloacetic Transaminase	UK	United Kingdom
SGPT	Serum Glutamic Pyruvic Transaminase	UMC	Uppsala Monitoring Centre
SLE	Systemic Lupus Erythematosis	UNESCO	United Nations Educational, Scientific, and Cultural Organization
SmPC	Summary of Product Characteristics	URL	Uniform Resource Locator
SMT	Safety Management Team	US	United States
SNOMED	Systematized Nomenclature of Medicine	USAN	United States Adopted Name
SOC	System Organ Class	USP	United States Pharmacopoeia
SOP	Standard Operating Procedure(s)	VAERS	Vaccine Adverse Event Reporting System
SPC	Summary of Product Characteristics	WHO	World Health Organization
SPL	Structured Product Labeling	XML	Extensible Markup Language
SQL	Structured Query Language		

Index